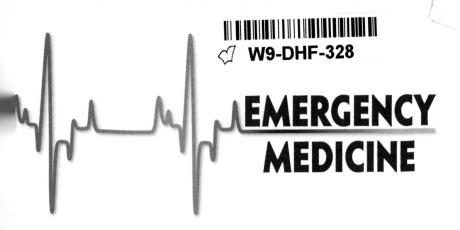

EMERGENCY MEDICINE

The Medical Student Survival Guide

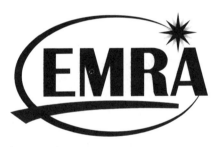

A Comprehensive Guide to The Specialty

Edited by
Kristin E. Harkin, MD, FACEP and Jeremy T. Cushman, MD, MS

A publication of the
Emergency Medicine Residents' Association
Medical Student Committee

Introduction

Kristin E. Harkin, MD, FACEP

Past President, EMRA; Assistant Professor of Medicine, Division of Emergency Medicine, Weill Medical College of Cornell University, New York-Presbyterian Hospital

Jeremy T. Cushman, MD, MS

Past President, EMRA; Department of Emergency Medicine, University of Rochester, Rochester, New York

Emergency medicine continues to be the fastest growing specialty since its formal recognition in 1979. The success of the specialty can be measured by the number of residents graduating each year, the tremendous increase in research publications and grant support, and the burgeoning opportunities for subspecialty and fellowship training. The provision of emergency medical care has become an essential public service to the more than 110 million patients who visit emergency departments every year, and the attractiveness of this specialty continues to draw the best and brightest students from around the world.

The first edition of this text was published in 1991 with nearly a dozen chapters. Three editions and more than 15 years later, this text represents nearly 75 chapters and appendices providing the most comprehensive published reference available for medical students considering the practice of emergency medicine. We have significantly expanded the text to cover issues important to you beyond just getting into residency, including how to thrive and take advantage of the myriad of career opportunities that are available to a residency-trained emergency physician.

We strive to provide you with the most up-to-date information written by nationally recognized experts in the specialty and expect that *Emergency Medicine: The Medical Student Survival Guide* will provide you with the answers to your questions and the resources to prepare you for a promising career in emergency medicine.

Dedications

This edition is dedicated to my mother, Diane Harkin. Her love, support, and faith have made all the difference in my life. She has been the best example of unwavering strength for me to live by and her wisdom has helped me in countless ways.

I love you, Mom. Thanks for helping me appreciate the many special blessings in my life, find peace in moments of chaos, and never letting me think anything was impossible. You have the most extraordinary and giving heart, and your ability to find hope has never let me down.

—Kristin

To my wife, Susan, and my son, Riley, for your patience, trust, and support. This and previous editions would not have been possible without your love and understanding. The specialty of emergency medicine is full of individuals who are willing share their experiences and mentor others into this noble profession, and it is a tremendous honor to facilitate that through the editing of this book.

—Jeremy

Acknowledgements

The production of this book could not have been possible without the generous support of each author and their willingness to share their time, knowledge, and experience with medical students interested in emergency medicine. We are indebted to the EMRA staff, Michele Byers, and Barbara Voll for their work on this project. Further, the tireless support of the EMRA Board of Directors and the EMRA Medical Student Governing Council made *Emergency Medicine: The Medical Student Survival Guide* possible.

Editors

Kristin E. Harkin, MD, FACEP—Past President, EMRA; Assistant Professor of Medicine, Division of Emergency Medicine, Weill Medical College of Cornell University, New York-Presbyterian Hospital

Jeremy T. Cushman, MD, MS—Past President, EMRA; Department of Emergency Medicine, University of Rochester

2006-2007 EMRA Medical Student Committee

Joshua Moskovitz
Timothy Cheslock
Jennifer C. Anderson
Alexandra Greene
Cristi Vaughn
Marlow Macht
Laura Oh
Erica Douglass
Deno Gaultieri
Joseph Zito
Travis Watson
Parag W. Paranjpe
Ben Harris
Zach Patrick
Julian Jakubowski
Bernard Sowa
Roopa "Rashi" Dhawan

EMRA Staff

Michele Byers, CAE
Executive Director

Table of Contents

section one

Emergency Medicine
The Specialty

chapter 1

Evolution of Emergency Medicine as a Specialty

Judith E. Tintinalli, MD, MS, FACEP
Professor and Chair Department of Emergency Medicine, University of North Carolina at Chapel Hill
Past President, American Board of Emergency Medicine
President-Elect, Association of Academic Chairs of Emergency Medicine

Last I remembered, Dave Wagner, John Wiegenstein, Ron Krome, and George Podgorny were welcoming a new generation of emergency physicians into the field of emergency medicine and mentoring us in the art of leadership.

From Dave Wagner, we learned vision—he lit the fire of pediatric emergency medicine, about 25 years ago when everybody else could only focus their near-sighted eyes on the immediate emergency medicineemergency medicine development tasks.

From Ron Krome, we learned when to be aggressive and how to stand up for our rights as emergency physicians.

From John Wiegenstein, we learned about statesmanship and diplomacy, and how to develop partnerships with physicians in other specialties. He is remembered by the Wiegenstein Award given each year by the American College of Emergency Physicians (ACEP).

From George Podgorny, we learned about tough love as the way to deal with the obstructions other specialties put in the way of the development of our specialty.

We all owe a debt to those first emergency physicians, and many others whom I do not have the opportunity to name here, for they made it possible for us to have wonderful medical careers in this exciting and challenging specialty.

Emergency medicine really began in the 1960s in Alexandria, Virginia, where a group of physicians led by James Mills, MD, organized themselves as the first emergency medicine specialists. Jim served as president of both ACEP and ABEM and was smart, calm, and politically very savvy. He practiced emergency medicine in Alexandria until the end of his career, and is remembered by the James Mills Award given by ACEP each year. The "'Alexandria Plan'" produced a set of physicians who devoted their practice to staffing the emergency department 24 hours a day. Previously, U.S. hospitals used a system of rotating medical staff to cover the emergency department as part of their responsibilities for hospital privileges. That meant dermatologists, ophthalmologists, otolaryngologists, etc., were expected to diagnose and treat all emergencies, or find suitable individuals to help them out.

About the same time, physicians throughout the United States interested in emergency care founded ACEP, and a group of academic surgeons responsible for trauma organized the University Association for Emergency Medical Services (UA/EMS) in Ann Arbor. This organization, UA/emergency medicine, evolved into the SAEM of today. By 1970, The University of Cincinnati developed the first emergency medicine residency. Its first graduate, Bruce Janiak, became president of both ABEM and ACEP. In 1973, the federal government demonstrated the importance of emergency medicine and emergency medical services to the nation by creating the Emergency Medical Services (EMS) Act. Federal funds provided seed money to develop emergency medicine residencies, and by the late 1970s there were about 50 emergency medicine residencies in the United States. As residencies proliferated, ACEP organized the Liaison Residency Endorsement Committee (LREC), which identified the essential components of an emergency medicine residency and developed criteria for residency approval. Bob Daley was the first LREC chairman, and we tried to balance a need for rapid growth of the specialty with a need for quality training programs. There were extremely heated discussions about whether or not academic emergency medicine could develop while providing 24-hour faculty coverage for our residents in the emergency medicine. I'm proud to say that the 24-hour rule won out. The essential components developed in the 1970s remain in the basic structure of the approval process we use today. When emergency medicine received official recognition as a primary specialty, the LREC was reorganized under the ACGME as the Residency Review Committee for Emergency Medicine (RRC-emergency medicine).

While emergency medicine was popular and rapidly accepted by community hospitals and private physicians, medical schools remained generally disinterested. Some traditional specialists were downright hostile to both the concept of, and individuals promulgating, emergency medicine. Many academicians thought that emergency medicine lacked a unique knowledge base. What finally persuaded them was the face that the administration, management, and operations of emergency medical services were functions unique to emergency medicine. So it was emergency medicine services that became the cornerstone of emergency medicine and was a leading factor in its eventual acceptance as a specialty. It is important for all of us to remember that.

Work was under way in earnest to develop a core curriculum. ABEM began developing a certification examination. That process was funded through voluntary donations from physicians practicing emergency medicine throughout the United States. Emergency medicine was the first specialty to develop a criterion-referenced examination (as opposed to norm-referenced examinations where the lowest percentiles fail). It was also the first specialty to require regular recertification examinations. The board examination was actually written, validated, and ready for administration before emergency medicine was approved by the ABMS (American Board of Medical Specialties). Some fiercely advocated going ahead, giving the exam, and forging our own course. Moderate views prevailed, because it was necessary to follow the rules of organized medicine in order to ensure the future of the specialty.

The first American Board of Emergency Medicine approved by the ABMS in 1979 was a conjoint board. This board consisted of a majority of emergency physicians but also had membership from other specialty boards, including internal medicine, obstetrics and gynecology, family practice, psychiatry, and otolaryngology, to guide and advise the emergency medicine directors. While the concept of a conjoint board was difficult to swallow, it did allow for a much smoother entry of emergency medicine into the world of the ABMS. In 1989, the ABMS voted to change ABEM into a primary board. The last vestiges of that first conjoint board disappeared about 2 years ago when all non-emergency medicine specialties ended their participation in ABEM. To me, this was a great milestone, but it occurred with barely a whimper. I thought it should have been heralded by fireworks and parades; it was that significant an event.

Obviously the very first emergency physicians developed the specialty by "bootstrapping." That is, they developed emergency medicine residencies when they themselves did not have the opportunity for such training. It was for this reason that a time-limited practice track for board eligibility was designed when the specialty originated. Time-limited practice tracks were not an innovation unique to emergency medicine—they were the mechanisms also used by other specialties such as internal medicine and family medicine, when those specialties originated. The practice track was phased out in 1989.

From about 1989 on, emergency medicine moved on a fast track. Emergency medicine residencies are thriving in many nations. I have visited many of these programs and find the practice, problems, and vision of emergency medicine are very much the same all around the world. It is amazing that emergency medicine has come so far in so short a time. We are compassionate and energized physicians who really make a difference. My own enthusiasm for the practice, research, and teaching of emergency medicine continues, as I know yours will in this fascinating, demanding, and fun specialty.

chapter 2

Emergency Medicine: A National Perspective

Brian F. Keaton, MD, FACEP
Department of Emergency Medicine, Summa Health System, Akron, Ohio
President, American College of Emergency Physicians

Our specialty was born out of adversity a little over three decades ago in places like Lansing, Michigan, and Alexandria, Virginia. Americans had a better chance of surviving serious illness and injury on the battlefields of Vietnam than on the streets of our major cities. The physicians who staffed the "emergency rooms" of the day were there as punishment. The workforce was made up of physicians who were at the beginning, end, or low point of their careers. How times have changed. We are now the most sought-after specialty, and our residency graduates are the best and the brightest American medicine has to offer.

When we look at the external environment, we're faced with unprecedented challenges. With them come opportunities to transform our health care system into one that can provide high-quality care for all Americans, regardless of their age, sex, race, creed, color, primary language, or ability to pay. When the government or organized medicine puts together a team to take on a tough challenge, emergency physicians are among the first to be asked to step forward. Instead of being a fly on the wall, we have a seat at the table, often a seat at the head of the table. Although we are relatively small in number compared to other specialties, we are disproportionately represented in leadership roles.

The same skills set that makes us good at what we do clinically makes us the perfect docs to bridge the gaps between medicine, business, and the government. Our knowledge base is miles wide, and we're able to speak intelligently about almost any aspect of medicine. We see the big picture and are good at cutting through the minutiae to focus on what is really important. We thrive in stressful environments where decisions must be made with less than complete information. We're good stewards of precious resources. We tend to be good politicians. We're seen by the public as healers more concerned about doing what's in their best interest than ours. There's a universal connection to what we do and a natural desire to associate with us because every person we meet is just a heartbeat from being one of our patients. We heal sick people, band-aid sick systems, and hold the greatest promise to resuscitate our flawed health care system.

Economic, demographic, and social factors are forcing fundamental change in our health care system. Emergency medicine has long been the safety net, and as a result has borne the brunt of the health care system's woes. Concerns to our specialty include: ensuring universal access to emergency medical services; ensuring the highest quality of care is provided to all our patients; improving the liability climate to ensure both emergency physicians, and the consultants who they rely on, can provide needed emergency care; easing the crowded conditions in which emergency physicians provide care; improving our emergency department's and hospital's ability to respond to natural and terrorist disasters; and ensuring adequate reimbursement for the services provided by physicians, much of which is uncompensated.

The spectrum of disease witnessed by the emergency physician is unparalleled and is often the draw for medical students choosing a career in emergency medicine. Your future training goes well beyond the bedside, however. As suggested, the challenges before the American health care system are significant. However, there is no group better prepared to lead this transformation than emergency physicians.

Patients have spoken with their feet, seeking our care in unprecedented numbers. We are the ones you come to when you're really sick, possibly sick, or kind of sick and in need of rapid evaluation, diagnosis, and treatment. We are the place you come to when you cannot or will not wait for others to find a place in their schedules for you, and the site of medical refuge when you don't know where else to turn. Despite limited resources, unrealistic expectations, and impossible demand, emergency medicine delivers on our promise to provide the best possible care to every patient regardless of their ability to pay or what time of day they choose to seek care.

Alan Kay once said, "The best way to predict the future is to invent it." We're in an inventing mode and are being presented with a historic opportunity to define both the future of our specialty and of American medicine. The opportunities in emergency medicine are endless and by choosing this career you will become a leader and a champion for the health care needs of your patients. The challenges before our health care system and emergency medicine are significant, but the rewards and honor of providing care to our communities are limitless.

chapter 3

Choosing a Career in Emergency Medicine

Kristin E. Harkin, MD, FACEP
Past President, EMRA
Assistant Professor of Medicine, Division of Emergency Medicine
Weill Medical College of Cornell University; New York-Presbyterian Hospital

Choosing a specialty is a lifelong commitment. Your specialty choice will define your future career and even your life. It will influence the way you spend the majority of your time and the people with whom you will most often interact. As a result, the decision of choosing a specialty often necessitates much soul searching and honest introspection.

Emergency medicine is indeed a unique specialty. Emergency medicine involves the initial evaluation, resuscitation, and stabilization of all patients presenting to the emergency department. Emergency medicine is a relatively young specialty with the first residency implemented in 1970. The American Board of Medical Specialties recognized emergency medicine as an official specialty in 1979.

Emergency departments are open 24 hours a day and demand that physicians work their best at all hours. The unique body of knowledge and breadth of medicine that the specialty incorporate requires emergency physicians to possess a decisive and quick mind, the ability to function with incomplete information, excellent physical diagnostic skills, adept manual dexterity, calm level-headedness, perseverance and dedication, and a good sense of humor.

The management of patients in the emergency department is a "team" approach. Therefore, emergency physicians need to work effectively as team members in cooperation with emergency medical services personnel, fire and police departments, nursing and ancillary staff, consultants, and most importantly with patients and their families. Emergency physicians also have special communication skills, to establish a rapport quickly with patients in often the most stressful conditions. Emergency physicians must be able to make split-second decisions with limited information about patients' past history. Furthermore, emergency physicians use their hands a great deal in performing procedures, such as airway intubations and the insertion of thoracostomy tubes.

Emergency care is a fundamental right and is available to all who seek help. Federal law protects patients' access to emergency departments without prior authorization from insurance companies and independent of their financial resources. Patients in the emergency department are, thus, from all walks of life. Patients are from diverse socioeconomic, racial, and ethnic backgrounds. They are from all ages with a wide range of medical and surgical conditions. As a result, the pace in the emergency department is unpredictable, and the high acuteness of care provides an unparalleled continuing educational experience. The order in which patients are seen is solely dependent on the severity of their conditions.

One of the most gratifying aspects of emergency medicine is being the first to examine, work up, diagnose, and treat patients with undifferentiated presenting problems. A typical day in the emergency department is never typical! The intellectual content of the specialty allows one never to get bored, because the diagnostic perplexities are challenging daily. Recognizing who is sick and needs emergent resuscitation in a large emergency department filled with patients requires skill, determination, and special training. One should expect the unexpected. The novelty of emergency medicine really never ends.

Patients present to the emergency department with a broad spectrum of problems. Complaints range from poisonings and drug overdoses, automobile crash injuries, heart attacks, penetrating trauma from gunshot wounds or stabbings, rape, child abuse, and pregnancy complications to seemingly minor issues such as colds. It is indeed a privilege to be with patients during some of the most important times in their lives. It is also a difficult, sometimes heartbreaking specialty. One will see things that one never dreamed possible before. It is amazing sometimes to see what human beings can do to each other. It is not easy. But, one does make a difference every day, every shift in the emergency department. To be the one who runs the resuscitation and orchestrates the code is a tremendous feeling of satisfaction.

Few careers are as satisfying as emergency medicine from the perspective of making an impact every day. Emergency physicians are fortunate enough to feel the incredible, unrivaled rewards of relieving someone's pain every day. It really does not get any better than that!

Emergency physicians are in the unique position of serving as a patient's best advocate. Emergency physicians are ultimately responsible for designing a plan for patient care and admitting patients to the appropriate setting to execute that plan. This requires great self-confidence, and emergency physicians must have the presence to interact with many consultants whose goals may be different. Admissions and discharges from the emergency department may be areas of disagreement between emergency physicians and other specialists, but emergency physicians see more patients with varying presentations by the very nature and hours of the specialty. Debating these issues may be tedious, but it also forces one to grow as a stronger clinician.

A significant amount of clinical autonomy exists in emergency medicine. Federal law gives emergency physicians the authority to pursue diagnostic testing to determine whether an "emergency medical condition" exists. Reimbursement, however, is decreasing in every specialty, and the pressure to provide cost-effective care is present in emergency medicine as well. Emergency physicians help control the utilization of hospital resources. Emergency medicine is highly valued by the public.

Emergency medicine is practiced in shifts of varying lengths at all hours. Emergency physicians work a significant number of nights, weekends, and holidays. Yet, the benefits of shift work include the ability truly to have time off with no clinical responsibilities from being "on-call." One is able to schedule shifts to accommodate family and childcare needs, to pursue other interests (such as other degrees), and to allow travel. However, the physical demands of shift work are intense. During a shift, there is often little time to sit or take a meal break. Working different hours constantly disrupts circadian rhythm. Thus, even though the work schedule is flexible, it is by no means "typical."

Emergency medicine does have its perceived downsides as well. The emergency department truly is a fishbowl. No one can really relate to it unless they have been swimming in it! Physicians in the other departments often 'second guess" clinical decisions made in the emergency department without appreciating the special circumstances that may have existed with a particular patient. It is easy to criticize the department when one does not work within its unique pressures. Furthermore, not all patients present with the need for emergency care. Some seek their primary care in the emergency department because they have no other access to medical care, and the emergency department does not turn anyone away. Moreover, some patients who present to the emergency department are difficult to manage. Intravenous drug users, intoxicated patients, and abusive patients may make the job frustrating. Caring for an indigent or a homeless population with limited social service resources is trying. The lack of follow-up for continuity of care and feedback about a patient's outcome are significant drawbacks. Financial pressures also contribute to stress.

All of these factors contribute to burnout in the specialty. Yet, it is important to remember that burnout is more prevalent for those who entered emergency medicine as a second career and for those who entered the specialty for the wrong reasons. Keeping a regular work schedule, not spending more than you can afford, and knowing when to take a vacation will contribute to long-term happiness and the ability to maintain your perspective and positive outlook.

This chapter was intended to provide you with an overview of a career in emergency medicine. However, the most important measure in deciding if emergency medicine is truly for you is by doing an elective in the emergency department. Nothing can substitute for clinical experience and time in the department. It is the best litmus test. You should talk personally to board-certified, residency-trained emergency physicians in your community in addition to physicians in academic teaching centers. This will help you better understand the broad spectrum of career opportunities in emergency medicine. Moreover, ask an emergency physician whom you trust to serve as your mentor throughout this process. Having a personal advisor guide you in your career path and academic training will help you make a wise decision.

You should sincerely love the specialty you choose. You will spend a tremendous amount of time training, and you deserve to be happy. So, take your time in making the right decision. You should look forward to going to work every day and feel good about the job that you do. Otherwise, it is not fun, and you will not last. Invest in long-term happiness. Delay some immediate rewards for bigger, better ones down the road after training. You will succeed if you spend the time carefully thinking through your decision for a specialty choice and focus on a balance between your professional and personal goals. Residency is not something that you just want to endure. It is a long road, but the pay off makes it all worthwhile!

Your career should bring out the BEST within you. You should feel direction, purpose, challenge, and motivation about your work. The right specialty for you is right because it makes you happy inside, because it matters to you. At times, it encourages you to do better and ultimately enables you to know that you are doing your very best.

This is, in the end, the most important thing you need to ask yourself. Does this specialty really bring out the best in you? If the answer is yes, then you've found it!

chapter 4

Practice Patterns in Emergency Medicine

Cherri Hobgood, MD, FACEP
Associate Professor Department of Emergency Medicine
Associate Dean for Curriculum and Educational Development
University of North Carolina School of Medicine

Contemplating a career in emergency medicine? One of the major attractions to a career in emergency medicine is your ability to grow and evolve in the profession as your personal and professional needs change. This is due to the variety and flexibility of practice patterns available. In this chapter, we discuss the two major career paths in emergency medicine and discuss academic and nonacademic practices. We list the pros and cons of each of these practice types as well as the significant considerations you should contemplate before deciding on a particular option. One of the most refreshing things about choosing a career in emergency medicine is the multitude of choices. This chapter will help you begin the process of thinking about which of these choices is best for you.

Types of Practice

The variety of practice options in emergency medicine is quite diverse. Section IV discusses the multiple fellowship options available to emergency medicine-trained physicians. In this chapter, we focus on the primary branch point for most physicians: deciding to pursue a practice in academics or a private group setting. Each of these may be located in urban, suburban, or rural environments. Physicians with military requirements will find emergency medicine to be a highly valued career choice within the armed services, and they have many professional opportunities from which to choose. As you evaluate practice patterns for their potential fit with your personal goals, it is helpful to list the pros and cons of each type. We evaluate each of the major practice types in this way.

Academic Practice

For many physicians, the academic practice is the ideal pattern. The opportunity to teach and influence the development of future emergency physicians is very rewarding. However, the academic practice has many other positive attributes. Many academic physicians rate the opportunity to make a lasting contribution to medicine as the single most important reason for selecting an academic practice. Others highly value the teaching environment, research opportunities, or the lifelong personal learning. In general, academic practices are larger than many community practices and may see a slightly different patient mix. This depends largely on the location and affiliation of the practice. Many emergency medicine teaching programs are located in busy community hospitals, while others are located within large tertiary or quaternary care facilities. These tertiary care referral hospitals are rich with subspecialists and frequently associated with medical schools. These hospitals tend to see a more complex patient population and more patients are referred from outside institutions.

Many students or residents are deterred from contemplating a career in academics by several perceived drawbacks. Many cite a lower academic pay scale as a reason not to enter an academic career. This difference in academic salary may seem quite substantial in the first few years out of practice; however, as academic stature and promotion occur, the salary scales become more comparable to those in the community. In addition, academic practices frequently come with very strong benefit packages that may not be calculated into the quoted salaries in community practice. All in all, you will probably make less at least initially; however, over the life of your career, this will probably not be substantially less. The most commonly stated reason for not considering an academic practice is the perception that research is required. Others state the structured advancement process for promotion and tenure as a deterrent. These obligations are very institution specific. Many institutions have developed special career paths designed to value the clinical educator, teacher, or administrator and have no research requirement. In order to dispel these myths, let's evaluate the basics of an academic career structure.

The traditional academic tenure path is organized along three components: teaching, research, and administration. Traditionally, individuals who were successful in this type of practice had to develop expertise in all three areas, that is, the "tenure track." This type of academic track has an "up or out" promotion standard, and if the individual does not complete the institution-specific requirements for tenure, he or she is forced to seek employment elsewhere. Because of the large number of talented individuals who were excluded by this process, many institutions have developed very broad and diverse "clinical tracks." These tracks were designed by institutions to recognize the importance of individuals who were specifically devoted to just one or two of these areas of expertise. The general premise is that mastery of one venue does not require demonstration of success in all three areas. The two most common content areas for clinical track faculty are education and clinical excellence. Emergency physicians are prime candidates for these areas of academic focus because our excellent clinical case diversity and 24-7 attending coverage in the emergency department make the teaching environment very rich. Faculty whose primary focus is research are generally on the tenure track; as success in a research career lends itself to publishing and successful grant writing. These two items significantly weighted in tenure track application.

Success in academics can lead to a rewarding career and all of these different academic career paths are available in emergency medicine, and if you believe your interest lies in an academic career, further information is available from EMRA and SAEM in *Emergency Medicine: An Academic Career Guide,* edited by Hobgood and Zink. This publication is available on the Web at www.emra.org and www.saem.org.

Private Group Practice

Just as there are many types of academic practice, the group practice in emergency medicine is changing to meet the needs of the practicing physician, as well as the hospitals that employ them. The type of practice most residents and practicing physicians find most appealing is the democratic group. Just as the name implies, these groups are founded on the principle that all members are created equal, and that all members should have a voice in the operating decisions of the group. This is appealing on the surface, but in real life one often finds that a committee is not the best format for managing the day-to-day operations of a dynamic emergency medicine practice. The reality of most of these types of group practice is that the group membership elects a leader who is responsible for the day-to-day operations of the practice. Ideally, major decisions are evaluated, and options formulated by the leadership then are presented to the group for approval. This typically allows for smooth day-to-day operations and ongoing investment by the membership in group functions. Because membership in emergency medicine group practice is dynamic, many groups have developed methods to increase the value of members who have a substantial investment in the practice. This traditionally takes the form of a partnership track.

Partners in emergency medicine groups are analogous to partners in a law firm. They represent the senior members of the group who may have years of investment in building hospital relationships, acquiring contracts, managing the group, and many, many night shifts. The most common rewards are enhanced pay scales, larger distributions of the bonus pool, or better schedules. The policies governing partnership status, rewards of partnership, and the terms for becoming a partner are established in the group's corporate bylaws or partnership agreements. These should be fully disclosed to any member seeking employment with the group. Nonpartnership democratic groups are usually smaller and function either as entirely democratic; that is, all decisions are made by the group, or all group members hold an equal administrative role or responsibility for which they are accountable.

Most democratic groups will hire only board-certified emergency physicians; therefore, most members are fairly equal as to their educational status. These groups have a sense of ownership and commitment to the hospital, leading to integration of the group into the medical staff and equal recognition by other hospital physicians. If the group functions well and it has a good business structure, it can be quite profitable.

Being a member of a private group is not always a "perfect 10." This type of group structure also has some drawbacks, and a few of these are elucidated below. Private groups are responsible for maintaining all of the components of a successful practice. The group members may or may not have skills in this area. The group must negotiate the contract with the hospital and keep the relationship with both the medical staff and hospital administration viable in order to maintain their employment contract on favorable terms. The group is also independently responsible for their own financial management. This includes the assumption of both positive and negative risk. When one considers the implications of paying all physician salaries and benefits while maintaining a positive cash flow from patient billing, it can become a stressful full-time job. For this reason, many groups hire management experts to ensure all of their financial goals are met in a timely manner. In smaller groups, this extra salary or contractual expenditure may have significant implications for the bonus pool. In this case, physicians may be delegated to assume additional business functions while maintaining their clinical assignments. As you can see from the previous discussion, this may require a substantial amount of physician time and require acquisition of additional management skills.

Contract Management Groups

In the previous business model, the physicians of the group directly contracted with the hospital to provide emergency medicine services for the hospital. The physicians functioned as a private practice and were responsible for all components of the practice. Another style of emergency medicine practice is employment by a contract management group. Just as the name implies, a corporate group holds the contract with the hospital to provide physician services, and it employs physicians to meet these needs. Typically, the contract management group is responsible for all the financial management of the practice and is either paid a flat fee by the hospital to provide physician staffing or negotiates a fee plus collections based on the group's billing.

Another important consideration is the manner in which you are hired. You may be hired as an employee with benefits such as life and health insurance, or you may be hired as an independent contractor, which means you are individually responsible for your own benefit package. This has significant personal tax implications as well as placing limitations on the way you collect your professional fees from federal insurance programs like Medicare and Medicaid. A complete discussion of the intricacies of physician contracting is beyond the scope of this article; however, further reading on this topic is available from EMRA in *Contract Issues for Emergency Physicians,* edited by Joseph P. Wood, MD, JD.

Continued education on these important topics is encouraged. As either an independent contractor or employee, the physician is solely responsible for providing clinical care and has no input into the financial management of the practice. This type of practice may not be for all emergency physicians, and it has distinct pros and cons.

One of the most positive attributes of the contract management group is its management expertise. These groups are very well versed in the day-to-day management of an emergency medicine practice. They can provide an economy of scale when hiring support staff to manage the financial resources of the group and acquire benefits for the physicians if these are offered. They may be able to enhance the negotiation with managed care organizations by providing large patient numbers through grouping all its contracted practices together to obtain a better rate of return for the care delivered by its physicians. Physicians with leadership potential may be able to move up within the corporate structure of the group to medical directors at the regional and national level.

On the flip side, there is very little room to advance within the individual practice, as there are limited leadership positions available. Physicians who work for contract management groups do not develop the financial management skills of those physicians involved in private group practices. Contracted physicians may not have input into the hiring or firing of physicians employed by the corporate contract management team. The contract management group may not hire all board-certified emergency physicians to meet its staffing requirements. This may lead to a poor fit between the individual physicians staffing a particular facility. It is important to understand the hiring philosophy of any corporate group before you agree to employment so this does not create personal conflict after you are hired. The major consideration here is that you are an employee of a corporate entity. When you walk out at the end of the day, you are not responsible for the function of the corporate group, the maintenance of the contract, the cash flow, or the billing. By agreeing to employment with a contract management group, you relinquish your responsibility to the practice with the exception of your clinical duties, but you also forfeit your ability to influence the way the practice functions. In addition to the contract management style of group practice, there are other types of employment practice options available to the emergency physician. One of the most popular and growing models is the hospital employee.

Hospital Employee

The emergency physician may be hired directly by the hospital administrator to staff the emergency department. This allows each individual physician to negotiate an individual contract with the hospital administrator. This is opposed to a corporate management team or leadership from the group negotiating collectively for all physicians, which occurs in the previously described models. This allows you, the physician, to strike the best deal possible for yourself. Much like the employee status of the physician hired by a contract management group, hospital employment alleviates the financial management side of emergency medicine practice. The physician is not responsible for billing or collecting, contract maintenance, or other administrative duties; they are simply charged with patient care and maintenance of a good relationship with the hospital administrator.

The down side of this practice pattern should be clear. You are not vested in the practice; you are an employee of the hospital. Each physician in the practice is independent of the other. This may be very functional or lead to a lack of cohesion and a high variability in clinical practice. The physician employed in this manner may have little opportunity to advance into leadership roles within the group or even within the corporate structure. Typically, there is little or no bonus or incentive plan, and you may or may not be viewed as an "equal" member of the medical staff by your colleagues in other specialties.

Career Development

No matter what choice you make as to practice format, it is important that you continue to grow and develop in your profession. Therefore, an important consideration when evaluating a position should be its opportunity for personal and professional development. This may take the form of simply seeing lots of patients and solidifying your personal clinical practice standards. Much of that will occur just by seeing patients independently and developing your own style of practice. Other aspects should be more conscientiously cultivated.

Opportunities to assume leadership within the group structure are an important consideration. Does the group rotate leadership or has the same individual served as group leader for an extensive period? If the leadership is rotated, how are the individuals prepared to lead? Many groups have developed specific tracks that lead to leadership, such as an executive committee with orderly progression through each of the positions. Individuals may start as members at large, progress to secretary, treasurer, vice president, and then finally president of the group before returning to regular group membership.

Mentoring opportunities within the group are also important to consider. This is important not only within academic practices but also within private groups as well. Individuals who are willing to teach the skills they have learned through years of successful practice are critical to the successful development of younger physicians. This mentoring can take many forms and is an important way to develop the professional skills needed for career longevity.

Fellowship training, which will be discussed in Section IV, is one venue for expanding the horizons of your career in emergency medicine. Other degrees, such as the MBA, MPH, or PhD, may also be considered. The important caveat to remember is that emergency medicine allows one the flexibility to enhance his or her personal education without the sacrifice of one's clinical career. This allows one to maintain clinical skills, as well as an income stream. As with all additional training, one should consider the long-term benefit of the extra degree before investing considerable time and energy in the process.

Perhaps one of the most rewarding opportunities to grow and develop as an emergency physician comes through membership in the American College of Emergency Physicians (ACEP). ACEP is a professional organization that provides a variety of member benefits. Continuing medical education, critical to your long-term viability in practice, is premier among ACEP benefits. Continuing education keeps you abreast of the latest issues in patient management, connects you with your peers, and allows you to explore new areas of interest within the specialty. Membership in ACEP also keeps you informed about legislative and regulatory issues that affect the practice of emergency medicine. Part of the commitment an individual makes to a profession, as opposed to just a job, is staying involved; and a high-quality professional organization is mandatory to maintaining this important component of your professional life.

What Is the Right Opportunity for You?

How do you decide what is the right career opportunity for you? These decisions are complex, multifactorial analyses that can only be decided on by you and your family. Some of the most important considerations for you will be your personal values when you choose a group. Is it important for you to work only with ABEM and AOBEM board-certified emergency physicians? Do you need or want to be a partner? How long are you willing to work to obtain partnership status? If these are very important considerations to you, then you will be evaluating groups based on their hiring practices and not location or salary. Other considerations may be more important. Do you want an urban, suburban, or rural environment? What patient mix interests you most? Do you just love trauma? Maybe you should consider an inner-city site. Your partner's job or profession may be the most significant factor in your choice of position. Does he or she require a large city or a college campus, or is he or she flexible? Is your family, church, or civic activity more important than your career? Do you need to be in a particular location for family or personal reasons? Maybe you just feel better at the beach.

In this era of high tuition and long periods of incumbency before repayment, physician debt after graduation from medical school has soared. In addition to your debt load, however, consider how much money you will need to live comfortably while you retire that debt. If you have a significant amount of debt, then you may want to choose a high paying position that will allow you to work as much as possible. Other options are debt repayment plans generated by some hospitals to assist them in recruiting and retaining high-quality physicians.

All of these personal considerations should play a part in your analysis. Only you can rank these issues as to their relative importance and only you can decide what, in the final analysis, is the best fit for you and your family. Start formulating your thoughts now on these issues as you to begin to select your specialty, your residency, and ultimately your first practice.

Conclusion

Training in emergency medicine opens the door to many exciting and challenging professional opportunities. The variety of practice patterns and locations provides options for almost everyone. The flexibility of scheduling and the diverse needs of many groups allow individuals the opportunity to pursue many other personal and professional interests while maintaining a viable clinical practice. The clinical practice is stimulating and provides a constant intellectual challenge. In addition, few careers are as satisfying as emergency medicine from the perspective of making an impact everyday. Emergency medicine is indeed the best of all worlds and provides its practitioners with all the components for a long and successful career.

chapter 5

Career Paths in Emergency Medicine

Kristin E. Harkin, MD, FACEP
Past President, EMRA
Assistant Professor of Medicine, Division of Emergency Medicine
Weill Medical College of Cornell University; New York-Presbyterian Hospital

One of the attractive aspects of emergency medicine is the ability to practice in a diverse variety of settings, literally anywhere. It is relatively easy to move because one does not necessarily have to establish a group practice, like cardiologists, for example. It is possible to do locum tenens work in emergency medicine, even internationally.

In short, opportunities in emergency medicine abound. You just have to be open to them. There are expanded types of practice and many different career paths in emergency medicine that you may not have thought of, and some of them are even outside the emergency department itself! You need to decide in which setting you will flourish the most and be happiest.

Most emergency physicians work as employees of hospitals or medical groups. Possible settings include academic teaching centers, tertiary care referral centers, trauma centers, community hospitals in suburban areas, rural hospitals, military hospitals, and urgent care clinics. Many work in academic positions at teaching centers or in corporate groups.

Other choices for careers in emergency medicine involve paths in pediatric emergency medicine, international relief missions, occupational industries, sports medicine, hyperbaric medicine, burn centers, emergency medical services, air medical services, disaster planning, toxicology, cruise ship medicine, health policy, and medical education to name a few! Emergency physicians also serve in different roles of hospital administration, community relations, or even public office. Emergency physicians serve as physicians at mass gatherings, such as concerts and stadium events, as well.

Many of the career options require formal fellowship training as a prerequisite. These are discussed in Section IV. Emergency medicine research is another important element for career development. Some career paths require additional credentials, such as an MBA, MPH, or JD. Information about these alternative career paths may be found by joining an ACEP Section or SAEM Interest Group. Look to societies outside of emergency medicine as well to help foster your development. Find a good mentor. A career counselor may be of particular help too.

Listed below is an outline of alternative career paths in emergency medicine that others have pursued and greatly enjoyed. The sky is the limit!

Expanded Types of Emergency Medicine Practice

- Administration: Medical director, CQI, risk management, clinical policies, schedule, finance, patient satisfaction
- Academics: Medical school (dean, course director), residency (director), fellowship (director)
- Fast-track/urgent care
- Occupational health/workers compensation
- Student health
- Pediatric emergency medicine
- Geriatric emergency medicine
- Nursing homes
- Toxicology/poison control centers
- Burn centers
- Hyperbarics
- Observational medicine
- Hospitalists
- Critical care
- Ultrasound
- Cruise ship physician
- Resort/hotel physician
- Sports medicine
- Injury control
- Wilderness emergency medicine
- EMS/disaster medicine/mass gatherings (concerts, games, events)
- International relief
- Aeroflight medicine/astronaut
- Entrepreneur: CME, inventor
- Locum tenens
- Operations consultant
- Medical-legal consultant, attorney
- Pharmaceutical consultant
- Medical stock analyst
- Medical informatics
- Patient safety consultant
- Designer of medical office space
- Physician recruitment
- Billing
- Transcription service
- Forensic medicine
- Military
- Government employee (Veterans Administration, prison physician, public health officer, OEM, NTSA, homeland security)
- Organized medicine
- Speaker
- Legislator
- Novelist/playwright
- Medical journalist
- Television/motion picture/news/media consultant

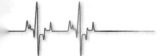

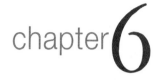

chapter 6

Emergency Physician Workforce: Current Needs and Future Requirements

David Guss, MD, FACEP
Chair, Department of Emergency Medicine, University of California, San Diego

Emergency medicine is still a relatively young specialty that remains in its ascendancy. Since its inception in the late 1960's through the first certification exam in 1979 and on into the present day, the number of training programs and the breadth of the specialty have consistently expanded. There are currently over 130 approved residency training programs with subspecialty training and certification offered in medical toxicology, hyperbaric medicine, sports medicine, and pediatric emergency medicine. Additional, noncertified training is available in research, administration, emergency medical services, and ultrasound.

Although not endorsed by this author as the basis on which to choose a specialty of study or a future career path, it is reasonable to query, What are the prospects for current and future employment in the field of emergency medicine? The determination of the physician workforce needs and projections for future needs can be quite complex and fraught with error. The reasons for this relate to the numerous variables that factor into the calculation and the capricious nature of the assumptions that must be made. In addition, workforce needs can vary significantly by region. Urban areas in general provide for more physicians per capita than rural areas, and this is often more dramatically so for specialists.

The first assumption, whether determining current or future needs, is that only board-certified or prepared physicians will provide medical services in the emergency department. The next assumption relates to whether specifically trained physician extenders in the form of physician assistants and nurse practitioners will play a part and then to what degree. For the purposes of this analysis, we exclude the physician extenders from the equation. The key variables are number of emergency department visits, number of emergency departments, number of emergency department beds, scope of emergency department services to be offered, patient mix with respect to acuity, current number of practicing physicians, percent clinical time for those currently practicing, physician productivity, workforce attrition through death, retirement, and reduction in clinical workload, and the number of new physicians coming into the workforce. Finally, there is the issue of subspecialty training and the impact pursuit of specialty services will have on overall manpower needs. Of course, after all of these factors are employed to determine current manpower needs the assumptions, and variables must be adjusted as they are projected into the future.

In 1992 the National Hospital Ambulatory Medical Care Survey (NHAMCS) reported that there were 89.2 million emergency department visits, for a visit rate of 35.7 visits per 100 persons. In 2004, there were 110.2 million visits and the visit rate had increased to 38.2 per 100 persons. Of note, for the first time since 1992, the visit rate dropped in the interval between surveys conducted in 2002 and 2004 from 38.9 to 38.2 per 100 persons. The number of active emergency department beds is not reported in this survey; however, the number of emergency departments was reported to have declined by 15% in the interval between 1992 and 2002.

In 2005, there were 22,376 active diplomats of the American Board of Emergency Medicine (certified emergency medicine specialists). In this same year, 1233 candidates passed the oral board examination and became certified emergency physicians. In the 2006-2007 academic year, there were 139 accredited programs in emergency medicine with positions for 4400 residents. This compares to 122 programs and 3652 positions in the 2000-2001 academic year.

The American Board of Emergency Medicine has been conducting a longitudinal survey of physicians for over a decade. This survey is designed to assess emergency physician practice pattern, job satisfaction, and future plans. In 2003, in the most recent report from this ongoing project, 85% of respondents indicated they were satisfied or very satisfied with their job. Satisfaction was greatest for those in practice for 2 to 3 years, at 95%, and lowest for those working over 30 years, at 82%. The best estimate for current attrition rate for certified emergency physicians comes from this survey where 8% of respondents indicated they had retired in the 5 years since the prior survey. Response rates for the most recent survey was 93%, and it is not known what percentage of those not responding were a consequence of retirement, death, or other.

Using some common assumptions and limiting the variables under consideration, we can conduct a simplified exercise of calculating the current and future emergency physician manpower needs. The current U.S. population, not including undocumented immigrants, has just crossed the 300 million mark. If there are 38.2 visits per 100 patients per year, then we might expect 114,00,000 emergency department visits in 2006. If an average emergency physician can see between 2.0 to 2.5 patients per hour, then we would need between 57 million to 45.6 million hours of physician coverage. If we assume the average emergency physician works 32 clinical hours per week for 48 weeks per year or 1536 hours per year, then we would need 37,110 to 29,688 emergency physicians. Factors calling for upward adjustment include number of emergency physicians working fewer clinical hours as a result of subspecialty work, administration, research and teaching, and the changing scope of patient evaluations. Downward adjustment would be introduced by utilization of physician extenders as they would likely displace the need for some emergency physicians or at least could be viewed as enhancing the estimated physician productivity estimates. Given the current pool of certified emergency physicians in 2006, we could credibly proffer that the current shortage of emergency physicians is between 7000 and 15,000.

Now, looking into the future, we would need to make some assumptions about population growth, number of new emergency physicians coming into the workforce, physician attrition, patterns of emergency department utilization, populations characteristics, emergency department overcrowding, and physician productivity. As many of these issues are particularly speculative, we will only consider population growth, the number of new emergency physician entries, and the likely rate of attrition. The NHAMCS projects the U.S. population to be 335 million in 2020 and estimates there will be 127 million emergency department visits. Applying our productivity estimates, the need for emergency physicians in the year 2020 will be in the range of 33,000 to 41,000. Based on the longitudinal survey results, we will estimate yearly attrition at 1.6% per year, which roughly correlates with estimates from other sources. The estimate for the number of new specialist entering the field will be based on the observed growth during the same 5-year interval as included in the longitudinal survey, is approximately 5% per year. The combination of attrition and entry of new physicians provides for an addition of about 950 additional emergency physicians per year. Using this figure in a linear fashion would mean that in the year 2020, there will be between an excess of 2,000 to a shortage of 6,000 physicians in the workforce. While the low range of this estimate may prove troubling to some medical students with a long-range view for their career, it should be remembered that the estimate for attrition is based on 2006 data and is reflective of a relatively young

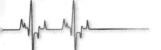

workforce. As this workforce ages, the attrition rate is certain to rise. Furthermore, the growth in new emergency physicians entering the workforce is predicated on a specialty in or near its maximal growth phase and the number of new entries into the field is likely to slow between now and 2020. Therefore, the likelihood is that a shortage rather than excess of emergency physicians will continue well out past 2020.

In comparing the above workforce estimates to recent publications, there is generally good correlation despite utilization of different methodology. The largest study was conducted by John Moorehead and colleagues and published in a 2002 edition of the *Annals of Emergency Medicine*. In that report, they projected a workforce need of approximately 31,700 physicians in 1999, which compares to the 29,000 to 37,000 mentioned here for the year 2006. There was no long-term number provided.

The most important caveat is that the projections provided are based on national estimates and the workforce needs of a particular community can vary significantly. In general, there is a tendency for the more desirable urban and metropolitan locales to have tighter job markets.

So, what is the take-home message? Accepting a reasonable degree of error, whether accepting the approach used in this offering or those published by others, there is presently a significant shortage of emergency physicians and this manpower shortfall is likely to continue into the foreseeable future.

chapter 7

Emergency Medicine Lifestyle

J. Mark Meredith III, MD, FACEP
Past Chair, ACEP Wellness Section

Residency is over, what is the real life like?

Now that residency is over, the long hours will get better. No more nights, no more holidays and weekends. No more on-call. Well, that might be true, but it may not. That might not be a reasonable expectation. Most groups will have a full-time position working 144 to 180 hours per month. That is, if the group is full. If there are gaps in the physician staff, then everyone works more. The schedule has to be full. So your hours may be a little higher. They will still probably be less than your residency days. That will be less than the 80 hours per week of residency.

We have a practice that is 24/7/365. That means that someone is always on duty. Weekdays, weekends, nights, holidays; that includes birthdays, anniversaries, and graduations. The upside is you will be on duty or off. You will not be on-call, maybe. When you are off, you are off.

In some larger groups, there may be an on-call physician to cover busy times or call outs. You might be with a group that has an on-call process for sick calls or for high volume days. The days of on-call may not be over. They will likely be less than those as a resident and less stressful.

The fact is the schedule needs to be complete and full and we need to cover the department. How this responsibility is shared will vary. Most groups will rotate weekdays, weekends, holidays, evenings, and nights. This is the fair way to treat colleagues and the fair way for an emergency department group to share the load. As we age individually and as a specialty, a group may opt to recognize time with the group or in the specialty by reducing or limiting the less desirable shifts. Not a completely unreasonable plan. You will all get there at some point.

Shift work is the bane of emergency medicine; it might be the only downside to the specialty. The main stressor of emergency medicine is no doubt the fact that we are 24/7/365 and that to do this we rotate shifts. Shift work brings with it an increase in depression, hypertension, miscarriages, infertility, divorce, ulcers, accidents, and errors. How you adapt to rotating shifts will vary.

In terms of nights, there is good evidence that younger physicians can better tolerate the rigors of night shifts, the stress of circadian disruption. Some groups will pay a premium rate for the night shifts to encourage those who tolerate night shifts better to be willing to work the night shifts.

In working night shifts, there are some things you can do to better tolerate this attack on your circadian rhythm. Schedule rotation should always be in a clockwise rotation. Counterclockwise (southern swing) rotations are more disruptive to our normal circadian rhythms. Another strategy used to cope with rotating shifts is isolated night shifts. Physicians work a single night shift and do not work several in a row. They do not disrupt their normal circadian rhythm. This is especially good if the group does have a physician or two working all nights or uses the night float concept. It works less well with small groups if all members are doing an equal number of nights.

Night float is yet another potential solution to the night work dilemma. With this concept, a physician lumps all of their nights into a 6-week (or longer) time frame. This allows for their circadian rhythm to be shifted to a nighthawk mode for this period of time. For this to work, the physician needs to convert their day lifestyle to a night lifestyle during this time frame. Days off need to be lived with morning sleep and evening awake times. This can be difficult or impossible for those with a family.

Moreover, another concept proposed is shorter night shifts. Six-hour night shifts coupled with 10-hour day shifts and 8-hour evening shifts has been considered. A recent development is the concept to split the night shift so that there is a break at 3 or 4 A.M. A variation of this is a typical 8- or 12-hour shift that ends at 4 A.M. This also has the effect of allowing each physician to get some normal sleep time.

Furthermore, the debate about shift length continues. One important issue to remember is that 12-hour shifts do not give any opportunity for adjusting your circadian rhythm gently. You are always shifting 180 degrees when you shift from 12-hour shifts.

Other suggestions for coping with night shifts include napping before a night shift, eating high-protein meals before a night shift, exercising before a night shift, and using bright lights while at work during the night shift. Often times, other staff members prefer dimming the lights, but that does not promote an alert mental state

Burnout is a real concern for emergency medicine. When I started in emergency medicine, there was an adage that a physician could only do emergency medicine for 10 years or until age 40. It is a high-stress, high-activity practice. We are constantly multitasking and have constant interruptions in our day. Thankfully, that was not correct. The longevity study by the American Board of Emergency Medicine has rebuked this idea. We do have physicians who practice emergency medicine full-time into their 60's. They may take fewer or shorter shifts. They may be allowed to drop night shifts but they continue to practice. They are often a valued asset to their departments and communities. One strategy for staying focused and sane is to remember, "It is your job, not your life." Be sure to develop outside interests outside of work. Develop and cultivate friendships. Explore and refine hobbies that give you rest and relaxation. Exercise!

We as physicians all too often allow our identity as a physician to become our sole identity as a person. We may lose our distinction as the doctor by injury, illness, or retirement, but that should not mean we have lost our identity as a person. Burnout is real. We all need to protect ourselves and guard against this. Develop outside interests.

You have chosen a specialty that demands 24/7/365 coverage. Every group has found ways to deal with this fact. In some, as the new person, you will get a larger share of the weekends, holidays, and nights. In some groups, you will be compensated for that. In others, you may not be monetarily compensated but may reap some other benefit. In some groups, it may be the way you pay your dues, prove your worth.

You have chosen a great specialty. It will be a fulfilling, active, simulating lifelong career. This is a marathon, not a sprint. Pace yourself and enjoy your career.

chapter 8

Urban Emergency Medicine

Jordan Moskoff, MD

Clinical Instructor, Department of Emergency Medicine/Rush Medical College, Cook County Hospital

When most people think of urban emergency medicine, they generally envision a scene from television or the movies. A large, chaotic, overcrowded room full of the sick and dying staffed by good looking, overworked, dedicated doctors working under the most difficult and extreme conditions. To the dismay of the many people who ask me "Is you job really like *E.R.*?" I have to answer, "No, there is a big difference. Actors on television and in the movies are generally better looking than most ER docs." The surprising reality is that working in an urban emergency department is not that different from what is portrayed in the media. We see an incredibly large volume of patients, many of whom are very sick, under difficult conditions, although if you lose your cool and yell "STAT" at a seasoned emergency department nurse, you'll be lucky if all you get is a nasty look.

One of the factors that distinguishes the urban emergency department from its suburban and rural counterparts is its role as a social safety net. Urban emergency departments are generally situated within working poor and immigrant neighborhoods whose populations have limited access to health care. For this reason, many of the medically underserved have no choice but to resort to the emergency department for their only means of medical care.

The most obvious consequence of this is the large patient populations that present to many urban emergency departments, creating enormous patient volumes. The immediate downsides are clear. The waiting room is always full and long waits are not uncommon. On rare occasions this can lead to disgruntled patients. We all have stories of patients calling 911 from the waiting room thinking that will get them in faster, or of angry patients threatening to riot and throwing soda cans and garbage at the triage nurses. Disgruntled patients aside, the real danger of long waiting times is the possibility of a time bomb like a missed myocardial infarction or a patient with gastrointestinal bleeding who looked good at first only to decompensate in the middle of the waiting room.

Of course the wait isn't over once the patients are in the emergency department. Patients wait for tests to come back and lab results and, longest of all, they wait for beds upstairs. A large volume in the emergency department means a large volume upstairs on the medicine wards. Patients will often wait in the halls for up to 2 or 3 days. Beyond the stress this places on patients and family members, this of course puts an additional stress onto the physicians and nurses as we must monitor and care for patients well past their initial treatment and disposition. Often I find myself starting a shift with ventilator rounds or antibiotic rounds to make sure patients are continuing to be cared for as they wait. But caring for patients in the hallway is just part of the job; we do our best and hope no one deteriorates unnoticed, as, unfortunately, time bombs are not limited to the waiting room.

There is, of course, an upside to the incredibly large volume of patients who we see. And that is that urban emergency department docs have seen it all—immigrants' fresh to the United States with malaria, dock workers with scorpion bites they got unpacking crates from the Middle East, uremic frost on a dialysis patient. And of course we see every kind of trauma imaginable.

But the real beauty of the urban emergency department is that every time I'm foolish enough to think I've seen it all, something truly new comes through the door—a jockey with a posterior hip dislocation after being kicked by a horse, a pancytopenic cancer patient in disseminated intravascular coagulation presenting in both hypovolemic and septic shock, or a patient with thoracic aortic dissection presenting with one episode of vomiting and some leg tingling. These, of course, are the moments that keep us humble as well as the moments we live for, the reason that we work in urban emergency departments. The large volume brings with it the strange, the bizarre, and the high acuity cases that make my job so interesting and enjoyable. I love the acuity, I love the difficult cases, and the greatest moments are when multiple sick patients come in at the same time. Without the incredibly large volume of patients, we wouldn't get these cases and work might actually become, dare I say it, routine.

Another effect of our role as a social safety net is that many people in the community with minor complaints and chronic problems have nowhere else to go but the emergency department, or what I once heard a patient refer to as the "24-hour clinic." This, of course, has the deleterious effect of turning emergency docs into primary docs, something for which I have neither the training nor the temperament. I admit sometimes this puts me in a less than generous mood, causing me to ask patients "Are you sure your arm only ever hurts on Tuesdays? How does your arm know it's Tuesday?" or "If this has been bothering you for six months, why did you pick today during my shift to present." But fortunately, these lapses are rare, and I can usually handle these chronic minor complaints with the respect they deserve and smile as I dispense Motrin and a clinic referral.

Knowing that many of our patients use us as their primary care physicians also often makes us do more than we otherwise would in just treating their emergent complaint. For example, I often draw off screening labs on patients with an obvious gastroenteritis because I know no one else will, or I might be quicker to admit a patient purely for social reasons. A visit to the emergency department may be a patient's only chance to get plugged into the system or receive the screening they need. Although I hate to say it, it is often in the best interest of our patients to forget we are an emergency department and play the role of 24-hour clinic.

Beyond the social safety net, the other factor that differentiates the urban emergency department is the type of patients we see. After working in several urban emergency departments, I've begun to notice that a vast number of patients we see often fall into just a few categories. The first group is by far the largest and my favorite. These are the patients who have nowhere else to go and really need us. Often they are the elderly, newly arrived immigrants, or the working poor doing their best to make ends meet with no where else to turn. These patients take their health care seriously, are active participants in their care, and follow our advice by following up in the clinics and taking their medicine as prescribed. It is really a pleasure to care for them knowing they have no one else to turn to and that as an emergency department doc, I am making a real and lasting impact not just on their immediate needs but on their overall health.

The next group is made of the patients who make our days harder. These are the patients who don't take responsibility for their care. When asked what medication they take, often they will tell me "Why should I know? You're the doctor. Look it up in my chart." The worst moments with this group are when I ask them who their primary care physician is, only to be handed an empty pill bottle. It's a real disappointment when I look down to see that the physician's name on the pill bottle is mine. This is the group of patients who doesn't follow up in the clinics and regularly run out of medicine, returning to the emergency department time after time seeking refills. By shunning all responsibility and not actively participating in their care, they hurt themselves and blame us. A couple of these patients in the same shift can make for a bad day.

The next group is my least favorite but absolutely unavoidable in any urban emergency department. These are the drug, warm bed, and sandwich seekers. Living on the streets and trying to scrounge by day to day, they haunt urban emergency departments looking for soft touches. These are the patients who abuse the system and try to get everything out of us they can. I've actually had a patient leave the emergency department against medical advice only to go and rob the hospital's coffee shop. Adding insult to injury, while in custody he was brought back to the emergency department demanding pain medication and claiming the hospital police beat him up. Fortunately, this group is relatively small in number.

The last group that typically inhabits urban emergency departments is strangely enough one of my favorites. These are the alcoholics and addicts that make their homes in our waiting room and hallways, the regulars. It's a symbiotic relationship. We provide a warm place for them to sleep and the occasional sandwich, and they serve as our unofficial greeters. I've actually overheard a regular defending us to a patient complaining about the long wait by telling the irate patient about all the amazing things he had seen us do and what great doctors we were. The regulars serve as a constant reminder for me why I do this job, to take care of those who need it most. There is a real pride in helping those who have no other options and who have been turned away by everyone else. It's nice to know that when they have lost absolutely everything else, there is still a place they can go where someone will take care of them.

The urban emergency department is defined by its role as a social safety net and by the patients who require our services. The large volume of patients ensures that we regularly see both the best and worst parts of human nature. Working in an urban emergency department means we see lots of chronic minor complaints, but we also see the oddities and high acuity cases that get our adrenaline pumping. It means working in an environment with a frenetic pace where decisions must be made quickly, many times without all the puzzle pieces in place. It means we function with or without all the equipment we need, depending on the latest round of budget cuts, but that we always function because we know that if we don't, then there is no one else. Working in an urban emergency department fosters a true feeling of collegiality with everyone on our team. Like soldiers in the trenches, we rely on each other for help and support, without which we would never be able to consistently provide such a high level of care under such difficult conditions to such an incredible volume of sick patients. This is the reason they make television shows and movies about us.

chapter 9

Emergency Medicine in Community Hospitals

Dan Murphy, MD, MBA, FACEP
Director of Emergency Services, Mercy Medical Center
President, Long Island Emergency Care, PC

One of the most profound choices for an emergency medicine resident is whether to pursue an academic teaching career or whether to practice emergency medicine "out in the community," away from the residency program, medical school, and university.

This decision exists in all specialties and is layered with personal value considerations of public service, fame, fortune, family, and lifestyle.

The majority of emergency physicians spend their career or a portion of their career practicing in community hospitals. Hospitals in the United States vary significantly, but the basic components are consistent. In smaller community hospitals, these components tend to be less layered, more "horizontal," and thus easier to grasp.

An understanding of the management, operations and constraints of community hospitals is fundamentally crucial to achieving job satisfaction in emergency medicine, because so much of our care and performance rely on other people and other processes that we may not directly manage.

This chapter is intended to be a brief description of the inner workings of a community hospital and its emergency department. Picture a place with 200 to 300 inpatient beds, no fellows, no residents, and no medical students. The inpatient medical orders are written by private physicians, hospitalists, consultants, or physicians assistants. Nurses and their assistants are the primary patient caregivers.

Management and Governance

A hospital is the only regulated health care unit that can fully support the complete practice of emergency medicine. A hospital is a corporation governed by a board of directors or board of trustees. The laws governing corporations require that it is accountable to its owners. Owners can be for-profit stockholders or the nonprofit public. The accountability is accomplished through the guidance and oversight of the board of directors. A community hospital's board of directors should include leaders and other representatives who live or work within its community.

In most community hospitals, the operations and management of day-to-day operations involves the inputs of three major stakeholders: administration, nursing, and the medical staff. A balance of power between these groups exists that varies from hospital to hospital and is significantly influenced by the history, vision, and personality of the community, the board, and the chief executive of the hospital.

The nursing department has its own management, hierarchy, and academic tradition. It is usually the largest and most expensive employee pool in the hospital. Nursing often finds itself strategically positioned between administration and the medical staff physicians when it comes to operational and patient care issues.

Nurses are crucial to the medical staff because of their clinical knowledge and abilities.

They are important to administration because they have the most consistent responsibilities at the patients' bedside and the best understanding of how to deliver attention and care efficiently. Nursing staff provides a valid and important perspective with respect to the clinical performance and intentions of the medical staff, something administration is not always qualified to do. The nursing department also often manages various unit-based ancillary staff such as unit secretaries and patient care technicians, the other people that emergency physicians work with and rely on each shift.

The administrators are the operational managers of the hospital. While an executive director or chief executive officer oversees the financial and operational functions of the hospital, the medical staff leadership and nursing leadership also report to the CEO. A CEO answers to the board of directors or a higher corporate office if the hospital is not independent.

A hospital "credentials'" a medical staff to work within its walls. The relationship between a hospital and its medical staff is very symbiotic. The community hospital depends on private, community-based practitioners to refer patients to the hospital instead of to a competing hospital. It also depends on capable intensivists, surgeons, and consultants to oversee care and perform procedures with a competitive length of stay. The practitioners need a hospital that provides good care for their patients and is a source of new patients or consults.

Finance

No matter how municipal or how charitable a hospital's mission, ultimately "form follows finance." Like any business, hospitals are dependent on customer volume and profitable delivery of services for financial viability and success. A hospital needs to collect more revenue than it spends delivering care, or else its mission to the community will be compromised and at risk.

In geographic areas where the community has less wealth and less health care insurance, the hospital is more dependent on government payers and subsidies while independent community-based private physician practices are more difficult to sustain.

The governments and commercial insurers recognize two major payees for any given clinical encounter—the hospital and the professionals. Academic centers have a mission of teaching and research, which create an additional source of reimbursement, funding, career development, and image enhancement. Community hospitals compensate for a lack of an academic "brand" through affiliation, quality care, community awareness, customer service, and efficiency.

The Emergency Department

Emergency services have become more critical to the successful operation of hospitals as more than half of any hospital's admissions come through the emergency department. When there are no office or clinic hours, we are often a patient's only alternative. To the uninsured or underinsured, we are always the only alternative. When a practitioner in an office or clinic has a patient who requires hospital care, a direct admission bed is often unavailable or difficult to secure. Furthermore, the modern emergency department has resources and priority access to diagnostic tools and a highly skilled clinical workforce with broader diagnostic perspectives. The emergency department may even have an observation unit that could obviate the need for a hospitalization.

Unfortunately, these qualities (and federal law) have created increasing and poorly controllable demand and a serious lack of capacity in our nation's emergency departments. Crowding, ambulance diversion and very significant waits for inpatient beds are now common. Ironically, to patients and their advocates, the caring, cleanliness, efficiency, and service experienced during an emergency department encounter are a direct reflection of the quality of the hospital.

An effective and empowered emergency medicine group works collaboratively with hospital management to maximize care and service and to inform the administration of what is required. This collaboration requires a mature understanding of the financial constraints and priorities of the hospital in the context of the institutional mission. The administration must be open and inclusive in order for this to happen.

Emergency physicians can be contracted to work as employees, as independent contractors, or as part of a group practice. As with any human enterprise, the performance of key operational decision makers and rate limiters (that would be us) are best when incentives exist that are aligned with transparent and objective measures of quality and efficiency. Shared group ownership is the strongest of motivators.

The Community Hospital Emergency Department Shift

There are no residents. There are only a few physicians, perhaps some physician assistants, along with nurses, patient care technicians, and a unit secretary or two.

There may be a room or an area for "behavioral" cases but probably not a separate and secure psychiatric zone. There may be a separate pediatric emergency department, but whether it stays open 24 hours depends on volume.

There is backup by specialists on-call, but they could live some distance away or be stuck in the operating room for a while. You have to be self-sufficient, but such is the nature of emergency medicine.

The ambulances keep coming, a combination of municipal and volunteer ambulance company rigs. It is important not to ignore these first-responders. Their opinions of you matter a great deal to your future emergency department volume. In addition, the smart emergency groups facilitate regular lectures for the prehospital providers so that relationships solidify and ongoing training and education requirements are satisfied.

You must remember to ask the patient if they have a doctor. You must remember to ask again when family or friends arrive, especially if your patient is elderly. You must remember to document this on the chart. I stress this because in a community hospital the emergency physician is held highly accountable to honor previously established patient-physician relationships. The private physicians and surgeons are trying to make a living, too. Furthermore, many patients or their families assume that we know who their doctor is. There is nothing more humiliating and angering to a private practice physician than to encounter a family in a hospital hallway on a Monday morning demanding to know why their mother, who was admitted Friday night, has not been visited by their real doctor instead of the assigned doctor.

It is a worthy attribute to be a good communicator with a winning personality.

An emergency department is much, much more than its physicians. The quality of care and the job satisfaction of the emergency physicians and nurses are highly dependent on how organized and efficient the department is. There are many models and theories and best practices to emulate and customize, but, in the end, all stakeholders must realize that the nurses and physicians are overseeing a dynamic process that requires steady throughput and output. We are at our best when our attention is on the new arrivals and those being worked up and stabilized. When we are preoccupied with boarding inpatients, traditional emergency care suffers.

In an academic center, there is satisfaction and joy associated with watching a steady stream of residents and fellows learn their craft in a highly specialized clinical setting. In a community hospital, the clinicians may be a bit more focused on the people who are their patients, satisfied with holding their hands, knowing their neighbors and neighborhood, and in delivering quality emergency medicine diagnostics and therapy.

chapter 10

Rural Emergency Medicine

George Molzen, MD, FACEP
Past President, American College of Emergency Physicians; Presbyterian Healthcare Services

Imagine you are on duty one night in a rural emergency department. The local EMS crew brings in a patient with an anaphylactic reaction. You have only minutes to institute the proper lifesaving treatment; all decisions are up to you. There are no other physicians in the hospital who can help you. You hold this patient's life in your hands. This is the adrenaline rush you frequently face when practicing in a rural emergency department!

The practice of emergency medicine in a rural setting is unlike practice in urban environments and quite unlike practice you are used to in an academic institution. The first and most important difference is that you are often the only physician present in your hospital. The patient load of rural emergency departments is such that most hospitals have only single physician coverage in their emergency department's. As such, often you will not have the luxury of another emergency physician on duty with you. You may not have a specialist on your medical staff whom you can call. Many rural medical staffs are made up of primary care physicians and few specialists; a urologist, an ENT specialist, or even an orthopedist is not likely to be on-call at your hospital. Your back-up in many cases will be a general internist, a family medicine physician, or a general surgeon. Becausee these physicians will have busy office practices, they will prefer to come to the hospital only if it is clear the patient needs admission to your hospital. Their ability to provide emergency department consultation on "interesting or puzzling cases" will be very limited.

If you do have a consultant, he or she is often the only one in town and may not always be available. In many cases, specialty consultation must be made by calling a regional referral hospital. This means you alone will need to decide the answers to questions like, Does the patient need intubation? What medicines should be given? Can the patient be admitted at your hospital, or does the patient need rapid transport to a tertiary facility?

These types of situations can cause you to be a bit uncomfortable at times. This is normal. The good news is that if you are confident in your skills and knowledge, you can manage these patients on your own. You can provide care that patients in rural areas might otherwise not receive. You can make a real difference in the lives of the patients in your community. Many times, you can save a life. Because saving a life is the ultimate gratification for an emergency physician and one of the reasons we love our work, you have experienced one of the joys of a rural emergency medicine practice.

Rewards

Even if you are not saving a life, there are many joys in being a "go to" physician in the community. Your ability to perform extensive diagnostic workups, not only diagnose but treat many illnesses, and relieve pain and discomfort, all are a part of rural experience that is not as easily available in an urban setting. Unlike urban settings, with their availability of specialists, you will become the one to diagnose and treat many problems that would be referred out in an urban setting.

There are many other rewards of a rural practice. For those with the right personality, training, confidence and mindset, rural emergency medicine can be the best possible practice. While the rewards of a rural practice are many, there are some that stand out. You are likely to have a good lifestyle, especially if you like to be out and about in a rural setting. Farming, raising livestock, hiking, and other activities are some of the many areas that may be more easily pursued in a rural setting. The pace of life in a rural setting is often more relaxed and low key.

You will be more likely to have shifts that are longer, giving you more days off. In addition, you may have more shifts where the patient load is less and the number of really sick patients is less. You may see problems that are not common in urban emergency departments. Skills such as removing fishhooks and ticks are quickly developed. Environmental injuries from pesticides and other farming chemicals may be seen with some regularity.

You will also have more ability (and expectations from the community) to participate in hospital activities such as medical staff office and leadership. You will be expected to assist in community efforts as well such as medical direction for the local emergency medical services system, volunteer medical staffing at high school events, etc. For those interested in these activities, it is easier to become involved in a rural hospital and community.

You will become close friends with many of your co-workers (nurses, technicians, emergency medical technicians, etc.), as well as members of the medical staff. Because a rural hospital tends to be smaller, almost everyone knows each other on a personal basis. You often may have a personal relationship with those you see as patients. You will run into patients you saw in the emergency department last week while you are shopping or picking up your children at school. For this reason, a rural emergency medicine practice can often be close to a primary care practice with the ability to interact with your patients on a more personal level

Of most importance is the care you can provide to your patients. Having a well-trained emergency physician can often be the difference between a good patient outcome and a bad one; often it can mean the difference between life and death. Your ability to provide care that makes this difference is the best reward a physician can have.

Challenges

The practice of emergency medicine in a rural area can be stressful while at the same time very rewarding. You may well be the physician at the hospital with the most up-to-date skills on resuscitation and stabilization of critical patients. In addition, you may have more up-to-date information on the management of diseases and processes than other hospital staff physicians.

You must be very comfortable practicing in an environment where you must make decisions without much back-up or consultation. Many of your patients may need transfer to referral hospitals once they are stabilized. Your hospital should have referral agreements in place with tertiary hospitals so transfers are as routine as possible. It is also helpful to discuss with the other physicians in the community their use of consultants as they may have developed good referral patterns. Developing relationships with specialists by providing routine referrals may make it easier when emergent transfers are necessary.

You must become comfortable with interpreting electrocardiograms and imaging studies because you often will not have anyone else to help you interpret them. In addition, you may not have easy access to magnetic resonance imagers, Doppler imagers, interventional radiology imaiging, or other diagnostic and therapeutic resources that you may be used to from your training in an academic medical center. This will require more use of your clinical skills and judgment to compensate for this lack.

You must have very good "people skills" because the emergency department staff, nursing support, and administration may have weaknesses that you can help address. These personnel have also chosen a rural lifestyle and cannot and should not be easily replaced. If you have a nurse who is weak in clinical skills, you will have to work with the nurse to improve the skills because the ability to recruit a new nurse is probably limited. In addition, because the volume of patients is probably lower, your nurses may not be as familiar with unusual cases and you will need to guide them in their care of these patients.

The other side of the coin is that you may do more urgent care, minor emergencies, and even some primary care than you would in a city. Your emergency department may be the only option for care in evening hours for your patients. Your emergency department may also be the only option for those without adequate health insurance. You will need to learn to embrace patients with minor illnesses or emergencies and realize you are often their only health care option.

Depending on whether your setting has tourist attractions, you may have seasonal influxes of patients. In warmer climates, you may see 'snowbirds" who spend most of the winter in your area and then disappear in the summer. In areas with seasonal activities such as skiing, fishing, hunting, etc., you will also see periodic influxes of visitors who at times can make your emergency department quite busy. As you know, the lack of previous medical records on these transient visitors can make your job more difficult.

Finally, you are likely to be exposed to a 'small town atmosphere" where many people know each other, making confidentiality a difficult issue. If you are single, opportunities for relationships may be diminished. If you have a significant other, you must make sure that he or she also will be happy in a rural environment. Theater, concerts, even shopping, and movies will be less available. Your family must also be willing to accept living in a 'small town" environment. If they are not happy, you will not be happy.

Closing

A rural emergency medicine practice is not for everyone. The benefits of a rural community and rural practice must be balanced with the downsides. For those who wish to live in a rural setting and have the right mind set and confidence in their abilities, rural emergency medicine can be a wonderful way to practice.

There has been recent development of combined emergency medicine/family practice residency programs to go along with the traditional emergency medicine/internal medicine and emergency medicine/pediatrics residencies. These require extra years of training but could be helpful to someone who is sure he or she wants to practice in a rural environment.

chapter 11

Academic Emergency Medicine

Sandra M. Schneider, MD, FACEP

Professor and Chair, Department of Emergency Medicine, University of Rochester

Unlike most specialties, emergency medicine emerged from the need for clinical service rather than from a unique body of knowledge or skills. The need to serve the large numbers of undifferentiated patients presenting to emergency departments gave rise to the specialty but also deterred the development of a rich research direction. Given the diversity of clinical problems, the challenges of a 24/7 operation, and the overlap of clinical territory with already established specialties; emergency medicine initially struggled to develop a solid academic presence. Despite these early challenges, academic emergency medicine has made great stride to develop its place in academia.

A career in academic emergency medicine can be as varied as it is rewarding. Unlike other areas of emergency medicine practice, academia has a defined ladder of success, with clear standards for advancement (which are not uniform from school to school). Success is measured by promotion—assistant professor to associate professor to professor. There are several tracks that the individual can work in and successfully be promoted.

Clinician in the Teaching Hospital

Teaching residents at the bedside can be rewarding and is often appealing to new graduates. In addition, many teaching hospitals have interesting patient populations that create a stimulating practice. The clinician working in a teaching hospital will generally work 32 to 40 hours per week staffing the emergency department. There may be other administrative tasks and interactions with residents/medical students. It is unlikely that individuals with this clinical load will have traditional academic careers (publications, grants).

Clinician-Educator

Most academic institutions offer promotion within a teaching track. These are the dedicated teachers who are involved in curriculum development, who are course directors for the medical school, and who develop new techniques in education such as simulation and virtual reality. Emergency medicine has embraced many of these new techniques as our field incorporates many nontraditional skills such as leadership and teamwork.

In many institutions, it is possible to enter a faculty position in this track without further training. However, just being a good teacher is usually not enough. Specific work in education, including graduate work, may be useful. Volunteering for tasks within the dean's office is a good way to get involved—curriculum reform, student promotion, etc. While less than with the traditional academic tracks, there are opportunities for travel and networking with other experts in the field. There are opportunities for research and publications, but these are a bit more limited than those for traditional academic roles.

Clinician-Teacher-Scholar

This role incorporates patient care, teaching, and research. Ideally, this academician balances all three. Most academic emergency physicians currently reside in this track. Although scholarship and research are required, the need for federal funding is less.

Few, if any, graduating residents have the necessary skills to be successful in this track. Research must be done rigorously whether funded or not. Most of the research done by individuals in this track is clinically or epidemiologically based. Therefore, successful clinician-teacher-scholars should strongly consider additional training, including obtaining an MPH. In some institutions, this can be done (and paid for) during the first few years on faculty.

To be successful, there must be adequate protected time for reading and reflection. The average clinical schedule for this track is generally 24 hours per week, with another 25 hours per week devoted to teaching and research. Salary is often tied to clinical time and therefore is often less than for the two previous tracks. However, the thrill of presenting your material at national meetings, of travel, and of networking with experts is well worth the time spent. Individuals in this track are often the leaders of our national organizations.

Researcher-Teacher-Clinician

There is enormous need for traditional researchers in emergency medicine. Our field has something most other clinical fields do not have—flexibility. It is possible to schedule your clinical time around the needs of the laboratory. This factor is attracting many traditional MD/PhDs into emergency medicine.

To be successful, a faculty member must obtain independent federal funding. This requires extensive training and years of working under the mentorship of an established and funded researcher. Choosing that mentor and institution is paramount. The flexibility to move from site to site usually afforded to emergency physicians is more limited. However, for the dedicated physician-scientist, emergency medicine offers unique advantages.

Currently, the National Institutes of Health offers a loan forgiveness program for dedicated researchers in their early years, about $35,000 per year. This incentive may make it easier to pursue the necessary training. In addition, there are grants available from the Society for Academic Emergency Medicine, American College of Emergency Physicians (Emergency Medicine Foundation), and AHRQ and NIH to support training. These grants not only supply funds to support research costs but also supply salary support to decrease clinical time requirement.

Selecting an Institution

Emergency medicine as a career offers the ability to move and change jobs more easily than other fields. With the exception of the research track, this flexibility continues in academia. In addition, there exists the ability to move in and out of academia. Community practitioners can become clinicians in a teaching hospital, and teachers and scholars can move into the community.

Once you are committed to a traditional academic career, the selection of an institution can be critical. It is important to understand both the track you are in and the requirements for promotion. Some institutions have less rigorous requirements, which may be problematic if one moves to an institution with more rigorous requirements.

Obtaining an Advanced Degree

Tomorrow's leaders in emergency medicine will clearly have training beyond residency. Given the flexibility of emergency medicine practice, it is often possible to integrate courses into clinical care requirements and obtain an MPH or MBA while being an effective faculty member. Many universities support these efforts with tuition rebates. In addition, some universities have K30 or CTSA training grants from the NIH that facilitate training.

Obtaining training in basic science is more difficult and requires a supportive mentor and laboratory. Here selecting the correct location is paramount. Funding from the NIH has in the past been very difficult, but that is changing significantly.

Closing Thoughts

Emergency medicine offers many possible careers ranging from running an EMS system to community practice, to administration, to an inner-city practice, to teaching and research as an academic physician. The flexibility of our field and practice removes many of the barriers found in other specialties.

Academic emergency medicine combines the excitement and challenge of clinical care in the emergency department with the thrill of new discovery. Because the number of academic emergency physicians is somewhat limited, networking is easy. This network provides advice, professional support, and friendship. Travel is an important component of this field, primarily in the United States but also internationally. Travel allows one to have a greater perspective on your own career. Although traditionally academic emergency medicine does not pay as well as community practice, the perks and professional satisfaction make up for the lower salary.

chapter 12

Government Opportunities in Emergency Medicine

Ricardo Martinez, MD, FACEP
Executive Vice President Health Affairs, The Schumacher Group

Training experiences and traditional pathways for emergency physicians do not often include government services, except for military training and the public health services. However, there are many exciting opportunities in government, for both traditional and nontraditional physician roles.

Mention the word "government" and many people roll their eyes, have visions of bloated bureaucracies, and assume that government work means just pushing paper, but is a mistake. Working in the government can be very rewarding on both personal and professional levels and can be the foundation of a stimulating career.

Public service is just that. It truly is service to your fellow countrymen, women, and families. Governments are institutions that are set up "of the people, by the people, for the people" in order for society to have resources to meet the needs of the population that these governments serve. In these roles, each day that you go to work may provide an opportunity to not just serve one person but to affect the policies, resources, and organizations that shape the lives of hundreds to millions of people.

There are government roles in military (described elsewhere), public health, and health departments that allow emergency physicians to practice pure clinical care in a variety of settings, to provide medical oversight and leadership to EMS and clinical services, and to respond to disasters, outbreaks, and medical incidents. These sorts of traditional health care positions allow emergency physicians to use their training and expertise in important ways and in a range of circumstances. The public health services also provide opportunities for emergency physicians to identify and respond to emerging threats to health, to work with a host of partners to provide solutions, and to track health trends in the population that is served.

Not all positions have to be in the realm of health care. Brushing up on your civics lessons may be of value here. There are three branches of government—the executive branch, the judicial branch, and the legislative branch. In truth, no one is in charge in American governments. Democracies work with blunt instruments based on power. The interplay between the three branches is robust and constant. Emergency physicians can work in any of these three branches of government at the local, state, and federal levels.

My own experience was in the federal Department of Transportation. Because my focus was motor vehicle trauma and injury prevention, working on transportation issues nationally was much more effective than just seeing patients one at a time. And the experiences that I had throughout the United States and around the world were opened to me solely because of my government role. Physicians also play major roles in other government agencies that focus on a myriad of issues such as environmental health issues, homeland security and disaster response, labor health and safety, school health and safety, energy-related health and safety, aviation and aerospace medicine, and the food supply. Emergency physicians are often effective members of these expert teams and provide insights and leadership for these issues.

Many of the more challenging government roles require a greater focus on policy and politics. Both of these arenas can be complex and demanding, but these positions can certainly be intellectually stimulating and professionally fulfilling. Government organizations, by their very design, are political in structure, with elected officials or their appointees providing the policy guidance and funding resources for the agencies to do their work.

Making policy is almost the opposite as practicing good medicine. At the bedside, a good physician can ask the right questions to determine the variables pertaining to the patient's social status, financial status, domestic situation, transportation issues, etc. Once those are identified and considered, the best solution for that patient is determined. With policy, you have to make decisions that affect a large number of people across a spectrum of circumstances. A democracy gives many interested parties a say in the decision-making process and whether a decision will even work once the policy is implemented. Needless to say, good intentions and good policy are not necessarily the same thing. To paraphrase a famous quote that making policy is like making sausage—If you saw how it was made, you would never want to eat it!

The government arena can be a difficult place, too. In the regular world, if you have a bad day, you go home and perhaps visit with the family and drink a glass of wine in the evening. In many government roles, if you have a bad day, you read about it in the paper the next day. Being a public servant does come with public scrutiny, and it should. A democracy requires transparency, and those in government are accountable for decisions and stewardship of resources that you oversee. What can be truly maddening is to find that facts may be less relevant than perceptions. The public discussions are very different from medical training in which facts are king. In public policy, sometimes one feels that the facts are interesting artifacts that interfere with a political agenda. Trying to "do the right thing" in this environment can be frustrating, but it can be done.

Having said that, those who worked together during my tenure in the Department of Transportation can point to tangible effects of policies that were implemented, including improved side impact protection, improved airbag designs, enhanced head injury protection, universal child seat restraints, higher child seat and seatbelt use, and the development of the CIREN Network, the EMS Agenda for the Future, and the National Advanced Driving Simulator—to name a few. Other emergency physicians have improved disaster response and EMS care, mobilized national resources against drunk driving, made our schools safer, and developed better treatments for difficult diseases both nationally and globally. The government arena can provide the resources needed to develop and implement such worthy programs, and leave a legacy long after you are gone.

So how does one get a government job? One recommended method is to work with government agencies on various committees or advisory councils so that you can understand the agency and its workings. If you would like to work with it more closely, there are often consultant roles available for specific projects or areas of expertise. All of these become valuable experience when later applying for a position. Most all agencies advertise positions on their Websites or the government Website. And it may be useful to take a position in the agency or other department as a starter position, because existing employees can often more readily transfer to other positions.

Many agencies offer internships or fellowships that can provide valuable experiences and relationships or open the door to important jobs in government. Jeff Runge, the first chief medical officer for the Department of Homeland Security, was first a fellow at the National Highway Traffic Safety Administration. A few years after that, he was appointed by President Bush to be the agency's admininstrator!

One other route to consider is to apply to be a White House Fellow, which has been bestowed on senior residents in the past. The White House Fellows program, started in 1964, is a 1-year intensive fellowship program that provides successful candidates with extensive experiences with the White House and Cabinet, working on national and global policy issues. The White House Fellowship "often requires long hours and, at times, unglamorous duties that require as much perseverance as ability on the Fellows' part." It is hard work but life changing for those who make it. Over 1000 candidates are narrowed down through regional interviews to 30 or so candidates. Only 11 to 19 are eventually named for this valuable position. More information can be found at http://www.whitehouse.gov/fellows/.

There are many ways to serve our country, our communities, and our patients. Government service provides a unique and valuable contribution opportunity for the emergency physician, whether it is working with and in support of government agencies, working inside them as a government employee, or providing insight and guidance to those making the decisions. By doing so, you will not only become a better emergency physician but a more effective one, too.

chapter 13

Military Opportunities in Emergency Medicine

Linda L. Lawrence, MD, FACEP, Col, USAF, MC
Chief of Medical Staff, David Grant Medical Center, Travis AFB
Chief Emergency Medicine Consultant to Air Force Surgeon General
Associate Professor Department of Military and Emergency Medicine, Uniformed Services University of the Health Sciences; President-Elect, American College of Emergency Physicians

Wait! Do not skip this chapter, thinking that it has no interest for you—I almost did that over 20 years ago and I might have missed what has proved to be an exciting career as a military emergency physician. My career as a military emergency physician has been full of unique opportunities and has opened more doors than I ever would have imagined. Even after 20 years, those opportunities keep coming. As emergency physicians, we tend to like change and diversity; we do not want the certainty of a clinic schedule but instead thrive on the excitement of a good challenge and unpredictability. A military career has provided me this not just in my day-to-day practice but also in job opportunities laced with travel and leadership opportunities I never would have pursued on my own.

Practice Environment

Most military emergency departments are synonymous with community hospital emergency departments. Patients comprise the full age spectrum and present with the same disease patterns seen in community hospitals. Depending on where you practice, this might vary slightly because of the number of retirees in the immediate vicinity of your hospital, but that is no different than the demographic variance seen in different communities. Depending on the size of your hospital, you may have a broader panel of on-call specialists, making life simpler, but for those areas not covered, it is no different than working in a community hospital where you find the need to transfer some acutely ill patients to tertiary referral centers.

However, there are some real advantages to treating patients in the military, and one of them is you do not need to worry whether they can afford your treatment, can pay for prescriptions, or will be able to seek follow-up care. The only reason my patients fail to fill the prescription I write is they are too lazy to walk down the hall to the pharmacy, as there is no cost for them. Immunizations are also a fully covered benefit for military patients along with comprehensive preventive care programs. In the military, all staff members work for the hospital commander, so we are on the same team. That means if my on-call specialist does not want to help, there are clear and easy channels by which to quickly resolve the dispute and provide the care necessary for patients. The reality is that this rarely happens and that all staff members—physicians, nurses, and administrators—are part of a team that deliver true patient-centered care. Most military hospitals have adequate inpatient capacity and do not struggle with the challenges of boarding patients. When process problems affecting patient care are identified, I often find it easier to build collaboration across disciplines within the hospital to solve the issues, because we are all on the same team. One of the most enjoyable aspects of my clinical practice is my physician colleagues both in the department and throughout the hospital. As a more senior physician years removed from residency training, I enjoy the constant turnover of physicians with many recently completing residency or fellowship training. There is frequent professional sharing of ideas on new ways to manage patients and new treatments, helping one to remain current and constantly learning and improving your clinical practice.

All three military services also have academic hospitals with emergency medicine residency programs. Military academic programs are more clinically focused, as the faculty are not pressured with publish-or-perish tenure requirements and the need to secure grants. One of the main emphases for military faculty is to be an outstanding clinical teacher. This keeps clinical teaching as a priority. Research is conducted and it is important, but often it is clinical research or operational field research. The military also has a medical school with a robust curriculum in emergency medicine that provides unique opportunities for faculty.

Typically, recent emergency medicine graduates find themselves working in one of these two settings, but for the few who desire more challenge, they can be assigned to an operational tour. Emergency medicine has established itself as a highly sought-after specialty in all three services to support the operational mission. Commanders value our training because it has taught us to be flexible and adaptable to almost any setting, maintaining the ability to provide emergent medical and trauma care as well as nonurgent care. In an operational tour, you work with specialized military teams. You may be responsible for training medics and providing care in austere environments. Operational tour positions include Special Forces, flight medicine, dive officer, ship doctor, or troop doctor. You receive special training that helps you in these unique roles. For many seasoned emergency physicians, the operational opportunities become a reason to remain in the military, providing some diversity to practice, a change from the day-to-day shift work.

Opportunities for leadership often present themselves early in a military career, including serving as medical director, EMS director, or department chair. Frequently, you will be asked to serve on hospital committees or in other roles. All of these experiences will help you quickly mature as an emergency physician and will make you extremely marketable if you decide to leave the military. In addition, all services offer sponsored fellowship training opportunities that vary from year to year.

Locations for practice span the world and depend on the military branch of service. In most locations outside the United States, your family can accompany you and experience a different culture with most of the comforts of America still provided through the base. How long you remain at a base depends on the branch of service, location, and clinical setting, with academic assignments tending to have the most longevity. Receiving a new assignment every 3 to 4 years has provided me new professional opportunities and sometimes new geographic locations. These opportunities and locations frequently would not have been jobs or places I would have pursued on my own, but each one has been an outstanding opportunity and has significantly changed my professional and personal life in very positive ways. This is a theme that I hear repeated from many military emergency physicians whether they remain in the military for a few years or for their entire career.

Deployments

In recent years, deployments in support of military war operations have become a way of life for military emergency physicians. We have found ourselves at the center of military medical care, making a huge difference in the outcome of the wounded soldier, sailor, and airmen. Each military service has different wartime roles and thus some difference in where emergency physicians might find themselves.

All services have developed critical care/surgical teams that are more flexible and able to quickly respond to medical needs of troops. Emergency physicians are critical to these teams. Some emergency physicians deploy to trauma centers that are busier than most U.S. trauma centers. In addition to providing care to military service members, it is not uncommon to provide lifesaving emergency care to local citizens. In the Air Force, emergency physicians are part of Critical Care Air Transport Teams responsible for moving acutely injured and seriously ill patients for hours in the air to more definitive care. Most physicians will tell you that while the work can be hard and emotionally trying, there is also much personal satisfaction in getting to use some of our greatest skills to really make a difference. In addition, while deployed, you become very close with other deployed colleagues and develop long-lasting friendships.

Other travel opportunities within the military include helping Third World countries develop prehospital systems, teaching mass casualty response, and emergency and trauma care. Some emergency physicians have traveled the world with congressional delegations or other dignitaries to include tours as a White House physician. These types of short trips or tours can provide a welcome change to the day-to-day work as an emergency physician and provide a lifetime of memories.

How to Enter the Military and Residency Training

Most military emergency physicians enter through an ROTC or HPSP (Health Professions Scholarship Program) commitment. HPSP is a scholarship that pays for medical school in return for 3 to 4 years of service. Another program exists that can provide financial assistance during residency in return for a short service commitment. For those who enter after residency with no obligation, there are additional bonuses available. A medical recruiter can provide additional information.

If you are an HPSP or USU medical student, you must apply for residency through the Joint Services Graduate Medical Education Selection Board (JSGMESB). This board meets at the end of November with applications due early fall. For Navy students, it is typically required that applicants first complete an internship and serve at least 2 years as a general medical officer (GMO). The Army and Air Force offer opportunities for students to directly enter residency training. Each year, services will determine their future needs for emergency physicians, establishing the number of available residency positions in the military match. Usually, the positions are a mix of military training programs and deferred spots for civilian training. To be allowed to train in a civilian program, you must be awarded a deferred position through the JSGMESB. The level of competitiveness is typically similar to that seen in the civilian programs, and for the past several years emergency medicine has remained a competitive, highly sought-after specialty. Medical students not chosen for an emergency medicine position will be assigned to an internship year. The opportunity often exists for you to reapply during internship to start an emergency medicine residency immediately after internship. The scoring system provides additional credit for having completed an internship and even more points for serving in a GMO tour. If you are a solid candidate but not competitive enough as a medical student, you might be competitive after an internship and GMO tour, so don't give up.

The military emergency medicine residency programs in all three services are very strong, and each has its own special attributes. Similar to applying to civilian emergency medicine residencies, it is important for you to identify which program and location best suit your needs. It is very advantageous to rotate through at least one military emergency medicine residency program no later than November of your senior year. You must train in your service, with rare exceptions being granted for extreme circumstances. It is also highly recommended that you interview with all emergency medicine residency training programs for your service at least by telephone and ideally in person, if you want to secure a spot at that program.

Resources

One of the best ways to find out more about military emergency medicine is to speak with a military emergency physician. Each service has a specialty consultant or specialty leader. The Government Services Chapter of the American College of Emergency Physicians provides some resources through their Website about military emergency medicine, and the chapter office can place you in touch with consultants or other leaders in military emergency medicine (toll-free 877-531-3044; www.gsacep.org).

Conclusion

I entered the military as a naive college student accepting an HPSP scholarship on my way to medical school. Over more than two decades, I have watched my professional career take turns I never would have predicted and found myself in locations in the United States and the world that I otherwise might never have explored. Emergency medicine itself is a specialty with extreme diversity and a broad scope of career possibilities, as highlighted in this book. Multiply that by what the military can offer, and you will easily find yourself looking back amazed at where your professional career has gone and the richness of your life through travel and friendships.

chapter 14

Ethics in Emergency Medicine

Jim Adams, MD, FACEP

Professor and Chair, Department of Emergency Medicine, Northwestern University

Professionalism is the enactment of the values and ideals of individuals who are called, as physicians, to serve individuals and populations whose care is entrusted to them, prioritizing the interests of those they serve above their own.[1]

Professional and ethical issues are commonly encountered by medical students and residents, yet there is little formal education surrounding these topics. Professional behaviors include not only providing quality care but also honoring the deep social commitment that society places on the doctor-patient relationship. We are constantly influenced by outside factors such as personal desires, financial temptations, and the pressure of peers. Despite these distractions, physicians are obligated to act in the best interest of their patients. The role of medicine in society is dependent on this concept.[2,3]

In studying ethical and professional issues, caring for patients in the emergency department poses several unique challenges. The nature of our environment forces us to become masters at gaining trust, building therapeutic alliances with strangers, and helping guide patients to rapidly make difficult decisions. As emergency physicians, we have this unique opportunity to model the behaviors that exemplify the moral duties of our profession.

Principles of Ethics

Ethics is the study of the fundamental principles that define values and determine moral duties and obligations. The concept of "right and wrong" in medicine is not only a legal issue but also one of social custom. Treatment decisions are not based solely on medical information, and a truly "right" answer does not exist in every clinical situation. We instead use our knowledge and abilities to tailor the treatment of each individual patient. This requires us to act with respect and integrity as well as with compassion and understanding. Being technically adequate in medicine is insufficient.

Development of ethical and professional behaviors requires an understanding of basic ethics principals. Skills then develop over time as you gain clinical experience and incorporate new experiences into your framework of decision making. Beauchamp and Childress[4] proposed a standard approach to medical ethics that includes the following four principles: beneficence, nonmaleficence, respect of autonomy, and justice. These principles help to guide our discussions and actions when making decisions with patients regarding their care.

Beneficence/Nonmalifecence

Beneficence is the concept of acting in the best interest of the patient or "doing good," while *nonmalifecence* dictates that we "do no harm." In both cases, we are attempting to act in the patient's best interest. Our most obvious ethical responsibility is to act in the best interests of our patients. The motivation to help others should be a driving force in our daily interactions, but it is often is difficult because of outside influence.

In some situations, it is not possible to strictly honor both principles. For example, a patient who needs a central line for resuscitation may suffer a pneumothorax. In such a case, you are forced to weigh the risks and benefits of various actions and advise your patient accordingly. When presented with these difficult situations, we are obligated to perform the action that produces the most good.

Autonomy

Any person can make decisions about their life and health, even decisions to refuse care that physicians would identify as important or even life saving. Individual values guide a person's medical decisions. This autonomy is a core social value.

In order for patients to make informed decisions, the physician must provide sufficient, relevant information about the condition, treatment recommendations, benefits, risks, and alternatives. The patient's decisions must be based on their goals and values, not unduly influenced. It must be tailored to the patient's ability to comprehend. This is the process of informed consent. Informed consent is not a signature on a piece of paper, but the active and full process of information sharing and decision-making. One of the key obligations of a physician is to be able to carry out this process effectively.

Decision-making capacity is the ability to understand the nature and consequences of medical care, and to make and communicate decisions based on this information. This is a medical decision and is distinct from "competence." *Competency* is a legal determination by a court that a person is able to make decisions to adequately and safely handle their affairs. Decision-making capacity can be event and situation specific. For example, patients may have sufficient decisional capacity to consent to noninvasive evaluation for a possible cardiac disease but lack the ability to comprehend more complex matters, such as the risks and benefits of elective aortic valve repair for moderate aortic stenosis.[5]

In addition to capacity, the patient must be free from coercion or outside influence. He or she should possess a set of values and goals necessary for evaluating the different options and be able to make decisions accordingly. Physicians are not barred from giving opinions or relating personal experience but should be careful to avoid imposing their own personal or religious beliefs on the patient. We must be willing to accept that some patients will not agree with our recommendations, while still providing the best treatment possible within these limitations.

Justice

Ethical principles should prescribe actions that are fair to those involved. We have the duty to treat all fairly, distributing the risks and benefits equally. Patients in similar situations should be offered similar care unless extenuating circumstances are involved.

This concept includes both legal and moral principles and may create difficult decisions when limited resources are available. Justice also dictates that respect is granted equally to all.

Professionalism

These basic principles of ethics provide us with guidelines to use in patient interactions. These ethical principles must be matched to overarching professional obligations of duty, integrity, and respect. The discussion below divides duties and obligations into three categories: responsibilities to the patient, to the profession, and to ourselves. Sometimes there is conflict between interests and obligations. Such dilemmas are resolvable only when the physician has clear, deep understanding of professional obligations, good communication skills, and wisdom.

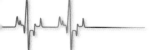

Duties to the Patient

Truth Telling

At the core of any successful doctor-patient interaction is trust. Integrity and honesty are necessary to achieve the trust of our patients. Without full honesty, the trust that is needed for a therapeutic relationship is unobtainable. Patients do not expect perfection of their care providers but do need to know that their physician is reliable and trustworthy.

For medical students, patients may overtly express a lack of trust. The student who reminds that patient that he or she is there as an addition to the care team, ideally as a patient advocate and aid, can quickly gain trust and acceptance. During more risky interventions, such as invasive procedures, the trainee must balance eagerness to perform skills with safety and proper supervision. Exaggerating skills and experience to gain autonomy serves nobody well. Knowing when to ask for help and understanding one's limits are hallmarks of integrity not just for the trainee but also for experienced clinicians. Such insight and honesty enhance trust.[6,7]

Confidentiality

As a member of the care team, you are entitled to a vast amount of private knowledge, yet with that knowledge comes the responsibility to maintain confidentiality. Some patients do not wish to share their medical information even with friends and family. As such, you should not discuss care issues with family members unless specifically instructed by the patient.

Patients should be aware that issues that cross legal or ethical boundaries will remain confidential as it pertains to their medical care. As a student, however, you should not be expected to hide or protect key medical information (i.e., substance abuse or HIV status) from other team members, but information should be shared only with those who have a direct obligation for the patient's care.

Some situations are of such importance that this obligation of confidentiality is superceded by the interests of others. For example, if child or elder abuse is suspected, an obligation to report for investigation is needed. No specific accusation needs to be made since society recognizes that protecting another person from harm is worth breaking confidentiality so that further information can be gathered by social agencies.[8,9]

Respect

The emergency department cares for patients from diverse socioeconomic, religious, and ethnic backgrounds. Differing values can create apparent conflict. For example, a patient who is a Jehovah's Witness may refuse blood transfusion despite life-threatening consequences. We first recognize that blood cannot be administered to an adult if there is an informed, autonomous refusal by a patient with decisional capacity. Respect, however, demands more. By understanding that the Jehovah's Witness believes that the administration of blood violates biblical teaching and, as such, violates their relationship with God and likely prevents them from achieving everlasting life, we can begin to understand why they believe that there are worse things than death. We can be genuinely respectful of these differences. The health care team is responsible for accommodating informed patient desires and, ideally, ensuring a mutually respectful encounter.

Emergency physicians are frequently required to care for patients with conditions that are self-inflicted (i.e., a skin abscess in an intravenous drug user) or that have resulted in harm to others (i.e., a drunk driver). In such situations when our instinct is to judge, criticize, or condemn, we must realize that negative judgment and condemnation serve no good goal; it only severs the respectful, trusting relationship. Medicine is not a transaction; it is a relationship. Even as we dislike individual behaviors, we must maintain an unconditional positive regard for the person as a human being. Maintaining respect for their humanity then allows our communication to be respectful and caring, even as we do advise against harmful behaviors and actions.

Suspension of Self-Interest

As we avoid letting our impulsive reactions dictate our therapeutic relationship with the patient and as we seek to understand patients' desires and limits for treatment, it becomes apparent that our own personal values must be suspended. It is quick and easy to say, "I would never want to live in that condition" or "It is crazy to refuse blood; that person could die." Projecting our wishes and values will lead to conflict and dissent. It is the patient's health that is at stake, so it is the patient's values that drive the encounter.

Duties to the Profession and Your Colleagues

Honesty

As with patients, being honest and respectful with colleagues is paramount, but reminders are still needed. In an effort to protect one's ego or advance personal interests, honesty is still sometimes threatened. In small ways, such as when a supervising physician asks if you completed a task, there is temptation to say "yes" first and then actually complete the task immediately afterward. Even these seemingly small events introduce catastrophic possibilities, not the least of which is to make the supervising physicians question core trustworthiness. It is necessary to always be fully and openly honest, even if negative consequences are possible. Reporting, "Sorry, I did not complete that yet, but I will do it immediately," then following through, is the way to build trust and respect.

Education

"Doctor" is derived from Latin root meaning "teacher," and this role is central. In addition to teaching our patients, we each have the responsibility to educate future physicians and other health care team members. This includes much more than simply sharing our medical knowledge. It also involves modeling professional behaviors and passing along the values and attitudes that are crucial to the success of the medical community. Every action, behavior, and attitude projected teaches subordinates, colleagues, and affiliated caregivers about your notion of proper behavior. You are now, even while still learning, a role model.

Duties to Self

Personal Well-being

Physicians devote large amounts of time and make huge personal sacrifices to complete training and take on the task of caring for our patients. This is only possible if the physician is physically, emotionally, and intellectually healthy. There is much stress, temptation, and demand. We must make a commitment to maintain physical health, mental health, and supportive social relationships. Early establishment of routines that allow for rest, exercise, and interactions with family and friends is essential.[10]

When addiction, depression, or significant threats develop to a physician's health and well-being, it is also essential to seek help, early and voluntarily. Fortunately, there are nonjudgmental and supportive ways to seek assistance. Physicians particularly are ill-suited to asking for help. Paradoxically, greater strength results when we realize that we do need the support of others.

When we are successful at maintaining ethical principles, professional duties, and personal well-being, we can achieve personal and professional fulfillment. We will feel effective, experience appreciation, and benefit from the knowledge that our care makes a difference in the lives of our patients. The professional and ethical duties are at the core of our happiness and success.

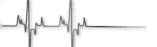

Summary

Although often overshadowed by the urgency to acquire and use medical knowledge, ethics and professionalism play a core, essential role in our professional lives. Difficult situations arise each day; some of the hardest decisions are ethical dilemmas. It is essential to gain deep insight to legal and ethical principles, understanding them not superficially but deeply, ensuring insight.

Aristotle noted that ethics is a rough and tumble business, not able to be understood only by thought and by reflection but requiring action, decisions, and implementation in the real world. Nowhere is this more true than in the emergency department, where goals, values, decisions, and time-urgency can collide. We must remain students of human nature, students of ethics, and gain wisdom, the mark of genuine excellence as a physician.

References

1. *AAMC professionalism task force,* 1998. Accessed at www.aamc.org, November 2006.
2. Adams J, Schmidt T, Sanders A; SAEM Ethics Committee, Society for Academic Emergency Medicine. Professionalism in emergency medicine. *Acad Emerg Med.* 1998;5:1193-1199.
3. Knopp R. The challenges of teaching professionalism comment]. *Ann Emerg Med.* 2006;48:538-539.
4. Beauchamp T, Childress J. *Principles of biomedical ethics,* 5th ed. Oxford: Oxford University Press; 2001.
5. Applebaum P, Grisso T. Assessing patients' capacities to consent to treatment. *N Engl J Med.* 1988;319:1635-1638.
6. Williams CT, Fost N. Ethical considerations surrounding first time procedures: a study and analysis of patient attitudes toward spinal taps by students. *Kennedy Inst Ethics J.* 1992;2:217-231.
7. Graber MA, Pierre J, Charlton M. Patient opinions and attitudes toward medical student procedures in the emergency department. *Acad Emerg Med.* 2003;10:1329-1333.
8. American College of Emergency Physicians. *Code of ethics for emergency physicians.* Dallas, TX: American College of Emergency Physicians; 2003.
9. Moskop JC, Marco CA, Larkin GL, Geiderman JM, Derse AR. From Hippocrates to HIPAA: privacy and confidentiality in emergency medicine—part I: conceptual, moral, and legal foundations. *Ann Emerg Med.* 2005;45:53-59.
10. Parkerson GR Jr, Broadhead WE, Tse CK. The health status and life satisfaction of first-year medical students. *Acad Med.* 1990;65:586-588.

chapter 15

Social Challenges in Emergency Medicine

Deirdre Anglin, MD, MPH
Professor of Emergency Medicine, Keck School of Medicine, University of Southern California

Gail D'Onofrio, MD, MS
Yale-New Haven Medical Center

Emergency medicine is a specialty that originally evolved around the care of the critically ill and injured patient. However, it has emerged as the specialty that provides access to care for any individual in need of medical services regardless of the ability to pay, race/ethnicity, or nationality. All patients are seen and evaluated 24 hours a day, 7 days a week. We as a profession have found ourselves, for better or worse, inexplicably entwined with public health, necessitating the incorporation of disease prevention into our daily practice.

The recent Institute of Medicine report *Future of Emergency Care: Hospital-Based Emergency Care at the Breaking Point* highlights the problems of overcrowding due to the failure of the larger health care system to cope with the uninsured and underinsured in providing both preventive care and chronic disease management. A November 2006 *Emergency Medicine Clinics of North America* issue was devoted to public health, and many of the social issues are outlined here. Often, making the diagnosis for a patient with a specific complaint is easy; it is then a challenge to provide the necessary treatment to that patient who may be homeless, unable to afford the prescribed medication, or suffering from a comorbid condition such as substance abuse or mental illness that may prevent compliance with a medical regimen. The old adage of "treat and street" can no longer apply. Emergency physicians have a responsibility to address these issues, and hospitals and emergency departments must find creative ways to assist with treatment plans. One such solution described by Gordon (1991) included the hospital emergency department as a social welfare institution. He writes about the emergency department as a sort of 'social triage" center to which emergency department patients with pressing social needs could be referred for screening, evaluation, and service coordination using community resources. He describes this center being located near or in the emergency department staffed by a social worker or service coordinator.

Specific Challenges
Homelessness

The Urban Institute estimates that 3.5 million people, including 1.35 million children, are homeless during a given year, which is probably an underestimate due to expected difficulties in surveying this population. Clearly, poor health is closely associated with homelessness, and homeless individuals are much more likely to use the emergency department as a source of care. One New York City hospital reported a 20% to 30% incidence of homelessness among its emergency department population. These patients averaged six emergency department visits per year and were more likely to be middle-aged men suffering from tuberculosis, HIV infection, depression, schizophrenia, alcoholism, poor dentition, or penetrating trauma.

Other factors influencing homelessness include domestic violence, mental illness, substance abuse, and lack of affordable health care. In a study of 777 homeless parents in 10 U.S. cities, 22% were homeless because of domestic violence and abusive relationships. Approximately 22% of the single adult homeless population has some form of severe and persistent mental illness, ranging from depression, bipolar disorder, and schizophrenia. There are high rates of alcohol and drug abuse among the homeless.

HIV and Homelessness

The prevalence of HIV infection among homeless persons ranges between 3% and 20%, and morbidity and mortality are higher as a result of the homelessness. The homeless die from AIDS more commonly than do other HIV-infected populations and have higher rates of tuberculosis. One study in Los Angeles found that two thirds of people with AIDS were homeless. Up to 50% of persons living with HIV infection and AIDS are expected to need housing assistance of some kind during their lifetime.

Homeless patients face many barriers to optimal care. It is difficult to adhere to even modest medical regimens without proper housing and basic needs such as food and clothing. High-risk behaviors in the homeless, such as drug use and risky sexual behavior, may increase the risk for HIV infection and other communicable diseases.

Mental Illness and Homelessness

A substantial proportion of the single adult homeless population, approximately 20% to 25%, suffers from some form of severe and persistent mental illness. According to the Federal Task Force on Homelessness and Severe Mental Illness (1992) only 5% to 7% of homeless persons with mental illness need to be institutionalized. Although most could live with supportive services and housing, there are not enough community-based mental health treatment programs and affordable housing to accommodate the number of people disabled by mental illness in the United States. Homeless people with mental disorders face many additional barriers compared with homeless individuals without mental disorders; they tend to be in poorer health and unemployed and to have more contact with the legal system.

Alcohol, Tobacco, and Other Drug Problems

Substance abuse is a major preventable public health problem affecting all racial, cultural, and socioeconomic groups, with total annual economic costs to the United States currently estimated at over $414 billion. Over 500,000 deaths annually are attributable to alcohol, tobacco, or illicit drug use: 107,000 related to alcohol, 435,000 to tobacco, and 25,000 to illicit drugs. Substance abuse is a risk factor for multiple diseases and a major risk factor for injury. Tobacco use, especially cigarette smoking, is the leading cause of preventable disease and a major risk factor for heart disease, stroke, lung cancer, and chronic lung diseases. It is responsible for more than 30% of all cancer deaths each year. An estimated 18 million people have alcohol abuse problems, whereas an additional 5 million abuse other drugs.

It is paramount that substance abuse issues be addressed in the emergency department as often this is the person's only entry to the health care system. Screening for alcohol, tobacco and other drugs can be performed quickly by a variety of persons, including nursing, physicians, or peer educators, or can be done creatively by kiosk or patient written surveys. Brief advice or intervention can be effective in changing behavior, and often a few minutes can make a large difference. The ACEP Website has a toolbox that is very helpful with training emergency physicians about alcohol screening, performing brief interventions and referral.

Mental Illness

According to the National Institute on Mental Health (NIH), an estimated 22.1% of American adults suffer from a mental disorder in any given year. Unipolar major depression ranks second as the source of global burden of disease, exceeded only by ischemic heart disease.

Data from the National Health Interview Survey indicate that approximately 2 million people visited emergency departments for mental disorders in 2002. Combinations of mental illness, alcohol and other drug problems, physical illness, and injury are common in this population. The elderly are a particular challenge as they may present with falls and medical illnesses compounded by issues of mental illness, particularly depression and/or alcohol problems. Obviously, it is often important to address each of the components of a patient's health problem to adequately treat the most evident and obvious problem. However, the constraints of an emergency department visit are well known and combinations of these problems can be very difficult to treat. Having social workers or continuity nurses available who can set up home evaluations and services is vital. A complex treatment plan is of no value if the patient's mental illness is not addressed.

Intimate Partner Violence

Intimate partner violence (IPV) affects up to 4 million women each year in the United States, with an estimated annual cost of $67 billion. *Intimate partner violence* is defined as the threat or infliction of physical or sexual abuse by adults or adolescents against their past or present intimate partners. The physical abuse is frequently associated with psychological abuse. Many terms have been used to refer to IPV, including *domestic violence, spouse abuse, wife beating, wife abuse,* and *battered woman.* The highest prevalence of IPV seen in clinical settings is in the emergency department. Based on several studies, 1% to 7% of all women who present to the emergency department for care do so because of an acute episode of abuse, 14% to 22% have experienced IPV in the past year, and up to 54% have experienced IPV at some time in their lifetime. While victims of IPV are most frequently females abused by male partners, females also abuse male partners, and IPV occurs in same-sex relationships. IPV occurs in all socioeconomic groups, racial groups, cultural groups, and religions.

IPV presents in the clinical setting in many ways, including injuries, chronic pain, nonspecific medical complaints, gastrointestinal problems, neurologic problems, sexualyy transmitted diseases, obstetric/gynecologic problems, depression, suicidal ideation and attempts, and alcohol and substance abuse. In addition to head and neck injuries, injuries that are bilateral, central, defensive (i.e., "night-stick" fracture), or patterned (resemble the pattern of an object, such a shoe print) are more likely to be intentional injuries. IPV results in numerous adverse physical and mental health sequelae. Children who witness IPV also experience adverse physical and mental health outcomes.

Conclusion

Social issues can overwhelm the emergency physician and the emergency department. However, we would be remiss if we do not address these issues at the time of the visit. Prescribed treatment plans do not have a chance of being followed if the patient has comorbidities that are not addressed or lacks basic needs such as safe shelter and food. Emergency physicians working with hospital administration are compelled to set up processes to aid in the screening, evaluation, and referral for all of these issues. A few moments spent in addressing these issues will promote the overall health of the patient and potentially prevent repeat emergency department visits.

Bibliography

1. Anglin D, Mitchell C. Intimate partner violence. In Pearlman MD, Tintinalli JE, Dyne PL (eds). *Obstetric and gynecologic emergencies.* New York, NY: McGraw-Hill; 2004: 486-510.

2. *Broadening the base of treatment for alcohol problems. Report of a study by a committee of the Institute of Medicine.* Washington, DC: National Academy Press; 1990.

3. Center for Disease Control and Prevention. Smoking-attributable mortality and years of potential life lost—United States, 1984. *MMWR Morbid Mort Wkly Rev.* 1997;46:444-451.

4. Centers for Disease Control and Prevention. *Chronic diseases and their risk factors: the nation's leading causes of death.* Atlanta: Centers for Disease Prevention and Control: 1999.

5. D'Amore J, Hung O, Chiang W, et al. The epidemiology of the homeless population and its impact on an urban emergency department. *Acad Emerg Med.* 2001;8:1051-1055.

6. D'Onofrio G, Woolard RH, Becker B. The impact of alcohol, tobacco, and other drug use and abuse in the emergency department. *Emerg Med Clin N Am.* 2006;24:925-967.

7. Department of Health and Human Services. *Ninth special report to Congress on alcohol and health.* Rockville, MD: National Institute on Alcohol Abuse and Alcoholism, Department of Health and Human Services; 1997.

8. Federal Task Force on Homelessness and Severe Mental Illness. *Outcasts on Main Street: a report of the Federal Task Force on Homelessness and Severe Mental Illness.* Delmar, NY: National Resource Center on Homelessness and Mental Illness; 1992.

9. Gerstein DR, Harwood HJ, Sutter N, et al. *Evaluation recovery services: the California drug and alcohol treatment assessment.* Sacramento: State of California Department of Alcohol and Drug Programs; 1994.

10. Gordon JA, Chudnofsky CR, Hayward RA. Where health and welfare meet: social deprivation among patients in the emergency department. *J Urban Health.* 2001;78:104-111

11. Gordon JA. The hospital emergency department as a social welfare institution. *Ann Emerg Med.* 1991;33:321-325.

12. Herman DB, Susser ES, Struening EL, et al. Are there risk factors for homelessness? *Am J Public Health.* 1997;87:249-255.

13. Institute of Medicine. *Pathways of addiction: opportunities in drug abuse research.* Washington, DC: National Academy Press; 1996.

14. Kleinman LC, Freeman H, Perlman J, et al. Homing in on the homeless: assessing the physical health of homeless adults in Los Angeles County using an original method to obtain physical examination data in a survey. *Health Serv Res.* 1996;31:533-549.

15. Morris DM, Gordon JA. The role of the emergency department in the care of the homeless and disadvantaged populations. *Emerg Med Clin N Am.* 2006;24:836-848.

16. National Coalition for the Homeless. *HIV/AIDS and homelessness.* Washington, DC: National Coalition for the Homeless; 1999.

17. National Coalition for the Homeless. *Mental illness and homelessness.* Washington, DC: National Coalition for the Homeless; 1999 (NCH #5).

18. *NIDA's economic costs of alcohol and drug abuse in the United States, 1992.* Accessed at http://www.nida.nih.gov/EconomicCosts/Chapter5.html#5.2.

19. *Reducing the health consequences of smoking: 25 years of progress. A report of the Surgeon General.* Washington, DC: Centers for Disease Control, National Center for Chronic Disease Prevention and Health Promotion, Office on Smoking and Health; 1989.

20. Schneider Institute for Health Policy. *Substance abuse: the nation's number one health problem.* Robert Wood Johnson Foundation, annual report; 2001.

21. Secretary of Health and Human Services. *Tenth special report to the US Congress on alcohol and health.* Washington, DC: U.S. Government Printing Office; 2000. NIH publication No. 00-1583.

22. Urban Institute. *A new look at homelessness in America.* Washington, DC: Urban Institute; 2001.

23. US Department of Health and Human Services, National Institutes of Health. *National Institute on Alcohol Abuse and Alcoholism. Helping patients with alcohol problems: a health practitioner's guide.* Washington, DC: U.S. Government Printing Office; 2004. NIH publication No. 04-3769.

24. Zorza J. Woman battering: a major cause of homelessness. *Clearinghouse Rev.* 1991;25:421-429.

section two

Emergency Medicine
The Training

chapter 16

Development of Emergency Medicine Residency Programs

Theodore R. Delbridge, MD, MPH, FACEP
Professor and Chair, Department of Emergency Medicine, East Carolina University

Efforts to prepare physicians to care exclusively for "emergency" patients are less than four decades old. Prior to this innovation in medical education, delivery of service, and care, a significant chasm variably existed between the needs of emergency patients and the experience and interests of physicians relegated to providing their care.

The first emergency departments in the United States were "accident rooms," which, in the 1940s, often existed in the back or remote areas of larger hospitals. These places soon became known as emergency rooms, where acutely ill and injured people could go for initial treatment. As a rule, emergency room staffing was inconsistent in terms of physician background and expertise. At larger hospitals, interns and residents from various training programs might staff the emergency room as part of their duties. In such cases, care of emergency patients was essentially delegated to the most junior physicians, those with the least knowledge and experience. At other hospitals, medical staff members might be required to occasionally "pull shifts" in the emergency room to maintain their hospital admitting privileges. This arrangement was probably acceptable when an emergency patient required the attention of the sort of specialist working in the emergency room at that moment. However, for other patients, the optimum quality of care for their problems could easily be lacking.

By the mid-1960s, there developed widespread appreciation for the lack of preparedness of the American health care system to care for emergency patients. This was especially true for injured people and for cardiac patients, for whom new therapeutic innovations were being developed. Hospitals began to invest resources to develop sophisticated emergency departments, where patients could receive improved service and optimal care. Additionally, physician groups, like the one in Alexandria, Va., began to organize themselves exclusively for the practice of emergency medicine. Recognition developed for the need to train the first generation of emergency physicians.

As a fourth-year medical student in 1968, the challenges found in the emergency department fascinated Dr. Bruce Janiak. He ultimately persuaded a neurosurgeon and internist at Cincinnati General Hospital to organize a residency program designed specifically to prepare emergency physicians. The curriculum, developed by Dr. Janiak and Dr. Thomas Blum, the first emergency medicine residency program director, included extensive experiences in medicine, surgery, pediatrics, obstetrics/gynecology, neurosurgery, and orthopedics and in intensive care units. Its goal was to provide the resident the necessary knowledge and skills to evaluate, resuscitate and stabilize any patient who entered the emergency department. Concurrently, similar programs were developed at the University of California-Los Angeles and the Medical College of Pennsylvania. In 1975, the LREC (later to become the Residency Review Committee) retroactively approved Cincinnati's program as an emergency medicine residency.

The first emergency medicine residency programs required residents to enter in the second postgraduate year. First, they would complete a rotating internship or at least 1 year of training in another specialty. At that time, emergency medicine residency was 2 years in duration, after which graduating residents were eligible for board certification. Currently, board certification in emergency medicine requires residents to spend at least 36 months in training under the direction of an emergency medicine residency program.

When EMRA published the initial predecessor of this book in 1991, fewer than 85 emergency medicine residency programs existed. Today, more than 135 programs are accredited, and the number continues to grow. The expansion of emergency medicine residency programs is just one indicator of the recognized importance of the specialty and the value emergency physicians bring to the medical care of more than 100 million people per year in the United States.

All emergency medicine residency programs use a common core curriculum as their education infrastructure. However, each program is unique and enjoys specific strengths and opportunities to provide emphases. To medical students contemplating emergency medicine residency, the most obvious differences among programs are their formats. Currently, emergency medicine residency programs are either 3 or 4 years in duration: PGY-I, -II, -III; PGY-II, -III, -IV; or PGY-I, -II, -III, -IV. Differences in formats most often reflect institutional needs, approaches to adjusting to board certification requirements that have evolved over time, or local philosophies regarding resident education. Each format undoubtedly has its advantages and disadvantages, which in all cases are subjective depending on personal preferences and points of view as faculty and residents. It is impossible to generalize extensively about differences among various programs. The most important consideration is how any residency program uses its resources, including the time each resident has dedicated to this phase of his or her career, to provide valuable and meaningful education and experiences.

The continuing need for emergency physicians has led to the development of residency programs in diverse locations throughout the United States. They exist in urban, suburban, and rural areas and at university and nonuniversity hospitals. Developing and funding any residency program is not a simple endeavor. Yet, many institutions make solo investments to support emergency medicine residency programs, and others forge extensive collaborative agreements in order to make emergency medicine resident programs a reality. Thus, prospective residents have myriad options in terms of the environment in which they wish to continue their education and live.

There are countless features to consider among emergency medicine resident programs. Some of the more obvious ones include the number of participating institutions, emphasis on academia, involvement in research, exposure to specific patient populations, and participation in the local EMS system. Many programs provide resident experiences predominantly at one hospital. Others, as a manifestation of institutional collaboration, require residents to rotate through several hospitals. In some cases, residents may travel to different cities in order to get specific experience. Each plan undoubtedly has strengths and weaknesses. When most emergency medicine experience is gained at one hospital, residents are more likely to develop intimate familiarity with the nuances of the emergency department, its staff, and the faculty. Thus, they are able to master their environment in order to focus on learning on providing care. When emergency medicine experience is provided by a number of hospitals, residents may benefit from the larger breadth of faculty expertise and interests and a more diverse exposure to patient populations.

As a matter of routine, each residency program requires its residents to pursue some sort of scholarly project. However, the relative emphasis on academic achievement for both faculty members and residents can vary significantly. Thus, expectations differ for residents to participate in meaningful research, deliver educational presentations, or contribute to the literature. Many residency programs have created rich environments, by virtue of faculty interests and accomplishments, for residents to become involved in pioneering basic or clinical research. In other programs, the focus may be on educational techniques, on excellence in delivering clinical service, or in administrative and public policy aspects of emergency health care.

Each emergency medicine residency program seeks to capitalize on local resources to meet core content objectives and develop valuable clinical experiences in diverse areas. For example, the availability and an excellent relationship with the pediatric intensive care service may lead to an outstanding pediatric critical care experience. At a program where there is also a burn unit, the program administrators might develop an excellent burn ICU rotation during which residents gain valuable experience to be used during their emergency medicine careers. Similar examples could be cited for a number of surgical and medical subspecialties as well as EMS systems. Resident participation in the EMS system exists in many forms, ranging from functioning as an EMS base station physician to serving as an EMS helicopter flight physician or responding in the field to EMS or disaster scenes. In all cases, the common threads are the relationships developed and maintained by emergency medicine leaders with others throughout the institution, the availability of enthusiastic educators available in other disciplines, and the dynamic nature of academic medical centers. These features mandate a continual self-evaluation of every residency program to ensure that it is all it can be.

The core curriculum that serves as the educational infrastructure at every emergency medicine residency program ensures that each resident gains the knowledge and experience necessary to become a competent emergency physician and master of six core competencies of graduate medical education. The environment created in each program and the mix of educational experience it provides further mold every physician who trains there. Diversity among emergency medicine resident programs with a common infrastructure is a great asset for residency applicants. It provides prospective residents with opportunities to explore each program's strengths and emphases and to consider these factors in the context of professional goals and aspirations.

During the past four decades, emergency medicine has made quantum leaps in terms of the sophistication of its science, the identification of its role in health care system, and the commitment and expertise of its practitioners. The need for empathetic physicians who are experts in emergency medicine is never ending. The growth and development of emergency medicine residency programs undoubtedly reflect these realities. The future of emergency medicine is secure and the potential for opportunity is almost limitless. Without question, emergency medicine and its residency programs will continue to offer a range of options for their applicants and strive to exceed the needs of emergency physicians in-training.

chapter 17

Choosing an Emergency Medicine Residency

Kristin E. Harkin, MD, FACEP
Past President, EMRA
Assistant Professor of Medicine, Division of Emergency Medicine
Weill Medical College of Cornell University; New York-Presbyterian Hospital

Choosing the right emergency medicine residency program for you is indeed a personal decision. There are many factors that influence this decision, but it is important to remember that this decision is yours (not your dean's, your advisor's, or your parents'!). Making this decision first requires some honest personal reflection. Overlooking this process may lead you to choose a program where you may not be satisfied and, most important, may not develop to your fullest potential. Next, you need to make an informed decision. Take the time to do your homework, and it will pay off. Choosing a residency can be a long and arduous process, but the return on your investment will be great. The rewards of making the right decision make it all worthwhile. The following outline reviews points to consider in evaluating each residency.

Philosophy of Program

It is not always easy to gauge the overall philosophy of a program on a first visit (particularly on the day of the interview), but you will get a general sense and flavor of a program. Is it sweet vanilla, cherry red, rocky road, or bitter almond? Ask yourself if it suits your personality and personal value system. One fundamental principle, which should be ingrained, is that the residency exists for resident education (not to serve as a cheap workforce and not to sustain departmental standing within the hospital institution). If this premise is firmly established, then everything else will fall into order.

Accreditation of Program

The Accreditation Council on Graduate Medical Education (ACGME) is a regulatory agency that oversees accreditation of graduate medical education (residency programs). The ACGME evaluates medical education in two divisions. It reviews the institution (the medical schools, hospitals, and clinics where one trains) through the Institutional Review Committee (IRC). The ACGME also accredits the residency programs that each institution sponsors through the Residency Review Committee (RRC). The RRC in Emergency Medicine is a peer-reviewed body composed of an ACGME-appointed executive director, three physicians appointed by the American College of Emergency Physicians (ACEP), three appointed by the American Board of Emergency Medicine (ABEM), three appointed by the American Medical Association (AMA), and one resident elected by EMRA. It should be noted that emergency medicine was the first specialty to include a full-voting resident member of the RRC through its representation from EMRA. The other specialties did not endorse this concept of resident representation until 20 years later.

Do not assume anything regarding the accreditation status of a program. This information can be found easily at www.acgme.org. Know the status of a program prior to interviewing there. An established program is either granted full accreditation or is on probation. Programs placed on probation are required to notify all applicants and residents of the change in status. New programs are granted provisional status and are subject to review at the end of year 3 or 4, depending on the length of the program. If the accreditation of a program is revoked or not conferred, then the residents in that program would have to find another accredited program in which to complete training. It is important to ensure that the residency provides adequate training and will continue to provide the education you need to graduate. Residency programs have not closed very often due to a loss of accreditation. The closing of a residency is a hardship, but the RRC will assist in placing those residents in alternate programs. You should directly ask the program director where the RRC found weaknesses in the program, when the next scheduled review is, and what changes are under way to improve the program's compliance.

Departmental Status and Age of Program

An independent academic department of emergency medicine within the university (medical school) and within the institution (hospital) is a good indication of the strength of a program. Freestanding departmental status reflects power at the bargaining table when the chairs of each department meet over budgetary considerations, admitting privileges, and consultant issues. When emergency medicine is housed in a different departmental division, such as medicine or surgery, there is a different "feel" at the institution in terms of autonomy (e.g., radiology "approving" use of ultrasound in the emergency department) and physician perspective within the hospital.

Another consideration is the age of a program. An older, more established program often runs like a well-oiled machine with few kinks. You know what you are getting in terms of a product—by looking at their graduated residents (where they are working [i.e., academic or community settings] and what the reputation of the program is locally and nationally). A younger program offers the excitement of shaping the residency to a certain extent by being a pioneer as an early graduate of a program. However, accreditation status is not certain because new programs are on provisional status. Each residency matures through time, like its residents. Furthermore, if the structure of a residency is strong, it will encourage residents to explore individual interests.

Length of Program

The length of a program one chooses can be an area of much debate and controversy in discussing the options of 1-2-3 programs, 1-2-3-4 programs, and 2-3-4 programs. Yet, the answer for you will be simplified if you focus on your own personal goals. The reality is that you will learn emergency medicine in all settings (the board scores of all groups are comparable). The key is finding the program where you will excel because you are happiest in meeting your goals.

Initially, residency training in emergency medicine was 2 years. Today, you may train in 3- or 4-year programs, with the majority being 3-year programs. Three-year programs are entered directly out of medical school. Four-year programs are composed of two types: 1-2-3-4, where one does all 4 years of training at that institution, or 2-3-4, where one does an internship (not necessarily at the home residency institution) and then enters the emergency medicine residency in the second year.

If one enters a 2-3-4 program, you may choose to do an internship in internal medicine, a transitional year, or a preliminary year in surgery. The advantage of a 2-3-4 program is that you can do a year of training anywhere in the United States in an accredited institution. Often, applicants choose to do a preliminary year of internal medicine as a solid foundation or a transitional year that affords one the opportunity to spend more elective time in rotations of critical care, cardiology, radiology, hand/plastic surgery, infectious disease, ophthalmology, dermatology, pediatrics, and obstetrics. Transitional years can be tailored toward your interests (and weaknesses), so that the added, broader knowledge and skills may be useful throughout your career. It is important to note that one applies to an internship program separately and at the same time as one applies for an emergency medicine residency. On match day, you will rank each program structure independently.

Proponents of 4 years of training state that the additional year allows one to enter an academic career more easily because the extra year offers more clinical experience, more time to develop teaching/supervisory skills, more flexibility in completing research, and the opportunity of designing "mini-fellowships" in areas of interest. The most important attribute of completing a fourth year is that of personal maturity and confidence that only come with more time. Emergency medicine is a unique fishbowl. One needs to be very comfortable in dealing with difficult patients and difficult consultants. Personal interactions are paramount, and clinical competence requires self-confidence. Self-confidence enables emergency physicians to be the strongest of patient advocates in getting patients admitted to the hospital when a service does not agree with the admission and in getting patients diagnostic tests and therapies (when other services disagree with performing them). However, make sure that fourth year is well spent for your education as opposed to offering the institution inexpensive labor.

Another factor to consider is that more 4-year programs will only hire graduates straight out of residency who have completed 4 years of training. Yet, the proponents of 3-year programs advocate that fellowships are an option if you want additional training.

Finally, the financial pressures of doing an additional year of training are real, especially for those with families. Keep these pressures in perspective, though, because it is only one more year and you will be making a very good salary once you complete your training. Others with the same financial pressures choose even longer training in disciplines such as surgery or the medical subspecialties. Do not base your entire decision on money or you will be paying for that decision for the rest of your life. Invest in long-term happiness.

Clinical Environment

The clinical environment of the residency is a huge consideration because nothing substitutes for patient care. Again, you will flourish in the environment where you are most comfortable and happiest. You need to be honest with yourself in deciding how you best learn. For example, do you like the busy, hands-on environment of a public facility, or do you feel overwhelmed with a large indigent patient population?

Tertiary care level I trauma referral centers offer the opportunities to train in an environment with diverse pathology, severe illness, and high activity in many patient populations (trauma, burn, hyperbarics, pediatrics, and neonates) with consult services readily available. Often those centers are located in urban areas. Community and rural training centers offer the ability to learn emergency medicine with fewer specialty consultants, as frequently the emergency physician is the only physician in the hospital. This setting encourages independence under the supervision of an emergency medicine attending. In either setting, you want to ensure that there are enough sick patients to support learning and excellent teachers who will teach. The following questions will help you understand the clinical environment of a program and will help you gauge where you will best learn emergency medicine:

- How would you describe the patient population?
- What is the patient volume and patient load per resident in the emergency department?
- Is there too much of one kind of patient?

- How busy does the emergency department get? How often does it go on diversion?
- What percentage of patients are admitted?
- What percentage of patients are admitted to intensive care units?
- How often are inpatient beds not available? Critical care and telemetry beds?
- What percentage of your patients are pediatrics and neonates?
- What percentage of your patients are trauma patients? Blunt versus penetrating?
- Who runs resuscitations (medical and surgical)? Do graduating residents feel comfortable running codes?
- Who controls the airway? Does anesthesia have to be called?
- Are there enough procedures to ensure adequate training?
- What percentage of your patients have drug- and alcohol-related illnesses? Psychiatric illness? How many are homeless?
- How often do you use thrombolytics in the emergency department? How accessible is the catheterization lab?
- What is the availability of radiology and studies? What is the role of ultrasound in the emergency department?
- Is there adequate supervision, or is the supervision from senior residents?
- What is the role of physician extenders (physician assistants and nurse practitioners) in the emergency department?
- What is the relationship of consultants with the emergency department?
- How difficult is it to get a patient admitted?
- How is the nursing and ancillary staff?
- Do residents often perform ancillary tasks (blood drawing, ECG, Foley line placement)?
- How available are social services?
- What are the follow-up capabilities of the emergency department?
- What percentage of your patients do not speak English? What is the availability of interpreters?
- Is there ready access to patient records?

It is important to note how much time you will be spending in the emergency department. Every program requires a basic minimum; however, pay attention to the amount of off-service time you have and where you spend it. Are you learning orthopedics by doing scut on the floor, scrubbing into a hip replacement, or taking call in the emergency department for orthopedic emergencies? As a second- or third-year resident, are you performing intern duties with intern responsibilities on these other services?

Faculty, Didactics, and Autonomy

It is impossible to learn medicine from books alone. You need patients and teachers as well. Good teachers make all the difference in the world. You need to like your faculty or you will not learn from them. Is the faculty happy? If not, why not? Are they approachable and available, or do inadequate staffing and overwhelming patient demands burden them? Is there enough attending supervision, or are you supervised and primarily trained by senior residents? Is the faculty productive and involved in the residency? Do they continue to "keep up" with the literature and latest advances? Do they get their hands dirty if needed, or is there a lot of "dead wood" on board?

Your residency director can be the greatest influence in your career. A residency director who will look out for your personal and professional development is key. What is his or her background and training? Do the residency director and medical director work clinically? Will you have adequate time to work with and learn from them or are they doing more administrative time? What is the chairperson like? Is he or she active in the department working clinically or is he/she too busy attending outside meetings and conferences? It is extremely important that the department leaders work clinically each week so that they understand the challenges and dilemmas you face each day working in the department.

Bedside teaching needs to be balanced with adequate formal lectures. What is the program's approach to teaching the core content of emergency medicine? How is the curriculum covered? What are grand rounds like? Who has lectured in the past? How much emphasis is placed on evidence based medicine in the residency? How often are journal clubs, trauma conferences, pediatrics conferences, radiology rounds, toxicology rounds, follow-up conferences, morbidity and mortality conferences, procedure labs, and board reviews? Do residents attend, participate in, and present at local and national conferences?

Another critical aspect of training is resident autonomy. There is often a fine line between adequate supervision and appropriate autonomy. Developing clinical acumen is dependent on being given graded responsibilities and increasing autonomy so that by the senior year of residency one is running resuscitations and making the "final decision" to admit or not to admit along with the support of an emergency medicine attending. Do graduating residents feel comfortable running the department? If not, then you do not want to train there.

Examination evaluations are also important. How do the residents do on the in-service exam? Do graduates do well on the board-certifying exam? Do they pass the written and the oral exams on the first try?

Are the residents taught good habits to continue medical education post residency? Medicine is a life-long commitment to study. Are residents encouraged to independently analyze the literature? It is difficult to "keep up" with the knowledge base of emergency medicine and remain proficient in clinical skills and procedures. Granted, good habits are developed early in one's education particularly during medical school, but they need to be fostered in residency as well.

Finally, and most important, how are the residents truly treated? The ACGME protects resident rights, but are these rights enforced at your prospective institution? Is your work appreciated? Are you just there to provide a workforce, or does the residency exist for resident education? Do residents have any role in the administrative or educational policy decisions of the department? Resident education is not easy to balance with the needs for cost-effective patient care in a time when health care costs are increasing and funding is cut back, but it is possible to succeed in both arenas if the commitment is strong from the faculty and administration.

Research

The opportunities for research in emergency medicine abound as the breadth of the specialty allows multidisciplinary research and the relative youth of the specialty provides a diverse area of investigation yet to be studied. The RRC in emergency medicine requires that residents complete a 'scholarly project" prior to graduation. Opportunities   are availablein basic science and laboratory research as well as in the clinical arena. Different programs place different emphasis on the role of research in residency. However, all teach critical evaluation of the literature, basic research design, and statistics. If research is an important area of interest for you, it is imperative that you consider institutional support (funding and protected time) and mentor relationships available in a specific program. Research fellowships also can expand one's education.

Special Interests

A solid residency will encourage you to follow your interests and develop your skills. For example, if you are an EMS or air medical transport "junkie," you may want to consider a program with a strong background in these areas so you can continue to develop them throughout residency and possibly fellowship. Other special interests include toxicology, wilderness medicine, hyperbarics, ultrasound, burns, sports medicine, pediatrics, critical care, trauma, cruise ship medicine, administration, and international emergency medicine. Basically, the sky is the limit, but you want to ensure that the program will be supportive of these other interests.

Schedule

There really is not much to say with regard to the schedule. Residency is tough on the body, mind, and soul. You will work long hours, get little sleep, and be overworked. It is a grueling circadian challenge working nights, weekends, and holidays. You will survive because the RRC is very good about enforcing strict compliance with work hours in emergency medicine. You cannot work more than 60 clinical hours per week in emergency medicine. Just remember, though, that it entails cycling the clock.

Lifestyle and Geography

Do not underestimate the role of lifestyle and the importance of geography in your personal life. After working long hours, you want to go home to a place you love. If you hate the city, chances are you will not have much free time to escape the city on your days off. If you abhor the country, then rural settings are not for you. Consider which locales you enjoy and what climates you prefer in choosing a residency. Otherwise, the residency will feel like the longest, most draining experience of your life. Equally important to consider are the preferences and needs of your significant other and family.

Perks and Benefits

These are all secondary considerations. Benefits for you and your family are a must, especially disability insurance, and you may consider buying an additional plan on your own. Possible perks offered by residencies include dues in EMRA, ACEP, and SAEM; stipends for attendance at national conferences; scrubs; meals when on call; and computerized educational modalities. Some residencies offer the opportunity to join the Council of Interns and Residents (CIR), a union that represents residents and provides benefits. However, all of these perks should not primarily enter into your decision process. They are, after all, "perks."

Conclusion

Choosing the right emergency medicine residency for you is a lot of hard work. It involves collecting and compiling a great deal of background information, but most importantly, it requires honest personal reflection, which is often the most difficult part of the process. The return on your long-term investment will be great, and you will be a much better physician for taking the time to think through the decision wisely.

In closing, here are some key evaluation questions to help you finalize this decision.

- What do the residents think of the training they are getting?
- How is the house staff's morale? Are they having a good time?
- Are the residents glad they attended this program?
- Do the residents consider the educational experience worthwhile?
- What are some of the residents' complaints?
- What are the strengths and weaknesses of the program?
- How are the weaknesses being addressed?
- What is the program known for?
- How does the program view itself?
- How would the program characterize their graduates?
- Finally, the most important questions to ask yourself are, Will you fit in there?

Will you be happy there for the next 3 or 4 years? Will you enjoy being up at 4 in the morning with these people? Is this truly the best learning environment for you?

Bibliography

1. Harkin KE. Choosing an emergency medicine residency. *Emergency Medicine: The Medical Student Survival Guide* 2001;27-31.

2. Katz GR. Evaluating a residency program: a resource for residents and medical students. *Emerg Med Res.* 1999;25:1, 4.

3. Koscove emergency medicine. Applicant evaluation of an emergency medicine residency. *Emerg Med Focus.* 1991;86-94.

4. Rosen P. Pro: four years are optimal. SAEM. Available at http://www.saem.org/inform/ provscon.htm.

5. Schlanger CM. Medical students urged to think carefully before applying to emergency medicine residencies. *Emerg Med Res.* 1998;24:8.

chapter 18

Combined Programs

Emergency Medicine/Pediatrics

Nathaniel Johnson, MD
Resident, Combined Emergency Medicine/Pediatric Residency Program, University of Arizona

Dale Woolridge, MD, PhD, FACEP
Director, Combined Emergency Medicine/Pediatric Residency Program, University of Arizona

Combined residencies in emergency medicine and pediatrics offer an exciting opportunity for dual board certification in a reduced training period. In 1989, the American Board of Emergency Medicine and the American Board of Pediatrics recognized training commonality and developed guidelines that offered graduates eligibility to both boards after completing an approved 5-year combined residency program. If done separately, training would take 6 to 7 years. In addition, graduates of these programs are fully eligible to pursue subspecialty fellowship training in either field.

Application Process

Application is made through the traditional Electronic Residency Application System (ERAS) and the National Residency Match Program (NRMP). The combined programs have a separate designation from their associated categorical programs in the NRMP. Therefore, an applicant can concurrently apply for a combined program and categorical programs at the same institution. Subsequent matching is based on the rankings of the applicant and program.

Typically, applicants interview with both departments when visiting an institution. These combined programs tend to be relatively competitive given the limited number of positions available in the match. For this reason, many applicants will concurrently apply to categorical emergency medicine and/or pediatric programs through the ERAS. At the time of printing, there are three emergency medicine/pediatric combined residencies: University of Arizona, University of Maryland, and Indiana University. Each of these programs has more detailed information on their Web sites.

Structure

The emergency medicine/pediatric programs are 5 years (60 months) in duration. The training is 3 months in each specialty and encompasses all of the requirements of each individual residency. At the time of printing, dual training programs are not overseen by the Residency Review Committee (RRC). Future oversight is anticipated for all dual training programs. Currently, RRC accreditation of dual training is through the individual categorical programs. For this reason, the curriculum of each dual training program varies slightly at each institution and is reflective of the differences between their affiliated categorical programs.

Why a Combined Program?

Completing a combined program offers the unique opportunity to become dual-board certified in a shorter period of time compared with training in series. Combining emergency medicine and pediatric training is ideal in that it limits redundancy while simultaneously allowing the strengths of each specialty to compliment the other. Combined training additionally opens up diverse opportunities for future practice that would not have otherwise been available after training in only categorical emergency medicine or pediatrics.

Past graduates of combined programs practice in both areas of training. Although most of these graduates emphasize adult and pediatric emergency medicine in their future careers, a variety of career combinations have been seen, which include concurrent emergency medicine services for children (EMSC), pediatric hospitalist practice, and pediatric clinic practice. In addition, graduates of emergency medicine/pediatric training programs have a high incidence of academic involvement; a recent survey of graduates showed 54% participation in academics. Of these graduates, all were involved with academic emergency medicine with half having joint appointments in pediatrics.[1]

Training in a combined program can also be used in the following ways:

Subspecialty Expertise

Emergency medicine/pediatric graduates demonstrate involvement and expertise in the subspecialty of pediatric emergency medicine. In fact, emergency medicine/pediatric physicians are the largest subgroup of emergency medicine-trained physicians associated with pediatric emergency medicine fellowship training programs (Murray, Unpublished Data) In addition, more emergency medicine/pediatric dual-trained physicians exist nationally than do emergency physicians who have entered pediatric emergency medicine fellowship training.[2] Many of the national experts in pediatric emergency medicine are dual board trained.

Hospitalist and Emergency Medicine Practice

Many residents pursue combined training programs because they want to practice in both fields when they have completed their training. The recent advent of the hospitalist system in pediatrics has given graduating combined residents new opportunities to practice in both fields. Community hospitals that have pediatric inpatient and emergency department services may hire such a physician to manage both pediatric inpatients and pediatric emergency department patients. The emergency medicine/pediatric physician who has the training to be credentialed to perform both duties is highly sought after for these settings.

Observation Units

Many emergency departments have developed observation units for patients who need extended treatment but may not need extended (longer than 24 hours) inpatient admission—the patient, for example, with dehydration in need of 18 to 24 hours of hydration but not necessarily admission. Physicians who have combined training are outstanding choices for directors and staffers of such units. They may also be able to assist in creating such units.

Rural and International Medicine

Primary care physicians in rural parts of the country and in international settings often are called on to manage adult and pediatric emergencies. Applicants who are interested in eventually practicing in either of these settings may benefit significantly from combined training as the combined emergency medicine/pediatric residency graduate is uniquely able to expertly address both the primary care and emergent health needs of these populations.

Is a Combined Residency the Right Path for You?

What is clear is that in order to be happy in these programs, one has to enjoy each specialty separately. Although most graduates have a greater focus on emergency medicine, they are also eager to practice pediatrics. With subspecialty fellowship training available in pediatric emergency medicine, however, a question arises: Is it better to complete a categorical emergency medicine or pediatric residency and then pursue fellowship training, or is it better to complete a combined emergency medicine/pediatric program? If your goal is to practice only pediatric emergency medicine, then fellowship training may be the better route. Having a clear picture of future goals will help to clarify whether a combined residency might be the right residency for you.

The combined emergency medicine/pediatrics residency is 5 years in length, 2 more years than categorical pediatric training and 1 to 2 more years than categorical emergency medicine training. Currently, fellowship training in pediatric emergency medicine is an additional 3 years following a categorical pediatric residency or 2 to 3 years following an emergency medicine residency (for a total of 5 to 7 years of training, depending on the track).

Graduates of an emergency medicine/pediatrics combined residency are a diverse group of individuals who go on to have diverse and interesting careers. Among graduates of combined residency programs, 93% reported that they would choose the combined training if faced with the decision again and 100% would recommend it to prospective candidates interested in emergency medicine and pediatrics.[1]

Emergency medicine and pediatrics are exciting, dynamic fields. Together, they form the basis for a diverse medical career with limitless opportunity.

References

1. Woolridge DP, Lichenstein R. A survey on the graduates from the combined emergency medicine/pediatric residency programs. *J Emerg Med.* 2007;32:137-140.
2. Medical Specialists Plus Database. American Board of Medical Specialists. Elsevier. December 2005.

Emergency Medicine/Internal Medicine

Michael E. Winters, MD
Assistant Professor of Emergency Medicine and Medicine, Program Director,
Combined Emergency Medicine/Internal Medicine Program, University of Maryland School of Medicine

In June 1989, the American Board of Emergency Medicine (ABEM) and the American Board of Internal Medicine (ABIM) announced the creation of a combined residency training program in emergency medicine and internal medicine. As outlined by both ABIM and ABEM, the goal of this combined program is to prepare physicians for an academic or community career that addresses the spectrum of disease from acute care through chronic illness. Emergency medicine/internal medicine programs are 5 years in length, with the resident completing 2½ years of training in each specialty. Graduates of an emergency medicine/internal medicine program are eligible for certification in both emergency medicine and internal medicine. Currently, there are 11 emergency medicine/internal medicine programs offering a total of 25 first-year positions.

Program Name	City, State	First-Year Positions
UCLA/San Fernando Valley	Los Angeles, CA	2
Christiana Care Health Services	Newark, DE	3
University of Illinois College of Medicine at Chicago	Chicago, IL	2
Louisiana State University	New Orleans, LA	2
University of Maryland	Baltimore, MD	2
Henry Ford Hospital	Detroit, MI	2
Hennepin County Medical Center	Minneapolis, MN	2
Pitt County Memorial Hospital/ East Carolina University	Greenville, NC	2
Albert Einstein College of Medicine at Long Island Jewish Medical Center	New Hyde Park, NY	2
SUNY Health Science Center at Brooklyn	Brooklyn, NY	4
Allegheny General Hospital	Pittsburgh, PA	2

It is important to note that emergency medicine/internal medicine programs, at present, are not independently accredited by the Accreditation Council for Graduate Medical Education (ACGME). Accreditation status for each emergency medicine/internal medicine program is determined by the status of the respective categorical programs in internal medicine and emergency medicine. Emergency medicine/internal medicine programs are not able to recruit new residents if one of the parent programs is on probationary status with the ACGME.

Structure

Emergency medicine/internal medicine residency programs consist of 5 years of integrated training. As stated, residents spend an equivalent amount of time within each specialty. Depending on the program, residents typically alternate between specialties in 3- to 6-month blocks. During these blocks, residents function exclusively within the department in which they are working and are not expected to perform duties for both fields simultaneously.

The emergency medicine component of emergency medicine/internal medicine training provides the resident with experience managing acutely ill patients of all ages. Emergency medicine/internal medicine residents can expect extensive experience managing a busy adult emergency department. In addition, each program must offer at least 4 months of dedicated pediatric emergency medicine training. Many emergency medicine/internal medicine programs also offer excellent training in emergency ultrasound, major trauma, obstetrics, anesthesia, toxicology, critical care, and emergency medical systems management.

The internal medicine component of combined training consists of a variety of inpatient and outpatient rotations. Typically, emergency medicine/internal medicine residents perform several rotations on general medical and subspecialty inpatient teams. Examples of subspecialty inpatient teams include oncology, cardiology (non-intensive care), and infectious disease. In addition to these inpatient teams, emergency medicine/internal medicine residents gain extensive critical care experience through numerous rotations in the intensive care unit (ICU). Depending on the program, ICU experience is usually composed of rotations in the medical and cardiac ICUs. Thirty-three percent of emergency medicine/internal medicine training in internal medicine must involve outpatient care. To achieve this, emergency medicine/internal medicine residents are required to have one half-day per week of continuity clinic and a variety of subspecialty clinic rotations. Examples of subspecialty clinic rotations include dermatology, endocrinology, rheumatology, and neurology.

Regardless of the program, all emergency medicine/internal medicine residents must demonstrate some form of scholarly activity. Examples of scholarly activity, as set for by ABIM and ABEM, include original research, comprehensive clinical reviews, or published case reports. In addition, emergency medicine/internal medicine programs have joint educational conferences involving residents and faculty in both categorical programs. These conferences are typically lead by an emergency medicine/internal medicine resident.

Careers for Emergency Medicine/Internal Medicine Graduates

Career opportunities for emergency medicine/internal medicine graduates have never been stronger. In contrast to early combined graduates, recent emergency medicine/internal medicine graduates are readily receiving dual departmental appointments that allow them to simultaneously practice both specialties. The success of recent graduates can be linked to career opportunities in hospitalist medicine, emergency department observation units, subspecialty training, and rural/international medicine. In addition to their clinical appointments, many recent combined graduates have assumed leadership/directorship positions despite being relatively early in their careers.

The hospitalist system has become increasingly popular in community and academic centers across the nation. Hospitalists are typically internal medicine-trained physicians who solely practice inpatient medicine. Depending on the institution, hospitalists typically work 12- to 24-hour shifts. There are usually no on-call, or outpatient, responsibilities. With this model, it is easy to construct a combined practice involving part-time hospitalist work with part-time emergency department care. In fact, several recent emergency medicine/internal medicine graduates are practicing both specialties using this system.

Many emergency departments have developed observations units for patients requiring extended emergency department care but not necessarily needing inpatient admission. Examples of patient conditions ideal for observation units include mild asthma exacerbations, dehydration, low-risk chest pain, cellulitis/soft tissue infections, transient ischemic attack, and hyperglycemia. Emergency medicine/internal medicine graduates are exceptionally qualified to establish, and direct, an observation unit.

With the depth and breadth of training, it is not surprising that some emergency medicine/internal medicine residents wish to pursue subspecialty training. With the epidemic of hospital and ICU crowding, many emergency medicine/internal medicine residents have developed interests in critical care medicine. Similar to the hospitalist model, physicians who become certified in critical care medicine typically divide their clinical time between the emergency department and the ICU. Emergency medicine/internal medicine graduates who pursue subspecialty training often become local and national experts in their field.

Rural and international medicine remains an underserved area desperately in need of qualified physicians. Because these physicians are likely to be the only physician within a certain geographic area, the physician must be comfortable managing acute and chronic illness. Emergency medicine/internal medicine physicians are ideal for these rural and/or international medicine initiatives.

Is an Emergency Medicine/Internal Medicine Program Right for You?

You should consider an emergency medicine/internal medicine program if you are truly passionate about *both* emergency medicine and internal medicine. You must enjoy the exciting, fast-paced environment of the emergency department along with the unique aspects of inpatient rounds and outpatient continuity clinic that characterize internal medicine. In addition to simply enjoying both specialties, it is crucial to consider career goals when deciding whether emergency medicine/internal medicine training is right for you. As discussed, emergency medicine/internal medicine training and certification are ideally suited for the physician who is interested in pursuing rural or international medicine, combining an emergency department practice with a hospitalist service, managing an emergency department observation unit, or pursuing subspecialty training in areas such as critical care medicine.

It is important that you also consider the challenges of combined training. Perhaps the most formidable is the simultaneous assimilation of two large knowledge bases. Because emergency medicine/internal medicine residents spend half of the year in each specialty, first- and second-year combined residents can become frustrated when comparing themselves to categorical residents of the same year. The fund of knowledge of combined residents typically surpasses that of categorical residents by the third and/or fourth years of training. In addition to the amount of information that must be learned, the length of training must be considered. A 5-year residency program is a considerable investment of your time. If you are only interested in practicing either internal medicine or emergency medicine, enduring a demanding 5-year residency may become overwhelming.

Poor reasons to pursue emergency medicine/internal medicine training include the inability to decide *between* each specialty and the desire to "become a better physician." Combined residents who are unable to decide which specialty they ultimately want to practice often withdraw within the first or second year of emergency medicine/internal medicine training to pursue a categorical program. Many students feel that an emergency medicine/internal medicine program would make them a "better physician." If your career goal is to truly practice *either* emergency medicine or internal medicine, an emergency medicine/internal medicine program would not be a valuable investment of your time. Excellent categorical residency programs exist in both specialties that would make you an outstanding emergency physician or internist. If you desire additional expertise, you can always pursue subspecialty/fellowship training.

Application Process

Students interested in combined training should apply to emergency medicine/internal medicine programs through the Electronic Residency Application System (ERAS). Applicants must interview with both departments while visiting an institution. Combined programs are ranked as a single program when submitting to the National Residency Match Program. Given the limited number of first-year positions in emergency medicine/internal medicine, many applicants also apply to categorical programs in internal medicine and/or emergency medicine. Applications to categorical programs must be indicated separately in ERAS.

Christopher Lewandowski, MD
Residency Program Director, Henry Ford Hospital

The combined emergency medicine/internal medicine/critical care residency program is designed to allow board certification in all three specialties by completing a 6-year integrated and coherent residency program. After the successful completion of 5 years in this program, residents are allowed to apply for their emergency medicine and internal medicine board certification exams. Completion of separate training in each of these programs would otherwise take 7 to 8 years or longer. This program requires 27 months of internal medicine supervised training, 27 months of emergency medicine supervised training, and 18 months of supervised critical care medicine training. In general, residents are expected to perform duties only in the department that they are working with at the time and will not have simultaneous duties in multiple departments.

The purpose of this training path is to allow residents to pursue academic careers or practice environments that involve a full spectrum of illness or injury from emergency presentation through intensive care unit (ICU) care to discharge.

The guidelines for this training path were approved in 1999 by the American Board of Emergency Medicine and the American Board of Internal Medicine. Accreditation of this program is provided through Accreditation Council for Graduate Medical Education (ACGME)-Residency Review Committee (RRC) accreditation of each of the sponsoring programs and fellowship; it does not receive independent accreditation. If any one of the three sponsoring programs receives probationary accreditation, no further residents can be admitted into the combined training path.

Is This Right for Me?

This program is for residents who have a strong interest in a career involving emergency medicine and critical care medicine and want to become board certified in each. Applicants generally have a strong interest in an academic career involving teaching, research, and providing advanced care to the critically ill or injured. The emergency medicine/internal medicine/critical care program prepares residents for academic careers by providing formal teaching opportunities and training in research including completion of a research project. To date, there is only one graduate of this combined track who is pursuing an academic career with dual appointments in emergency medicine and internal medicine/critical care medicine while practicing in both environments.

It can be very difficult to commit to a 6-year training program and a long-term career path after only 3 years of medical school, especially considering that the third year is the first year of clinical medicine. Residents can enter an emergency medicine/internal medicine/critical care program from a categorical emergency medicine or a categorical internal medicine program after 1 year of training or after 3 years in an emergency medicine/internal medicine program.

Couldn't I Just Do a Critical Care Fellowship?

Many emergency medicine-trained residents have completed a critical care medicine fellowship and have gone onto successful careers involving both specialties without gaining critical care medicine board certification.[1] Residents completing a categorical emergency medicine program, followed by an accredited critical care fellowship, are not eligible to apply for board certification in critical care medicine in the United States. It is unclear if and when a direct path from emergency medicine to critical care will result in critical care board eligibility.[2] Residents who complete a critical care medicine fellowship after a categorical emergency medicine residency are eligible to gain certification from the

European Society for Intensive Care Medicine.[3,4] These credentials will need to be accepted by each hospital or health system where privileges are requested. Residency training in internal medicine provides residents with the background required to provide longer-term care and is necessary to allow board certification in critical care medicine as the certifying exam is provided by the American Board of Internal Medicine (ABIM).

What Are the Advantages of This Type of Training?

Critical care medicine as defined by the Society of Critical Care Medicine is a multidisciplinary health care specialty that cares for patients with acute life-threatening illness or injury. As such there are great similarities between emergency medicine and critical care medicine in regard to patient care as well as the need to provide this care on a 24-hour/7-days-a-week basis. There is a shortage of critical care physicians combined with an increasing demand for these services. Only one in three critically ill or injured patients is provided care by an intensivist. This will be accentuated as the population ages.[5] Given this situation, the demand for well-trained physicians with this expertise will continue to rise. Formal board certification in all three specialties will be advantageous when applying for privileges after training and will prevent any limitation in career opportunities.

The combined emergency medicine/internal medicine/critical care program will facilitate an academic career in emergency medicine and critical care medicine. It will provide for a multidimensional career with increased professional satisfaction by incorporating teaching, research, and administrative duties that would expand and coordinate the role of emergency medicine in critical care medicine at institutional and national levels.[6] Further, multispecialty groups that staff both the emergency department and the ICUs would find those with emergency medicine/internal medicine/critical care training as ideal partners and future leaders. Finally, such broad subspecialty expertise can be used for a wide range of career options, including practice in any of the specialties alone or practice at their interface, such as a hospitalist, as an inpatient teaching attending, or in international medicine.

What Are the Disadvantages of This Type of Program?

Residents in combined programs need to realize that these are accelerated programs and do not provide more time to develop more knowledge; rather you must master three specialties in less time. Despite being off cycle with colleagues in categorical programs and having less experience in a single discipline, faculty and others still expect you to function at the same level as categorical residents in the same postgraduate year.

In addition, this program takes a very early commitment to a long training path. As a resident grows and develops, career paths become clearer and may change direction. It can be very difficult to realize that you are facing 2 to 3 more years of training when those you started residency with are embarking on new jobs and careers at much higher salaries. Therefore, it is extremely important that long-term career goals are well developed. If they are, this could be for you.

How Do I Apply?

Application can be submitted through the Electronic Residency Application System (ERAS), as for any other program. Some programs accept applications directly into the emergency medicine/internal medicine/critical care medicine program at the R-1 level, others may require initial application into the emergency medicine/internal medicine program and will support transfer before the start of the R-4 year, allowing the resident to consolidate future career decisions. All residents need to register with the National Residency Match Program (NRMP) as these programs participate in the match.

There are three programs as of this writing:

Henry Ford Hospital Program
Nikhil Goyal, MD (emergency medicine, internal medicine)
John Buckley, MD, MPH (internal medicine, critical care medicine)
2799 West Grand Boulevard
Detroit, MI 48202-2689
(313) 916-2421, Fax: (313) 916-9102

North Shore-Long Island Jewish Medical Center
Albert Einstein College of Medicine
Barbara Barnett, MD (emergency medicine, internal medicine)
Alan Multz, MD (internal medicine, critical care medicine)
27005 76th Avenue
New Hyde Park, NY 11040
718-470-7501, Fax: 718-470-9113

University of Maryland Medical Center
Michael E. Winters, MD (emergency medicine, internal medicine)
Pamela Amelung, MD (internal medicine, critical care medicine, pulmonary medicine)
Department of Medicine
110 South Paca Street
Baltimore, MD 21201
410-328-8025, Fax: 410-328-8028

References

1. Bozeman WP, Gaasch WR. Trauma resuscitation/critical care fellowship for emergency physicians: a necessary step for the future of academic emergency medicine. *Acad Emerg Med.* 1999;6:331-333.
2. Overton DT. Emergency medicine and critical care medicine: have the stars (finally) aligned? *Ann Emerg Med* 2005;46:225-227.
3. European Society for Intensive Care Medicine. Available at www.esicm.org.
4. Gunn S, Grenvik A. Emergency medicine and critical care certification. *Acad Emerg Med.* 2002;9:322-323.
5. Huang DT, et al. Critical care medicine and certification for emergency physicians. *Ann Emerg Med.* 2005;46:217-223.
6. Cawdry M, Burg M. Emergency medicine career paths less traveled. *Ann Emerg Med* 2004;44:79-83.

Emergency Medicine/Family Medicine

Robert E. O'Connor, MD, MPH, and Jennifer Naticchia, MD
Co-Program Directors, Combined Emergency Medicine/Family Medicine Residency Program,
Christiana Care Health System

In 2005, the American Board of Emergency Medicine (ABEM) and the American Board of Family Medicine (ABFM) announced that they would offer dual certification for candidates who enter and successfully complete the curriculum of the 5-year program. Combined training in emergency medicine/family medicine is the sole recognized pathway for emergency medicine residents to train in family medicine and the sole recognized pathway for family medicine residents to train in emergency medicine, other than completion of both categorical emergency medicine and family medicine residency programs accredited by the Accreditation Council for Graduate Medical Education (ACGME). Combined training in emergency medicine and family medicine will develop physicians who are fully qualified in both specialties. The strengths of the two residencies complement each other to provide an optimal educational experience.

Combined programs include components of categorical emergency medicine/family medicine residencies that are accredited respectively by the Residency Review Committee for Emergency Medicine (RRC-emergency medicine) and by the Residency Review Committee for Family Medicine (RRC-FM), both of which function under the auspices of the ACGME. Graduates of combined programs are eligible for board certification through the ABEM and the ABFM. The boards will not accept training in a combined program if the accreditation status of the residency in either primary discipline is probationary. If the residency in either discipline receives probationary accreditation after initiation of the combined training program, new residents may not be appointed to the combined training program until such time as the residency in the primary discipline is restored to full accreditation.

The objectives of the combined training in emergency medicine/family medicine include the training of physicians for practice or academic careers that address the spectrum of patient illness and injury from the emergent through the total health care of the individual and the family. Graduates of the combined training program may function as generalists, practice either or both disciplines, enter subspecialty training programs approved by either board, or undertake research. Within an institution, their perspective spanning two specialties has the potential to increase communication and understanding among the two disciplines.

Application Process

Applications are handled through the traditional Electronic Residency Application System (ERAS) and the National Residency Match Program (NRMP). The combined programs are ranked as a single program for the NRMP. Applicants interview with both departments when visiting an institution. If an applicant also wants to apply separately to a categorical emergency medicine or family medicine program, then an ERAS application would be required. These combined programs tend to be very competitive given the limited number of positions available in the match. At the time of printing, there is only one approved combined allopathic emergency medicine/family medicine residency, located at Christiana Care Health System in Delaware. There are five osteopathic combined programs and more detailed information is available on their Web sites.

Structure

The emergency medicine/family medicine programs are 5 years (60 months) in duration. The training is 30 months in each specialty and encompasses all of the minimum requirements of each individual residency. Residents traditionally alternate between emergency medicine and family medicine and function exclusively within the department in which they are working and are not expected to perform duties for both fields simultaneously.

Certification

To meet eligibility for dual certification, the resident must satisfactorily complete 60 months of combined training and this must be verified by the director or co-directors of the combined program. The emergency medicine and family medicine certifying examinations cannot be taken until all 5 years of training in the combined emergency medicine/family medicine residency program are satisfactorily completed.

Program Requirements

Guidelines from the ABFM and the ABEM stipulate that combined training provide 30 months of training under the direct supervision of each specialty for a total of 60 months. Program graduates can sit for certification in each specialty and practice as family physicians, emergency physicians, or both. They also can enter subspecialty training programs approved by either board or undertake research.

The combined training must be coordinated by a designated director or co-directors who can devote substantial time and effort to the educational program. An overall program director may be appointed from either specialty, or co-directors may be appointed from both specialties. If a single program director is appointed, an associate director from the other specialty must be named to ensure both integration of the program and supervision of each discipline. The two directors should embrace similar values and goals for their program. An exception to the above requirements would be a single director who is board certified in each discipline and has an academic appointment in each department.

Why a Combined Program?

If done separately, the training would take 6 to 7 years (depending on whether the emergency medicine residency is 3 or 4 years). Completing a combined program offers an opportunity to become dual-board certified in a shorter period of time than separate training would involve. Combined training opens up opportunities for certain types of future practice that might not be available after categorical emergency medicine or family medicine residency. This type of training program may be ideally suited for physicians seeking to practice both specialties either concurrently or sequentially. Such practice is thought to be ideally suited for rural settings, but practitioners seeking international or disaster response opportunities may also find the combined training beneficial.

Primary care physicians in very rural parts of the country and in international settings often are called on to manage adult and pediatric emergencies because of the lack of residency trained emergency physicians. Medical students who are interested in eventually practicing primary care in either of these types of settings may benefit significantly by combined training in order to treat all types of medical conditions, both chronic and acute.

chapter 19

Scheduling in the Third and Fourth Years of Medical School

David C. Gordon, MD
Division of Emergency Medicine, Duke University Medical Center

Susan B. Promes, MD, FACEP
Residency Program Director, University of California San Francisco-San Francisco General Hospital

Putting together a schedule for the clinical years of medical school raises a lot of questions. When is the best time to take one's first emergency medicine rotation? Which electives are most helpful in preparing for residency? How many away rotations should one do? In this chapter, we address these questions and others in providing both philosophical and practical advice in planning for a future career in emergency medicine.

Third Year–The Fundamentals

The third year of medical school is composed of the building blocks for your career in medicine. Core rotations in surgery, internal medicine, obstetrics/gynecology, and pediatrics will serve as the backbone of your early clinical development. The goal is to excel in everything you do. Emergency medicine encompasses a broad knowledge base, and while some areas of medicine will be more interesting than others, all will be used in taking care of patients in the emergency department. It would be great if you could perform at honors level on all of your third-year core rotations. The grades on these rotations, as well as your USMLE grades, are key to getting an interview at an emergency medicine residency program.

The timing of your first emergency medicine rotation in your third year is important. Ideally, the sooner the better with one caveat: your emergency medicine rotation must be balanced with already having achieved a certain level of clinical proficiency to be able to perform well on the rotation. Ideally, this will mean having completed rotations in both internal medicine and surgery. Emergency medicine is a broad specialty, and the more knowledge you bring with you to the rotation, the better you will do during your emergency medicine clerkship. Remember that you will see patients of all ages in the emergency department, so previous pediatric experience is helpful as well.

By scheduling your emergency medicine rotation as early as possible in your academic year, you not only will be able to confirm your interest in emergency medicine as a career choice but also will be able to identify mentors who can provide continued career guidance, write future letters of recommendation, and facilitate involvement with academic projects. If your school does not allow electives in the third year of medical school, it is imperative that you choose an emergency medicine elective as soon as possible in your fourth year. Remember, you can always spend some time shadowing emergency medicine faculty in the emergency department during your third year to get exposure to emergency medicine and start to network with the emergency medicine community in your institution.

Everyone's situation is unique, and if you are ever in doubt as to how to handle your particular situation, set up an appointment with the medical student coordinator or emergency medicine residency director at your institution; if you do not have an emergency medicine residency program at your institution, consider using the SAEM Virtual Advisor service.

Fourth Year

If you did not do an emergency medicine rotation as a third year, now is the time. You should schedule your rotation as soon as possible. As far as fourth-year electives are concerned, the electives you should take should in large part be guided by what you are interested in and want to learn more about during your final year of medical school. In addition, your medical school may have national expertise in a specialty that would offer a strong learning experience. There are, however, some electives that will provide skills particularly pertinent to the practice of emergency medicine and should be strongly considered:

- Anesthesia (airway assessment, bag-valve-mask ventilation, laryngoscopy, advanced airway techniques)
- Critical care (MICU/SICU) (principles of resuscitation, ventilator management, hemodynamic monitoring, vasoactive therapy)
- Dermatology (rash description, identification, and treatment)
- Ophthalmology (slit lamp exams, fundoscopy, ocular trauma)
- Orthopedics (fracture principles, splinting techniques, reductions, hand injuries)
- Radiology (interpretation and use of plain films, CT, MRI, and ultrasound)
- Sports medicine (diagnosis and treatment of sports related injuries)
- Toxicology (diagnosis of poisonings, decontamination, enhanced elimination, antidotes)
- Trauma surgery (assessment and management of traumatic injuries)

We recommend at least one rotation in anesthesia or critical care. Otherwise, allow your personal interest, clinical experience, and the reputed quality of the rotation guide your selection. You should also consider scheduling a light rotation or taking the month of December or January off to allow time and flexibility for interviewing for residency positions.

Fourth Year—Away Rotations

There are many benefits to an away emergency medicine rotation. Every hospital has its own culture and style of medicine. Stepping outside your home institution will allow you to experience a different practice environment and thereby help you better understand which elements are personally important. From the perspective of the residency application process, an away emergency medicine rotation can help facilitate an interview offer and, with a good performance, residency position. Program directors like certainty, and demonstrating your clinical skills and professionalism at their institution will help to reassure them that they will be getting an excellent resident in choosing you.

Overall, two rotations in emergency medicine—one at your home institution and one away—will suffice. There is no need to overdo it when it comes to emergency medicine rotations. In fact, doing more than two or possibly three rotations is not looked on favorably. You will be doing emergency medicine for the rest of your career; take this opportunity to broaden your knowledge base and clinical exposure to other specialties. Away rotations in specialized areas of emergency medicine like toxicology that may not be offered at your medical school can be very valuable to your training. Remember, however, that each medical school has its own policies on the number of away rotations permitted.

Planning for away rotation takes time and energy. Start early (winter or spring of your third year) and familiarize yourself with policies surrounding away rotations at your institution as well as the policies at the institutions at which you are interested in doing a rotation. Make sure you have malpractice coverage and a place to stay and that your immunization records are up to date.

Fourth Year—Final Preparations

Our discussion so far has centered on your academic preparation for residency. There are, however, other important considerations to be made in designing your schedule. While residency work-hour restrictions are now in place, residency is still no walk in the park. You will work hard and learn fast in what will ultimately be the most formative years of your professional development. As such, it is important to enter residency feeling mentally and emotionally refreshed.

If you anticipate making a big move between the end of medical school and the beginning of residency, make sure you will have plenty of time to make this transition. Once residency begins, you will have plenty of other issues to worry about other than which apartment to rent. If possible, consider scheduling vacation time at the end of your fourth year to allow plenty of time to get your personal affairs in order. Even if there is not a big move ahead, a vacation at the end of fourth year can help recharge your batteries.

Final Thoughts

We have provided you with some guiding principles in planning your last 2 years of medical school. Take a dedicated rotation in emergency medicine early but only after obtaining an appropriate degree of clinical skills. Certain electives will be particularly pertinent to emergency medicine, but your personal interests and the strengths of your medical school should also be part of the equation. Away rotations can take time and effort in arranging but offer great insight into other institutions as well as into what is important to you. Last, do not forget about the personal factors. Make sure you have scheduled enough free time to enter residency energized and excited for the rewarding career ahead of you.

chapter *20*

The Fourth-Year Medical Student Emergency Medicine Clerkship

Robert Brandt, MD
Synergy Medical Education Alliance/Michigan State University Emergency Medicine Residency Program
Resident Clinical Instructor, Program in Emergency Medicine
Michigan State University College of Human Medicine

Mary Jo Wagner, MD
Program Director, Synergy Medical Education, Alliance/Michigan State University Emergency Medicine
Residency Program, Associate Professor, Program in Emergency Medicine
Michigan State University College of Human Medicine

Before the Clerkship

Preparation is essential for success in your fourth-year emergency medicine rotation. Not only must you decide when and where to rotate, but also you must determine what to take with you, how you should dress, and with whom you will be working. This chapter will guide the decision-making process and help answer many of the questions you may have.

Where Should I Do My Rotation(s)?

Choosing the best location can be a difficult process. If your medical school has an emergency medicine residency program available, that makes it easy. Doing a clerkship there gives you the advantage of a familiar environment for your rotation, even if you have only seen the emergency department during your surgery or medicine rotation. You will know the systems of a hospital (including lab, radiology, and what the orders sheets look like), which makes it easier to 'shine" right away.

Programs differ greatly by location. Large, urban programs may offer more penetrating trauma cases, a large volume of patients, as well as multidisciplinarian coverage for specialties and possibly more autonomy. Smaller, rural hospitals may have the emergency department as the only available health care for many people. Such a setting may depend on emergency physicians for a more complete work-up of patients. This may also mean that residents and medical students are allowed to see and do more. University hospitals may offer an array of unique patients not seen in other facilities. Multiple specialists and subspecialists may offer a perspective toward medicine rarely seen elsewhere. At the same time, such programs might have several levels of residents and fellows, which may mean more consulting and less patient evaluation by students in the emergency department. Community hospitals can have a wide variety of patients with different types of trauma and a more varied difference in the level of responsibility given to the student. Obviously all programs have different levels of involvement for the medical student. Researching the location and opportunities at a possible rotation is important depending on your goals for that rotation.

If you do two (or three) emergency medicine rotations, you should try to vary the experience. If your first rotation is at community hospital, then try to do your next rotation at a large urban or university hospital. By varying your experiences, you will be a better judge of programs during your interviews, as well as learning which type of facility you may ultimately desire to work. Try to be realistic about your strengths, weaknesses, and expectations about the rotation. After weighing what you have experienced so far, try to determine which location would benefit you the most as an interview candidate, and as a future physician.

Also, before you begin your rotation at any hospital, go to the hospital Web site and research it. Read the entire Web site; your knowledge will definitely show your interest level in their program. Also, many Web sites will list the faculty you will be working with, and you will know their areas of expertise as well as a name and face before starting the rotation, which will give you a definite edge.

When Should I Do My Emergency Medicine Rotation?

If you are considering emergency medicine as your career, you should try to do two (not more than three) rotations in your first 4 months of the fourth year. In many medical students' minds, interview season starts in November. For the programs evaluating you, it starts the first day they see you. If there is one program for which you truly desire to have an interview, consider doing a rotation at that location.

What Supplies Do I Need Before the Start of the Rotation?

Certain supplies are invaluable in the emergency department. Because multiple people often require these supplies, they can be difficult to obtain when needed most.

- A *stethoscope* is needed for virtually every patient; have your name and contact information on it.
- *Trauma sheers* (which can be obtained at nearly all medical supply stores) are needed in most trauma cases and for other situations. Purchase a retractable name badge and use this to secure the sheers to your waist, so that you can have them easily accessible when needed but out of the way otherwise.
- *Hemoccult cards* and *solution* can often be difficult to find. Having a bottle handy as well as a few cards in your pocket if you are required to check for occult blood can save time and frustration.
- A *pocket pharmacy book* or a *PDA with a drug program* you are familiar with is required. The vast multidisciplinary involvement of emergency medicine requires knowledge in a wide variety of drugs.
- A *penlight* can be very helpful, especially if there are no convenient wall-mounted light sources.
- *Scrubs* are the most common attire in the emergency department, some programs supply them for you, and some do not. Be sure to find out if you need to bring your own scrubs, as well as what color scrubs are allowed or required, before you show up on the first day. Be sure to have an extra pair with you (or know where you can get an extra pair while at the hospital) in case you need to change during a shift. You should also inquire about whether you will need your white coat or any other specific attire.
- Pack at least one *interview outfit* if you are doing an away rotation and bring a copy of your CV if you have not yet submitted your ERAS application. If you are doing your rotation during interview season, it is possible that you will be asked to interview while you are there. Earlier in the year, these are sometimes labeled as "informal" interviews, but it is always best to look professional.

What Should I Read/Study Right Before the Start of the Clerkship?

The knowledge base required in emergency medicine is staggering, considering it covers all aspects of medicine. Emergency physicians are experts of resuscitation in the acute setting, so a thorough review of ACLS procedures would be of great help. You should also review any other procedures you are likely to be asked to perform, including the indications, contraindications, and complications. Being able to answer the question, "Do you know how to do this?" in a positive manner will give you more chances to do procedures.

During the Clerkship

Show Up on Time

You should be in the department, ready to work, 10 minutes BEFORE your shift begins. Showing up a few minutes late, unless excused, sets a bad tone for your work ethic and professionalism.

Work Hard

Most other rotations you have been involved in have breaks, but in emergency medicine, a fast pace and continuous activity are normal. In the emergency department, you may not get a single break in action for the entirety of your shift. Expect this and be prepared to work for the whole shift, and possibly a little longer. Depending on where you work, the attendings may sign out, or they may stay until all of their patients have been worked up and discharged/admitted. Be prepared to do the same.

Bringing your own food from home is encouraged so that if you do get a few minutes down time, you can get a bite to eat without having to take 20 minutes to go down to the cafeteria. Formal coffee breaks usually do not exist, but if you drink coffee, bring it from home so you have it for your shift if you need it.

Ask for Help

It is possible that you may be the first person to see a patient. It is also possible that the chart could be labeled with "nausea" and you will go into the room and see a patient who looks like he or she might be having an active myocardial infarction. If you go into a room and see a patient in acute distress or one who appears to be having a life-threatening problem, it is always better to excuse yourself and ask for a supervising physician immediately. Remember, in the emergency department, a patient has evolving symptoms. The patient who appeared stable in triage could be crashing a few minutes later in the room. Being overconfident and trying to handle too many things yourself is more likely to be viewed in a negative manner compared with asking for help appropriately.

Be an Active Learner

The emergency department can be an intimidating and chaotic place. However, this should not dissuade you from becoming involved in the action. If you have experience suturing, ask if you can do the sutures. The physician may just want you to watch at first, but if he or she sees you perform, the next time you could be doing it yourself. If you hear that a chest tube is going to be inserted, ask to watch or assist. If a patient with a gunshot wound to the chest is coming in, see if you can be part of the case. It is easy to slip into the background if you are shy or quiet; however, the proactive medical student not only learns more but also is perceived as a better student.

Talk with the residents and attendings about emergency medicine, not just about emergency patients. Find out from them what they think you should learn. Residents also have great insight into how the various programs work, as well as the interviewing process, which they just went through. Find out what they like and dislike about the programs they have seen. This can give you insight that is unobtainable anywhere else.

Keep Your Differential Diagnosis Broad

A patient may come into the emergency department with any disease that you have ever read about, and one of the tasks of an emergency physician is to quickly determine what could kill the patient in the next minute. Keep in mind the acronym "ROB," which stands for "Rule Out Badness." Sometimes patients arrive just a little short of breath, but you still have to think about the possibility of a tension pneumothorax or pulmonary emboli. An emergency medicine attending is likely to be more impressed that you have considered many possibilities (a broad differential diagnosis) than to have you give one definitive disease process.

Follow Up on the Details

One of the most helpful aspects of your care of patients in the emergency department is to follow up on patient care details. These include the little tasks like checking up on lab tests (were they drawn? are the results back?), checking on radiographs, or calling the nursing home for more information. Keeping on top of these aspects will impress the emergency department faculty with your organizational skills and ability to multitask.

Study Hard

Knowing everything about emergency medicine is impossible in a month. To be honest, it is impossible in a lifetime, because emergency medicine covers all medicine as a whole. However, if you have an interesting case, you should read about it and know about it for the next day. Even common complaints may be seen in a different light after studying about them. Whether you are caring for a child with a common cold, a 40-year-old with a kidney stone, or a 70-year-old with weakness, there is always more to learn and understand.

You may be on an away rotation in a new city with many new sights to see and activities in the area; however, you must balance your free time with studying. It is tempting to assume that after the shift is over one can turn off studying and relax till the next shift. Do not fall into that trap; try to study every day. Remember to consider the entire month as an interview for a job—you will need to impress all the emergency department staff at all times, and showing that you learned from yesterday's patients is a part of this. Socializing with the residents or staff provides a great time to see how everyone interacts and to ask some of the important nonmedical questions about the residency program. Be careful to continue to be polite, professional, and honest; do not allow your judgment to be impaired even at these social events.

Be Yourself

Throughout the entirety of your rotation, be true to yourself. Emergency physicians work in all types of settings, but all of them are trained to spot phonies. They will know if you are putting them on. Do not put on an act to hope to impress someone. Just be you. Also, do not put down any of the other programs. Talking down about surgery, family medicine, or any other program will only make you look arrogant or like you have a negative attitude. Even if you hear a physician griping or a resident complaining, resist the urge to put others down. By taking the high road you not only stay professional, you also avoid hurting yourself by insulting any individuals listening to the commentary.

After the Clerkship

Be sure to thank everyone with whom you worked. You may want to get the e-mail address of residents with whom you worked in case you have any new questions. You will also benefit from writing down the names of people you worked with, in case you go back to interview or call to ask questions.

Take notes either during or soon after the end of your rotation. This will help you to keep track of the people, the highlights, and the deficiencies that you observed of the program. It can be difficult after several rotations to try to remember the important details.

chapter 21

The Makings of the Ideal Emergency Medicine Resident Applicant

Stephen R. Hayden, MD, FACEP
Program Director, Emergency Medicine Residency, University of California, San Diego

To understand what makes for the ideal emergency medicine (emergency medicine) resident applicant, it may be helpful to identify a few qualities that distinguish the true emergency medicine specialist. Dr. William Menninger once said, "There are six essential qualities that are the key to success: sincerity, personal integrity, humility, courtesy, wisdom, and charity." It is hard to imagine a better description of the ideal emergency medicine specialist or applicant to an emergency medicine residency program. Beyond these basic qualities that identify success as a physician, one quality that distinguishes the emergency medicine specialist in particular is the capacity to make clinical decisions for critically ill and injured patients based on very limited information. Of course, the skill is to gather as much information as you can to make an educated decision in a timely manner. Another key characteristic is the ability to multitask and prioritize the needs of the patients under your care. Furthermore, emergency physicians must quickly be able to recognize who is ill and who is not. The first two skills develop from innate characteristics, the last from years of training and working with patients to develop the necessary pattern recognition. This is not an exhaustive list by any means; however, it frames well the discussion of what makes the ideal emergency medicine resident applicant.

What Characteristics in Emergency Medicine Applicants Predict Future Success as an Emergency Medicine Resident?

If you ask most emergency medicine program directors this question, you will probably get almost as many different answers as there are residency programs. There is actually a very good reason for this, and that is that each program takes a slightly different approach to emergency medicine resident training, emphasizes different things, and has a slightly different personality based on their specific resources and the individuals at that program. It is a "match" process, and it is important for applicants to assess a training program as much as it is important for programs to assess applicants so each can find the best fit.

There has been some research done in an attempt to enlighten us on this subject. In a survey of program directors in February 1998,[1] criteria that were reported to be most important in the selection of applicants were emergency medicine rotation grades, the interview, clinical grades, and letters of recommendation. Criteria that were judged to be of moderate importance in the selection process were whether or not an elective was done at the program's institution, USMLE Step II results, whether or not interest was expressed in the program, and awards or achievements. The least importance was placed on whether or not the applicant was elected to the Alpha Omega Alpha (AOA) Honor Society, the medical school attended, extracurricular activities, basic science grades, publications, and personal statement. In this same study, the most consistent criteria cited by program directors were emergency medicine rotation grade, interviews, and clinical grades. The least consistent criteria were whether or not an elective was done at the program director's institution, whether or not interest was expressed in the program director's institution, and AOA status.

In another study done at a single emergency medicine program,[2] a multivariate analysis attempted to define characteristics present in the initial applications of graduates from that program that predicted future success in residency defined by a global rating of the faculty categorized by percentiles (for example, graduate A is among the top 10% of all residents I have worked with). Characteristics that consistently predicted success in residency were the medical school attended, the rating of the applicant in the dean's letter (now called the medical student performance evaluation [MSPE]), and distinctive factors such high-level achievement in sports, music, service to the medical school or national organizations, and so on. Just an average level of involvement was not enough; rather, such achievements as being an Olympic medalist, high level black belt, accomplished musician, or president of an international medical student organization, for example, was necessary to meet these criteria. The grade on an emergency medicine rotation was not available in this study separate from the medical school record. The results may not be applicable to all residency programs. While other criteria such as interviews, letters of recommendation, USMLE scores, research, etc., did not predict success, they may still be considered important by many program directors and faculty.

What can we learn from these studies? On one hand, there is a survey of many emergency medicine program directors that studied what program directors think they want, and on the other hand, there is a study that identified a few characteristics that actually predicted success in a single residency program. Despite the diversity in the selection approach, there are a number of common elements. Most programs use some sort of scoring system that includes evaluation of the medical school attended and performance in medical school with a much heavier weighting toward clinical rotations including the emergency medicine rotation. In addition, they will score information from the MSPE, letters of recommendation (especially from experienced emergency medicine faculty or other emergency medicine program directors), USMLE scores, research or other academic experience, extracurricular activities or distinctive factors, the personal statement, and, finally, the interview. In the MSPE, most program directors will focus on performance in the clinical rotations and emergency medicine rotations. While few medical schools have formal ranking systems, the MSPE frequently will give some rough indication of where an applicant ranks relative to other medical students. The preclinical years are typically less important. For certain residency programs, class rank and election to the AOA Honor Society may be important. The board scores are used as a screening tool for some programs, yet for others, they are not emphasized. Most often the USMLE score will stand out if it falls greater than the 90th percentile or lower than the 50th percentile. For some programs, extracurricular activities such as volunteer work, language fluency, and international experience are less important, yet they still play a significant role because they demonstrate that you are well rounded. As mentioned previously, truly distinctive achievements are something that an applicant should emphasize. Experience as an emergency medical technician or paramedic may be important as it will be assumed that you are familiar with the unique aspects of emergency medicine as a specialty. Previous experience in business, law, and public health may be considered a benefit, but each program will have a different approach to this depending on the program emphasis. For example, a doctorate may make you more competitive at an academically oriented program. Along these lines, academic experience, including presentations at national meetings and publications, also are often sought. Most program directors like to see a commitment to research yielding a manuscript or presentation, rather than just spending a small amount of time as a research assistant. Finally, and least important, is the personal statement. The personal statement should be used to highlight what makes you different and give the reader a window into who you are.

The interview process is discussed in a separate chapter. Much of the purpose of the interview day is to determine if you are a good fit with the program. Do you get along well with the residents? Do you see yourself fitting in with the other residents and faculty? Most programs will have a luncheon, mixer, journal club, or other informal evening session arranged for you to meet the residents and sometimes faculty. This is the time to see if you like the people, determine if they are happy at the program, and see if you would fit in well with them and if you match with the personality and philosophy of the program.

What Do Program Directors Want?

Colin Powell advises us to "look for loyalty, integrity, a high energy drive, a balanced ego and the drive to get things done." Ideal applicants to residency will be professional, reliable, enthusiastic, and hard working. They should have a thirst for learning and be eminently educable. They should be self-motivated, self-confident, honest, and intelligent. You will notice that for most program directors "intelligent," although important, appears on the list behind some of the other qualities that denote a hard-working, balanced, educable resident. Ideal residents will pass the 3 A.M. test; when the proverbial you-know-what hits the fan in the emergency department at 3 A.M., "I want resident X to be by my side." Ideal applicants will be capable of rapidly establishing a rapport with patients and families, engender trust, and inspire confidence within a brief interaction. They will remain calm in difficult situations and inspire others through their leadership. They will be approachable by colleagues, staff, and patients. It is very important in the emergency department environment to be a team leader and to work with the nurses, technicians, and other staff as they will look to you as a role model and teacher, and you must inspire confidence in them. In dealing with consultants from other services, it is helpful to be a consummate diplomat while simultaneously being a strong patient advocate. In this regard, interpersonal skills and the ability to "win friends and influence people" are vital.

In addition to these qualities, program directors want applicants who are willing to become fully engaged in the program. To paraphrase John F. Kennedy, "Ask not what your residency can do for you but what you can contribute to your residency." Residency is a time for exploration, to find your passions within our specialty. Residency directors want applicants who will take full advantage of unique opportunities for learning that exist at a particular program. The paradigm shift toward competency based education ensures that residents will graduate with a certain minimum acceptable competency in clinical emergency medicine, but what makes our job rewarding is to train a resident that goes well beyond acceptable proficiency and has a drive to excel.

During the course of residency training, life events will occasionally intervene. A resident may become injured or ill, have a family emergency, get pregnant, etc. Residency programs work when residents are willing to help their classmates. Program directors look for characteristics in applicants that indicate a willingness to support fellow residents, to step up to the plate and do whatever needs to be done without necessarily expecting payback. Finally, program directors do not want whiners or complainers. Instead, they want problem solvers. A good residency program will encourage residents to be creative and make suggestions for improvement, but do not be the kind of person who brings up problems unless at the same time you offer a solution.

Summary

Harry Truman once said, "I studied the lives of great men and famous women; and I found that the men and women who got to the top were those who did the jobs they had in hand, with everything they had of energy, enthusiasm and hard work." More than raw intelligence alone, the ideal applicant to an emergency medicine residency will combine great character, a love of learning, a willingness to help colleagues, tremendous work ethic, professional attitude, diplomacy, and great leadership with a well-balanced personality both at work and after work. When I meet this person for the first time, I will let you know.

References

1. Crane JT, Ferraro C. Selection criteria for emergency medicine residency applicants. *Acad Emerg Med.* 2000;7:54-60.
2. Hayden SR, Hayden M, Gamst A. What characteristics of emergency medicine applicants will predict future performance as an emergency medicine resident? *Acad Emerg Med.* 2003;10(5):458.

chapter 22

The Application Process

Carlo L. Rosen, MD, FACEP
Program Director, Beth Israel Deaconess Medical Center
Harvard Affiliated Emergency Medicine Residency

Emergency medicine has become one of the more competitive specialties in medicine. The level of competition makes the application process a stressful one. This is complicated by the Electronic Residency Application Service (ERAS) that has decreased the amount of paperwork involved in the application process but may still be daunting to many applicants. The deadlines for the ERAS application, letters of recommendation, and the United States Medical Licensing Examination (USMLE) can also be anxiety provoking. This chapter presents a concise approach to the application process that will help you to focus on the important parts of the process and avoid pitfalls that will waste time and decrease your chances of matching at your first choice.

Selection Criteria

ERAS asks you to enter a lot of information, but it is important to consider how each part of your application is viewed by program directors. In a survey of program directors published in 2000,[1] criteria that were reported to be most important in the selection of applicants were emergency medicine rotation grades, the interview, clinical grades, and letters of recommendation. Criteria that were judged to be of moderate importance in the selection process were whether or not an elective was done at the program's institution, USMLE Step II results, whether or not interest was expressed in the program, and awards or achievements. The least importance was placed on whether or not the applicant was placed on Alpha Omega Alpha (AOA) Honor Society status, medical school attended, extracurricular activities, basic science grades, publications, and personal statement. In this same study, criteria that showed the highest consistency of responsiveness among program directors were emergency medicine rotation grade, interviews, and clinical grades. The least consistent criteria were whether or not an elective was done at the program director's institution, whether or not interest was expressed in the program director's institution, and AOA status.

Each program director has an idea of what parts of the ERAS application are actually important. A recent study in the emergency medicine literature[2] attempted to identify characteristics of applicants that predict future success in residency. This paper was based on one residency's experience. It is worth considering the results, because you have control over a few of these factors. The authors found that graduating from a "top-tier" medical school, the presence of "distinctive factors" (e.g., being a champion athlete, an officer of a national organization, or a medical school officer), and the dean's letter were predictors of overall success in residency.[2] Because some program directors may have read this article, it is important to highlight any distinctive factors that you have in your application.

The Curriculum Vitae

The curriculum vitae (CV) is a resume of your academic experience. It summarizes your education and any publications or other academic projects that you have completed. The CV should include undergraduate education, graduate education, medical education, medical school honors, employment, research experience, as well as a bibliography. For the bibliography, publications are listed as abstracts, published manuscripts, or manuscripts in press (accepted), and some institutions allow you to list submitted manuscripts. Research presentations should also be listed. It is important to be truthful on the CV, as well as the entire application. Publications should be listed only if you were an author; it is very easy for these to be checked with a literature search. It is also a good idea to bring copies of the published manuscripts to the interview. Program directors like to see that you have presented abstracts at emergency medicine meetings and that you have already made contributions to the specialty. At the early stage of the game, during medical school, it may be difficult to achieve a lot in this category. Some of the more academic programs will look for any research experience, not just in emergency medicine. Work experience should include recent employment that is relevant to emergency medicine such as work as an emergency medical technician or paramedic. If you have worked in another field such as business or the law, this should also be added. As mentioned above, distinctive factors are listed here. However, too much "fluff" or "padding" will not add to the CV and may actually detract from it. Your medical school will have its own official format for the CV, and you should be consistent with this format.

The Personal Statement

According to the survey of program directors,[1] the personal statement is one of the least important parts of the application. However, it requires the most amount of thought on your part and may cause anxiety. The personal statement should include an explanation of why you chose emergency medicine and what are your career goals. It should also include a description of other interests that you have that make you a unique candidate. If there are gaps in your medical school training or if you have a nonstandard academic background (time off from school to pursue another career), this should also be explained in the personal statement. The art of personal statement writing lies in your ability to make it interesting without being too creative. Remember that program directors read several hundred of these each year. My only word of advice is to use the spell check function on your computer and to have someone else read it for grammatical errors and content.

Letters of Recommendation

The letters of recommendation are an important part of the application process. These should ideally be from faculty members in emergency medicine and other specialties who know you well. It is much more meaningful and will be read more carefully if it is from someone who has done clinical work with you. In general, three letters should be obtained. Some applicants will have four. At least one, and preferably two or three, should be from emergency physicians. Program directors like to see letters from different faculty from the different emergency departments where you have rotated. This shows that you have done well, not just at your home institution but also on away rotations. Other service attendings in medicine or surgery or other specialties should write the third or fourth letter. The most highly ranked letters are those from academic emergency physicians such as a chairman, program director, or medical student rotation director. Anyone who is a known colleague of the person reading the letter is ideal as well. It will be obvious if the writer of the letter did not work with you, and these letters are less meaningful. When asking a faculty member to write a letter for you, provide them with a copy of your CV, personal statement, and cover letter. Ask for letters as early as possible, because the writer may be very busy writing letters for other students and you do not want these to be delayed.

Most emergency medicine faculty use the Council of Residency Directors' standard letter of recommendation (SLOR), which is available at cordem.org.[3] This replaces the traditional narrative letter of recommendation and represents an attempt to bring objectivity to the process of writing letters of recommendation. The SLOR is a more standardized letter that is easier for program directors to interpret. The first part of the SLOR asks the writer to provide information about how long and how well he or she knows the applicant and what grade the applicant received on the emergency medicine rotation. The SLOR then asks the writer to evaluate the student in several different categories, which include commitment to emergency medicine, work ethic, ability to develop a differential diagnosis and treatment plan, personality, how much guidance the applicant will need during residency, and a prediction of success in residency. The letter writer is also asked to make an overall global assessment of the candidate. Space for a narrative evaluation is included on the form. It is recommended that you ask someone to write you a letter who has worked in the emergency department with you and who will write a favorable letter.

The USMLE

The USMLE Step I examination is taken in the summer of second year. The Step II is more clinically relevant and may be taken in the summer and spring of the fourth year. If it is taken in the spring, the scores are not available in time for the application. This can work in your favor if you are not a good test-taker. However, if you are at risk of failing them, it is recommended that you take them earlier so that they are completed before graduation. For many medical schools, graduation is dependent on passing Step II.

In the study that surveyed all program directors, 39% of the programs had minimum cutoffs for USMLE Step I scores and 32% had cutoffs for Step II scores.[1] Because a significant number of programs have these minimum cutoffs, it is wise to do to as well as possible on these examinations.

The ERAS Application

The ERAS was developed by the Association of American Medical Colleges (AAMC) to transmit application materials including letters of recommendation, the CV, personal statement, dean's letters, and transcripts to residency programs via the Internet. Currently, all emergency medicine residencies use this system. There are three components to the service: the Web-based Applicant Webstation (AWS), the Dean's Office Workstation (DWS), and the Program Director's Workstation (PDWS). Applicants complete the application and select the programs to which they are applying. This is submitted to ERAS. The medical school dean's office scans in the applicant's transcripts, dean's letter, and letters of recommendation and transmits them to the ERAS post office. The final step occurs when program directors connect to the ERAS post office and download the application materials.

The ERAS application includes your general information (name, birthdate, etc.), medical licensure, medical education, medical school honors, graduate and undergraduate education, work experience, volunteer experience, research experience, publications, language fluency, hobbies, and "other accomplishments." My only piece of advice on the ERAS application is to be honest.

The ERAS processing fees are based on the number of programs to which you apply. Instructions for using ERAS as well as your individual passwords are distributed from your dean's office in late June of the third year. For more information, see the AAMC Web site (www.aamc.org).

The Timeline

The application process begins as early as the spring of third year when fourth-year electives are chosen. The summer of the fourth year is the time to do your first emergency medicine rotation and request letters of recommendation. It is also the time to work on your personal statement, CV, and ERAS materials. The ERAS application materials are available from the dean's office in late June. September 1 is the date when you can begin to upload ERAS materials. The application materials should be complete by the end of September at the latest. The Society for Academic Emergency Medicine Residency Catalogue is an invaluable resource for information about the programs (www.saem.org).

Although program directors receive the dean's letters on November 1, as early as October 1 some programs will begin to review applications based on your transcript, letters of recommendation, and the other materials. Many program directors will do an initial screen of the applications before the dean's letters arrive and begin to invite candidates. You will begin to receive invitations to interview as early as mid October. The deadline for applications is in mid to late December. However, this is very late in the process because most programs have already offered invitations and have been interviewing candidates. Because most programs have a limited number of interview slots, it is wise to get application materials in as early as possible. The interview season runs from mid November through the beginning of February. In February, the rank lists are due, and match day is in the middle of March.

Summary

The way to decrease the stress involved with the application process is to be as organized as possible. In assessing how competitive you are as an applicant, remember that the most important parts of the application are the dean's letter including third year clinical rotation grades and emergency medicine rotation grades, letters of recommendation, and the interview. Once you have decided on emergency medicine, there are two things you can do to bolster your chances of matching at your first choice program. The first is to do well on your emergency medicine rotations. The second is to get involved in a research project or other academic project if you have the time. Finally, it is important to apply to a generous number of programs because of the competitiveness of the specialty.

References

1. Crane JT, Ferraro C. Selection criteria for emergency medicine residency applicants. *Acad Emerg Med.* 2000;7:54-60.
2. Hayden SR, Hayden M, Gamst A. What characteristics of applicants to emergency medicine residency programs predict future success as an emergency medicine resident? *Acad Emerg Med.* 2005;12:206-210.
3. Kiem SM, Rein JA, Chisholm C, et al. A standardized letter of recommendation for residency application. *Acad Emerg Med.* 1999;6:1141-1146.

Timeline for the Application Process

Spring of third year	Choose away emergency medicine electives
Summer of fourth year	Request letters of recommendation and gather ERAS materials/emergency medicine rotations
September 1	Begin to submit ERAS materials
October 1	Complete ERAS submission process
Mid October	Programs begin to offer interviews
November 1	Dean's letters are sent
Mid November	Interview season begins
Mid December	Final deadline for ERAS materials
Third week of February	Rank lists are due
Mid March	Match day
Mid June	Intern orientation begins

chapter *23*

The Interview Process

Kai M. Stürmann, MD
Chairman, Department of Emergency Medicine, Brookhaven Memorial Hospital Medical Center

The residency interview begins when you send the last of your documents to the Electronic Residency Application Service (ERAS) and ends on the day you submit your rank order list. How you approach the interview will determine to a large extent the return on your investment of time and money. The number one rule: Be true to yourself. This is not an acting audition. You want to present the "real you" and present yourself as accurately as possible. Your goal is not to create any false impressions—negative, positive, or otherwise. This may seem basic, but understanding this key concept and approaching the interview day with that perspective in mind can do a lot to lower your anxiety level. It will also do a lot to help the program understand who you really are.

Maximizing Your Chances

Emergency medicine remains a competitive field. Advance planning (and work) is essential to increase the likelihood you will be invited for an interview. Apply early. Many programs will be unable to interview all desirable candidates simply for lack of time and resources. Early applicants have a better chance to schedule an interview. An early application means a complete application. The one letter of recommendation that you forgot to ask for until the last minute may keep your application in the "pending" file while other applicants are filling up the programs' interview schedules.

Be sure that you provide a way for program coordinators to reach you throughout the interview season. A "permanent" telephone number may not be the best way to get in touch with you during that wilderness medicine elective. For practical purposes ,easy global access means e-mail. The senior year of medical school is not a good time to change your e-mail address. Be sure to check your e-mail daily once ERAS has distributed your application. Programs generally issue interview invitations in groups. Early respondents will have a broader choice of available dates; late respondents may find their choices limited or no longer existent.

Scheduling

Geography, time, and money are usually the major considerations. You can save much of the latter two by doing your homework. Find out as much as possible about a program from the materials they sent you, the Internet, from conversations with your advisor and other emergency medicine faculty, and from networking with your friends. If you realize the program is not really what you are looking for and you have already been invited to 20 other interviews, perhaps you should decline. Taking a slot and simply not showing up is not advisable. If you already have scheduled an interview, which you cannot (or do not want to) attend, call the program as early as possible to inform the coordinator of your change in plans.

Match day is still 4 months away. When should you interview? Geography comes into play, so try to arrange your plans in order to achieve a minimum of travel time. The particular week that gives you the most interviews for the least number of miles traveled is the best time to see those programs.

What about interviewing too early or too late? Whether you interview in October or February makes little difference from the program's perspective.[1] From your perspective, however, it might. Schedule interviews for less desirable programs early. There is a learning curve to the interview process and you may not want to tackle the most competitive program while you are still on the bottom of that curve. If you can, schedule your most desirable programs somewhere in the middle. It is hard to maintain that "really enthusiastic look" after 3 months on the road.

Some caveats: Never schedule more than one interview per day. Never schedule an interview on a day when you will be post call. There are two reasons for this: you will not remember anything about your visit and the program will remember everything about your visit.

How many interviews should attend? Clearly, this depends on many factors. How competitive is your application? (Your advisor may be helpful here.) Do family and/or other commitments restrict you geographically? How much time and money do you have? As a rough guide, consider 5 interviews an absolute minimum, 10 about average, and 15 or more if you have doubts about your application.

Preparation

The more prepared you are for the interview, the more relaxed and confident you will be. Preparation begins well before the evening prior to your visit. Assemble your interview kit. The interview kit will travel with you and should include a copy of your application and all supporting materials. If you did not provide ERAS with a photograph, consider leaving one with the program to be placed into your file.

Inform yourself. No doubt you reviewed a brochure or Web page on the Internet, material that probably influenced your decision to apply to that particular program. Read it again. Augment this information by networking with your friends. Speak with faculty from your medical school; if possible, contact someone who trained at the program where you will be interviewing. Ask about strengths and weaknesses. If you are really compulsive (not necessarily a bad trait), run a literature search on the departmental chair, program director, research director, and other key people in the department. Your ability to discuss topics and research of interest to a particular program will leave little doubt that you are a serious candidate. Who knows, you may even approach patient care and didactic studies with the same foresight, diligence, planning, and enthusiasm.

Prepare a list of questions. Some questions may be generic, applicable to all programs, and some will be specific for the particular program with which you are interviewing.[2]

The Informal "Ice-breaker"

An increasing number of programs offer an opportunity to meet residents the night before the scheduled interview. That meeting may be in a restaurant or bar and attendance is decidedly optional. Go if you can. You may meet people who will not be around the next day and you may get a feel for group dynamics that will be less apparent or absent the following morning. Have fun, be inquisitive, but do not be stupid. This is not the time to demonstrate your expertise in beer-pong. Informal does not mean irresponsible.

The Interview

Arrive on time. Make sure you arrive on time. Remember that the weather may be uncooperative across much of the country during this time of year. If possible, arrive the evening before. When in a major city, avoid using a car unless you absolutely need to. Get a good night's sleep. Plan to arrive about 15 to 30 minutes early. Few things create an impression like sweat dripping off your face and a shirttail flapping in your wake. I know it has been said before, but it is worth repeating: You only have one chance to make a first impression.

Most interview days will begin with a general information session, perhaps over a cup of coffee or breakfast. Pay attention. Yes, you know all of this already. You have followed all of the previous suggestions, and you are better informed than perhaps even the program director. Pay attention still. The way information is presented may tell you as much about the program as the information itself. While this part of the day is less formal than the one-on-one interview, it is no less important. Do not act disinterested or bored, read a newspaper, read the program brochure for the first time, or treat anyone you meet with less respect than you would show for the program director. The last item is particularly true for the program coordinator or administrator.

You will likely be given an opportunity to review a sample resident contract and relevant departmental policies such as those that cover promotion, dismissal, and moonlighting. If you find it necessary, ask for a copy of this material to take home with you. A word about questions: Ask them when the time is right. Otherwise, save them for later. Take notes. They will help you remember what you will otherwise forget.

The tour through the emergency department and related areas is an opportunity for you to observe how well the area is designed and, to some degree, how it is equipped and staffed. The 15 to 20 minutes usually allotted to this part of the day is rarely sufficient to give you an accurate picture of what goes on. One way to approach the tour is to think in terms of patient process. Imagine a patient arriving by ambulance: How is the patient triaged and assigned to staff? How are x-ray and ancillary tests performed? Things should appear to be well organized, without undue anxiety on the part of the staff. If you have a question related to patient care, this is the time to ask. Note items you may want to explore in more detail later.

Sometime after the general information session, either before or after your tour of the emergency department, you will meet individually with members of the faculty and staff (the interview!). Contrary to what was said before, this may be your second opportunity to make a first impression. Shake hands. Smile. Make eye contact. Take your seat. Lean forward, reestablish eye contact, and listen. If you are sitting on the other side of the room or facing the wrong direction, take charge. Move. Move to where it is more comfortable to engage in conversation.

Allow the interviewer to make an opening statement. Listen carefully to the question the interviewer is asking. A good interview is an exchange of information and ideas that flows both ways. Before you trip over yourself in an attempt to answer the question, take a second or two to think about the question and reflect on why the interviewer is asking it. What information is the interviewer looking for? Sometimes things are straightforward, sometimes not. In any event, you must be prepared to answer obvious questions, such as why you are applying to emergency medicine, why you consider yourself a good candidate, a description of an interesting (gratifying) medical case, etc. Think about these before the interview. Your answers will depend on who you are. Approach your answers by highlighting your individuality (not to be confused with eccentricity) and, whenever possible, provide examples or (short) anecdotes. When you have answered the question, stop. Emergency physicians pride themselves on conveying the most information in the shortest period of time and demonstrating that you have this ability will be helpful. Find the middle ground between the yes and no answer and the run-on sentence.

When asked what you plan to do after completion of residency training: "I want to practice medicine in an emergency room" is not a good answer! By the way, the correct terms, and you should only use correct terms, are "emergency medicine," "emergency department," and "emergency physician." It is hard to take a candidate seriously who does not know the name of the specialty to which he or she is applying.

Be prepared to discuss in some detail items you listed as hobbies or extracurricular interests. It is likely that an interviewer may have similar interests (and expertise). Do not list cooking unless your talents go beyond TV dinners. If you indicated that you like to read, be prepared to discuss a book you have read (recently).

Just when you think the interview is over, you hear the question you hoped would not be asked: "What about the year between the third and the fourth year of medical school, or is that a misprint on your CV?" No, you think to yourself, it was the year I was making license plates. Well, what should you say? The truth. In whatever truthful way you can tell it. If there is an irregularity in your past, or a course you did not get honors in, own up to it. Try not to sound too defensive and emphasize the more recent past.

Verboten questions. Rarely, you may be placed into an uncomfortable position. The overwhelming majority (read: near 100%) of emergency medicine programs conduct themselves in a completely ethical fashion. That having been said, some questions and certain lines of questioning are illegal. Period. An obvious example: "When do you plan to have children?" A less obvious example: "Do you speak any foreign languages?" How you answer will depend on what you are comfortable with. If the question does not bother you and you think it was asked with good intent, by all means answer it honestly. If the question makes you feel uncomfortable and you would rather not answer it, politely decline.

There is one thing here that is important to know. Once you have brought something up, then it is acceptable for the interviewer to ask questions about that subject. For instance, while you cannot be asked about your marital status, if you volunteer information about your spouse, then you may be asked questions about your spouse's career plans and how they mesh with yours.

There are times when you have a responsibility to provide information even if you have not been asked. Although your religious beliefs and your medical history are not acceptable lines of inquiry, if something prevents you from doing your part as an emergency medicine resident it is your obligation to let the program know. If you require the same day off every week for religious observances or you cannot work night shifts because of a seizure disorder, the program may be able to make accommodations or may not. That needs to be discussed ahead of time, not after the match is over.

What about your opportunity to ask questions? Certain questions are right for the faculty interviewer, some are right for the resident assigned to have lunch with you, and some questions you should not ask at all. Common sense will tell you the difference. Questions you should ask: Fair game here (and important stuff, by the way) includes educational philosophy and objectives, didactic programs, and research. Where have previous graduates gone? Are they enjoying the kinds of careers (or continuing their education) in a way that you hope to enjoy yours? Questions you may not want to ask: How many hours can I moonlight? How many hours a day/week/month will I have to work? How many sick days can I take? Questions you should (absolutely) avoid: Anything stated in the program brochure/catalogue or detailed during the interview day information session. Questions regarding rank order (incidentally, it is also unacceptable for the program to ask you about rank order).[3] Questions that may appear to be condescending; for example, "You are a new program. Do you really think you'll fill on match day?" (Answer: Yes, we will, long before we get down to your name on our rank order list!) Remember, you will only have limited time to ask questions. What you ask about will be perceived as the aspect of training most important to you. Suggested questions have been published elsewhere.[2] Choose wisely but avoid looking like a geek going down the preflight checklist.

The Offer

The what?? Yes, that's right. There are not supposed to be any offers. Rarely (very rarely) a program might make a promise contingent on an agreement: "We'll rank you first if you rank us first." Although you are not likely to hear it, if you do, it constitutes a flagrant violation of NRMP rules. Decline, politely. When you return home, inform your medical school advisor of what happened and that person should take care of the rest. Similarly, in the unlikely event that you are asked questions that should not have been asked (see above), inform your advisor. Keep in mind that the majority of these rare infractions come from inexperienced and well-intentioned junior faculty without ill intent.

The NRMP does allow early offers to applicants outside of the match if the applicant is a graduate of a non-U.S. medical school. The rationale for this has always eluded me. Program directors who engage in this behavior claim to be acting in the best interests of the applicant, but my perspective is that all they are doing is limiting choices. If the program really wants you, all the program has to do is rank you in a "guaranteed match'" position and it can do that without forcing you to sign on a dotted line. If offered, do what you think is right and what is in your best interests. If you are a U.S. medical school graduate, signing outside of and then withdrawing from the match is not an acceptable option. Ever.

The Return Visit

Consider a return visit after the interview day is over. Many programs make this offer to all applicants; if you are interested and an offer is not forthcoming, ask about it before you leave. Several hours in the emergency department will tell you more about an institution than the 15-minute tour. This may even allow you to get the elusive "feel" for a program, something that may be more important than stats and figures. Decide on this option only if you are truly interested in a program and only after you make arrangements with the program coordinator. Dress appropriately and ask questions without getting in the way of patient care. Introduce yourself to the attending physician and other staff you may come into contact with. Do not give in to the temptation to grab a laryngoscope and assist in a quick intubation—you are there as an observer, not as a medical student. The way that staff members interact with each other (and naturally, with their patients) may be of particular importance.

Common Myths

The objective of the interview is to get the program to like you. Not true. The interview is for you to find the program that will be the best fit for you. When it comes down to it, that is what really matters. Keep this in mind. It takes time and an attentive and inquisitive approach on your part.

The blue suit. This, like everything here before it, applies to both sexes. Interview experts will tell you to wear a blue suit with a conservative tie, scarf, etc. Have you ever been in a room full of people all looking the same? Rather sedating. Wear what you feel comfortable in. Preferably something that allows some aspect of your personality (or at least good taste) to show through, but no fish ties or the latest in courtside footwear.

All truths will be revealed. A dangerous myth. Many truths (particularly unflattering ones) will not be revealed unless you seek them out. Take an active part in this day. You have invested much time and money in it. Make sure you leave with all the information to which you are entitled.

Closing Thoughts

Before you leave, make sure you have the names of people you have spoken to, particularly those who interviewed you, the program coordinator and one or two of the residents. Get addresses and telephone numbers when possible, in case you want to follow up with a letter or a telephone call.

Written notes will be of immense help 3 months from now when you compile your rank order list. When you get home, review your notes. Make more notes. Keep a running rank order list as you interview in various places. If additional questions come to mind, consider a telephone call back to a faculty member or resident. This will give you additional information and serve to communicate your interest. Thank-you letters are nice but should be written only if sincere. They are not likely to influence ranking.

The selection process from the program's perspective has been well described.[4-7] DeSantis and Marco reviewed selection factors from the candidates' perspectives.[8] You may gain valuable insight by reviewing this information. In addition, be sure to visit the Internet sites (medical student sections) described elsewhere in this book. Good luck!

References

1. Martin-Lee L, Park H, Overton DT. Does interview date affect match list position in the emergency medicine national residency matching program? *Acad Emerg Med.* 2000;7(9):1022-1026.
2. Kosgove emergency medicine. An applicant's evaluation of an emergency medicine internship and residency. *Ann Emerg Med.* 1990;19(7):774-780.
3. Wolford RW, Anderson KD. Emergency medicine residency director perceptions of the resident selection process. *Acad Emerg Med.* 2000;7(10):1170-1171.
4. Balentine J, Gaeta T, Spevack T. Evaluating applicants to emergency medicine residency programs. *J Emerg Med.* 1999;17(1):131-134.
5. Crane JT, Ferraro CM. Selection criteria for emergency medicine residency applicants. *Acad Emerg Med.* 2000;7(1):54-60.
6. Aghababian R, Tandberg D, Iserson K, Martin M, Sklar D. Selection of emergency medicine residents. *Ann Emerg Med.* 1993;22(11):1753-1761.
7. Hayden SR, Hayden M, Gamst A. What characteristics of applicants to emergency medicine residency programs predict future success as an emergency medicine resident? *Acad Emerg Med.* 2005;12(3):206-210.
8. DeSantis M, Marco CA. Emergency medicine residency selection: factors influencing candidate decisions. *Acad Emerg Med.* 2005;12(6):559-561.

chapter 24

The Match: An Overview

Wallace A. Carter, MD
Program Director, Emergency Medicine Residency, The New York-Presbyterian Hospital

Jeffrey A. Manko, MD
Associate Program Director, Emergency Medicine Residency,
New York University/Bellevue Medical Center

Welcome to the process that represents the culmination of all your hard work for the past three years in medical school, the *match*. Even the name gives the impression of a marriage or life-long commitment that will change the rest of your life like some internet dating service. However, once you understand the match, you will find it far less imposing. This chapter is here to help you navigate through the intricacies and nuances of the match.

First, the match represents the coupling of emergency medicine programs with prospective emergency medicine applicants to form mutually beneficial training relationships. The match is run by the National Residency Matching Program (NRMP), with all the rules, regulations, and information available at www.NRMP.org . A tremendous amount of time and energy are invested by both sides, applicants and program directors, into the process. It is extremely important to understand that as much as you want to be happy with your choice, the program directors want you to be happy with your choice (and theirs as well). The match is also geared toward the applicants' rank lists as opposed to the programs'. Therefore, you should feel free to choose your true preferences when it is time to create your rank list.

Emergency medicine as a specialty has been growing in popularity over the last decade. The number of students pursuing emergency medicine has risen, and so, too, has the number of emergency medicine programs and therefore emergency medicine spots. Currently, the ratio is very close to 1:1. In 2006, there were 135 emergency medicine programs with 1251 applicant spots for PGY-1s and 114 for PGY-2s. The program fill rate was 97.4% with 33 spots being unfilled among 14 programs. Emergency medicine represented 5.8% of applicant spots in the NRMP in 2006. Although emergency medicine is very competitive, you should be optimistic about your chances of landing a residency spot.

When deciding on a program to do your training, it is important to factor in many variables. All Accreditation Council for Graduate Medical Education-Residency Review Committee (ACGME-RRC)-accredited programs meet a standard to ensure you that you will be appropriately and adequately trained in emergency medicine to sit for the American Board of Emergency Medicine (ABEM) certification exams. Emergency medicine has three different program formats (1,2,3, 1,2,3,4, and 2,3,4), which only adds to the complexity of the decision making. Rest assured that all the formats train excellent emergency physicians. Whether you go to a small, rural program or a large, urban program, you will learn how to intubate, treat myocardial infarctions, and reduce fractures. The emergency medicine curriculum is amazingly similar, so other factors begin assuming a larger role in your decision-making.

A wise man once said, "happy wife, happy life." Certainly a bit dated and sexist, but the underlying message is a good one. Extrapolated to the 21st century, it would read as, "happy outside the hospital, happy inside the hospital." The idea is simple. If residents are satisfied with their geographic location and their personal lives, they are much more energetic and enthusiastic about their jobs and their work. As residents you will spend an inordinate amount of time in the hospital (even with the duty hour guidelines), but you should take into consideration the things you like to do outside the hospital when thinking about choosing programs.

A frequently cited reason as to why one program is chosen over another is geography. Never underestimate the influence of the significant other or the in-laws (to either be close to or farther away from). Proximity to family and friends can be an important component when choosing a program and can certainly make your 3- through 4-year training more enjoyable. If the need for year-round skiing is a deal breaker, do not go to southern Florida. However, if sailing and surfing are your passions, we would recommend a program near a coastline. All of these recommendations are assuming that you are doing this solo. If, however, during the course of your medical education you have managed to find the love of your life who is also in the same boat, then you will need to consider entering the *couple's match*. Here is what the NRMP says, "The NRMP accommodates applicants who wish to be matched as a couple by allowing two individuals to form pairs of choices on their primary rank order lists, which are then considered in order of preference when the matching algorithm is run." So what does that actually mean? Well, the devil is in the details. If, for example, your significant other is interested in neurosurgery and you both have your hearts set on a city with a single academic medical center that only takes two neurosurgery residents per year, then your chances will be less than looking for the same arrangement in New York City. The good news is that the numbers are on your side with the vast majority of couples being matched. If you are entering the couple's match, then you will need to be very thoughtful about your applications and should consult closely with your advisor, even having them talk with your partner's advisor so that they can make a realistic assessment of your joint candidacy.

Applying to residency programs is extremely easy now with the advent of the Electronic Residency Application Service (ERAS). All of your letters of recommendation, the dean's letter (MSPE), personal statement, your CV and transcripts, and USMLE scores are uploaded to the same site to be retrieved by whichever programs you designate. Just a click of a button (and a little more money), and you can apply to as many programs as you can afford. We would strongly recommend speaking to advisors, current residents, and former students to help narrow the field to those programs you might actually be interested in. There is no penalty to applying to programs that you feel may be a "reach" based on your medical school academic performance. However, it is critically important that you have a realistic idea about how competitive an applicant you are. Applying to only the most competitive and top-rated programs with only a marginal transcript and below-average board scores would not be considered realistic. This would be a good point to address the question of, "How many programs should I apply to"? Another wise man once said, "Only one since you can only train at one program." Seriously, though, this number will depend on your criteria. For example, if you are only interested in 4-year programs in public hospitals, then this number is predetermined. If, on the other hand, you have not done your homework and worked with your advisors and colleagues to identify the training characteristics that are most important in a training program to you, then you are potentially looking at a list that will become so large that it will be unmanageable. You need to be realistic and appropriate. Apply only to those programs that you feel you are interested in. Consider every application a potential interview that will cause you to throw more clothing into a bag and head out on the road again. It may sound like a nice idea in

September, but you will not be happy getting snowed in at O'Hare Airport in January trying to get to an interview that, in retrospect, is a program in which you have little interest.

The dean's letters (MSPE) are available on November 1 on ERAS. Program directors should have all your letters or recommendation, CV, and dean's letter by that time. At least one letter of recommendation should be from an emergency medicine rotation (most likely at your home institution). It has become extremely popular for students to do an away elective in emergency medicine as well. A letter should also be provided from that rotation, with the proviso that it be a letter of substance. Superficial letters from faculty members who have limited exposure to you except for one or two shifts offer little substantive help in advancing your candidacy. We refer to these as "1-month wonder letters." If possible, see if you can get a departmental consensus letter.

An away elective can serve two important purposes. The first is your chance to have a 1-month audition at a program you are considering strongly. This is an opportunity to show the residents and faculty first-hand why they should want you to join their program. Keep in mind, most residents are impressed by students who work very hard and are fun to be around. The litmus test is often "would I be happy working with this person at 2:00 A.M. when the emergency department is on fire?" Conversely, "if the emergency department were really quiet at 2:00 A.M., would I be comfortable sitting next to this person?"

The other side of the coin, however, is if you have a poor performance during the elective. Tardiness, absenteeism, arrogance, and laziness will certainly torpedo even the best applicant (on paper). Often a successful rotation will supplant an otherwise mediocre application and result in securing that coveted residency slot. Put your best foot forward and enjoy!

The elective also provides you with the opportunity to see the operation of the emergency department and residency program up close and personal. You can directly visualize the didactics, teaching, and relationships that exist at a particular program. Speak with the residents about any issues that concern you. All the beauty marks and all the warts will be apparent, and you can decide if it is a good fit for you. Remember, beauty is in the eyes of the beholder.

The second reason to do an away elective may be to see how emergency medicine is practiced in a totally different environment than your home institution (geographically or practice setting). If you know you want a big city urban hospital, try a different big city. If you want to try a suburban community hospital before committing to a big city hospital, now is your chance to compare. Remember, all accredited emergency medicine programs will provide you with excellent training toward board certification. The choice of setting is up to you.

For those students who want to do five away rotations and spend your entire fourth year of medical school touring the United States, DON'T. No one should do more than a total of three (one at home and two away), and two is just fine. Take the opportunities afforded by medical school to do electives in other specialties. You have the rest of your life to work in the emergency department.

Your application is now complete and all the supporting letters are in ERAS. The boxes have been clicked and the fees have been paid. Now you will be checking your e-mail incessantly, waiting for the invitations to interview. Then, the responses start to arrive, and your whirl-wind tour of the United States, on seven different airlines, will begin. Take some time now to reevaluate again which part of the country you want to live and how much money you have budgeted for travel. Try to group your interviews geographically to cut down on flying expenses (unless you need to accumulate a boatload of frequent flier miles). Find out if a program has an evening activity before the interview day that you might want to attend. To cut down on lodging expenses, this is a good time to look up old family and friends for a spot in the guest room or on the couch.

Hopefully you have received many interview invitations, and now you are feeling more confident that you will not have to 'scramble" for a spot. You do not have to go to every program that invites you, but you do have to show proper etiquette and withdraw your application in a timely manner if you decline. My pet peeve (as well as many other program directors) is the complete lack of courtesy and respect when applicants simply do not show up for a scheduled interview. I am sure someone on the waiting list would have gladly taken the spot to interview that someone else selfishly disregarded. A call in advance is expected and always appreciated by the program. If there are unforeseen circumstances (weather, traffic, illness), make sure you let the program coordinators know or leave a message as early as possible to see if your interview can be rescheduled.

On the interview day, you have only one chance to make a first impression. You are on display from the moment you arrive until the moment you leave. Everyone and anyone you encounter may play a role in your evaluation. Asking the program coordinator for a date that night might not be the most prudent decision and will likely torpedo your application. Dress conservatively, be prompt, and come with energy and enthusiasm.

Often we are asked about "thank-you" cards following an interview. We are split on this one: J.M. likes receiving them and W.C. does not. So what to do? Err on the side of being polite and send them unless you are told otherwise. If you do send them, please make sure that you send the right note to the right person. There is nothing more embarrassing than getting a letter meant for one of our colleagues.

Once all your interviews are completed and your bank account is depleted, it is time to sit down and make out your "rank list." Here are some very important recommendations:

1. Rank the programs based on your preference (based on whatever criteria you choose to use). Your number one program should be the one you would MOST like to attend, even if you consider it to be a "reach."

2. Your ranking of a program should have NO bearing on where you think the program will rank you. Assume you are at the top of everyone's list and make your list accordingly.

3. Rank ALL the programs you would be willing to attend. A program may not be your first choice, but you should still rank it if it is one you would not mind matching at. (Better than not matching at all.)

4. NEVER rank a program you absolutely do not want to go to. You should be thinking that you would rather not match and scramble afterward than go to that program. (Jail would seem like a viable alternative.)

5. The match is BINDING for both the applicants and the residency programs. Make your decisions accordingly.

6. Expressions of love and devotion between applicants and programs are NOT binding and NOT commitments. It is certainly acceptable for programs and applicants to exchange pleasantries to inform one another of their mutual interest in each other, but discussing where someone is on the rank list is forbidden. (If we only had a dollar for each time an applicant told us we were "number one" and then he or she matched elsewhere... .)

Speak with the important people in your life. Decide on your priorities and preferences and make your list. Once the list has been entered into the computer and certified, the waiting game begins. Unlike when you applied to college and medical school, and you waited by the door for each school's acceptance or rejection letter, there is only "match day." One day in mid March, all senior medical students will receive an envelope with only their matched program listed inside. Congratulations, and hopefully you are happy with the results.

If you unfortunately did not match, you will be notified a few days earlier and have to "scramble." This involves finding the programs that have unfilled spots and trying to secure positions with them. The process is frantic and nerve-racking for everyone. Once again, though, it is vitally important that you not go to a program you will absolutely hate. It may be worth waiting a year and reapplying. The dean's office at your school will notify you that you did not match and help you through the process. Fortunately, this does not happen often and can be mitigated by ranking more programs.

Hopefully, this has provided you with some tips on how to approach the match. This is an exciting time as you embark on your career in emergency medicine. There are currently 139 emergency medicine program choices available across the country, and the fun is finding the one that is just right for you. Good luck on this adventure, and we look forward to your contributions and future leadership in our growing specialty.

chapter 25

Osteopathic Emergency Medicine Residencies

Jerry Balentine, DO , FACEP, FACOEP
Senior Vice President and Chief Medical Officer, St. Barnabas Hospital

Mary Hughes, DO, FACEP, FACOEP
Professor of Emergency Medicine, Michigan State University College of Osteopathic Medicine
Department of Internal Medicine, Section of Emergency Medicine Program Director
MSU-COM Emergency Medicine Residency

During the 1970s, osteopathic emergency medicine residencies were established in response to a rising need for emergency medicine-trained physicians. Today, emergency medicine residencies comprise the second largest group of osteopathic postdoctoral education programs with 40 programs and over 700 approved residency positions.

Unlike allopathic (Accreditation Council for Graduate Medical Education [ACGME]-approved) residency programs, all osteopathic programs are 4 years in length. Traditionally, the first year was an internship year that could be either a traditional internship (similar to a transitional year) or an emergency medicine specialty internship (additional emergency medicine training rotations during the internship). As of the 2007 match, the internship will become the first year of the residency and the internship and residency years will be fully linked, requiring students to match into the first year and following years simultaneously. The length of training will remain 4 years.

The content and program requirements for an osteopathic emergency medicine residency are very similar to ACGME-approved programs. There are some additional requirements relating to a minimum number of faculty members being osteopathic physicians and the program director being certified by the American Board of Osteopathic Emergency Medicine (ABOEM).

Residents graduating from an osteopathic emergency medicine residency are eligible to be certified by the AOBEM. Several of the osteopathic programs are dually accredited by the ACGME and American Osteopathic Association (AOA). This makes graduates of these programs eligible to take the AOBEM as well as the American Board of Emergency Medicine (ABEM) certifying examinations.

After completion of an osteopathic emergency medicine residency, the graduate has 6 years to sit for the certifying examination, which includes a written test, an oral exam, and a chart review.

There are several options for combined programs in the osteopathic profession: emergency medicine/internal medicine, emergency medicine/family practice, and emergency medicine/pediatrics. These programs are 5 years in length and allow the graduate to be eligible to sit for both board exams.

Students interested in osteopathic emergency medicine residencies need to apply to the osteopathic match. This is a significant change from the past when residencies used a "rolling" admission process. Programs will usually conduct on-site interviews and generate a "rank list" similar to ACGME programs.

chapter 26

The International Medical School Graduate

Satchit Balsari, MD, MPH

Chief Resident Physician, Emergency Medicine Residency, The New York-Presbyterian Hospital

Each year, hundreds of international medical graduates are accepted into U.S. residency programs. Their distribution across specialties is highly varied. Traditionally, most international medical graduates match in internal medicine, with psychiatry and pediatrics following suit; surgical specialties, radiology, and emergency medicine have remained more challenging to match in. In 2005, international medical graduates filled a little more than half of the positions in internal medicine, and 37% and 30% of those in psychiatry and pediatrics, respectively. International medical graduates filled 22% positions in general surgery, 7% in radiology and only 5.7% in emergency medicine.[1] Of the 1308 PGY-1 filled entry positions in emergency medicine, in 2005, 44 positions were filled by U.S.-born international medical graduates, 6 were filled by foreign-born international medical graduates, 2 were filled by Canadian physicians, and 3 were filled by Fifth Pathway graduates.[2] In 2006, of the 1251 PGY-1 filled entry positions in emergency medicine, 49 were filled by U.S.-born international medical graduates, 25 were filled by foreign-born international medical graduates, 2 were filled by Canadian physicians, and 2 were filled by Fifth Pathway graduates.[3] Emergency medicine remains one of the most competitive specialties in the United States. While applying to an emergency medicine residency, the international medical graduate is competing with the strongest applicants in the country.

The Challenges

International medical graduates applying to a residency in the United States are usually cognizant of the hurdles they face. Much emphasis is placed on test scores, and a significant proportion of international medical graduates applying to competitive residency programs in the United States do score high on their USMLE Steps I and II. High board scores are, however, a small, though significant, factor influencing the selection process. While good board scores certainly strengthen an international medical graduate's application, at best they put an international medical graduate on par with others with similar test performance patterns. Major criteria that program directors examine while looking at an application, whether domestic or international, include the applicant's performance through medical school, especially the clinical years; the dean's letter; recommendations from faculty; evaluations during emergency medicine electives; research experience; and extracurricular activities. Herein lies the greatest challenge for an international medical graduate. International medical school transcripts and evaluations of clinical rotations are written in a format that U.S. program directors may be highly unfamiliar with. Not only is it difficult to gauge where an applicant ranks under in his or her medical school class, but it is almost impossible to compare that performance to our domestic indicators. Furthermore, letters of recommendations and publications are associated with faculty and journals that program directors may not be familiar with. This alien frame of reference often contributes to international medical graduate applications being rejected at the early stages of the screening process, even before an interview call.

Overcoming the Hurdles

Familiarity is the international medical graduate's friend. To help program directors better understand an international medical graduate's past record and their potential, an international medical graduate must offer performance indicators that U.S. faculty are familiar with: U.S.-based clinical rotations, U.S.-based research and academic experience, and recommendation letters from domestic emergency medicine faculty.

Clinical rotations for international medical graduates are broadly divided into two categories: fourth-year medical school electives and observerships. Fourth-year medical electives, although hard to come by for foreign graduates, are available. They allow the international medical graduate to be evaluated on the same clinical platform as U.S. medical students. It must be noted that fourth-year medical electives are pregraduation opportunities and can only be set up while the international medical graduate is still in medical school. On completion of medical school or the "pregraduate internship" included in the MBBS model in Commonwealth countries, an international medical graduate can apply only for an "observership." The observership is an abbreviated experience: the international medical graduate is given very limited clinical responsibilities, is not allowed to participate in bedside procedures, and may have restricted access to patient's computer charts and lab tests. Nevertheless, for those international medical graduates who choose to apply to emergency medicine later in their careers, an observership is a better option than having no U.S. clinical exposure at all. Although most domestic medical students are encouraged to complete one or two rotations in emergency medicine, international medical graduates may want to consider spending 2 or 3 months to allow adequate exposure to emergency medicine and to provide ample opportunity for faculty to evaluate the international medical graduate's skills in a domestic program. These electives are hard to plan in the face of visa restrictions and limitations placed by foreign and U.S. medical schools. Nevertheless, if an international medical graduate has the opportunity to rotate through more than one institution, it is advisable to rotate last in the program she or he is most likely to match with.

Finding emergency medicine programs that offer electives to international medical graduates can be daunting. The first set of programs to look at would be those that have historically accepted international medical graduates. An extensive search of Web home pages of emergency medicine residency programs will help cull this information.[4] Also, institutions that offer electives to international medical graduates in other specialties will be more familiar with the paperwork and logistics involved, and hence more likely to support the application. If applying to large academic centers that may not have accepted many international medical graduates, it may be worthwhile to volunteer research time to the department before requesting a rotation, giving the faculty the opportunity to better know the applicant. This strategy may be most advisable while requesting observerships.

Once accepted to a clinical elective, the international medical graduate should be dually focused. First, an international medical graduate must ensure that the specialty of emergency medicine meets his or her expectations. Often international medical graduates applying to emergency medicine have trained in countries where emergency medicine has not evolved as a specialty. Understanding the nature of emergency medicine, the scope of clinical practice, and the current challenges in the U.S. system is a prerequisite to avoiding disappointments in the future. The international medical graduate's second focus should be on clinical performance. The international medical graduate has 1 month or, more specifically, about 15 to 20 shifts to help emergency medicine faculty draw the connection between an international medical graduate's stellar resume and his or her clinical skills. Letters of recommendation from emergency medicine faculty that the international medical graduate has worked with can reset the frame of reference for an international medical graduate's application and are crucial to influencing an interview call.

The lifestyle that the specialty of emergency medicine allows attracts applicants with other academic, research, and administrative interests that they wish to pursue in parallel with their clinical careers. International medical graduates, while navigating through the cumbersome process of visa applications, USMLE tests, and CSA exams, often enroll in a health science allied master's degree program that offer an MS or MPH. While an additional degree buttresses the international medical graduate's application (just as does a high board score), it is not essential or unique to the international medical graduate. However, if this additional training has been, or can be, applied to emergency medicine, it creates a familiar context within which to evaluate the international medical graduate application. Emergency medicine-related research, presentations in academic emergency medicine organizations, or publications in reputed academic journals make the foreign applicant highly competitive. Program directors do understand the hurdles faced by international medical graduates, and demonstrating promising potential may earn the international medical graduate at least an interview call.

Value Added: Turing the Tables

Foreign training, while seemingly the biggest drawback in an international medical graduate's application, can be genuinely turned into an advantage. Most established foreign medical schools offer excellent clinical training and impart robust bedside skills. That foreign medical graduates are often good bedside clinicians is generally well accepted. However, taking the foreign-training experience beyond the bedside into the realm of systems development may be tremendously advantageous. If the international medical graduate has an earnest interest in capacity building, collaborative research, or international exchange and training programs, she or he can be a valuable conduit between local institutions and U.S. programs. Such collaborative work allows international medical graduates the opportunity to use the foreign training to shape their careers beyond the residency. International emergency medicine is a growing focus of interest in leading academic institutions in the country, with many programs now offering a 2-year fellowship opportunity. International medical graduates can certainly create a niche for themselves in the expansion of emergency medicine as a specialty internationally.

Summary

A familiar frame of reference is vital. An international medical graduate must take adequate steps to ensure that program directors can interpret the applicant's skill sets in a recognizable context. Clinical rotations that allow the forging of student-faculty relationships and demonstrate good clinical acumen and interpersonal skills are key. An academic bent illustrated through quality research and publications is very helpful, while strong letters of recommendations from emergency medicine faculty are invaluable. Time spent understanding the specialty in the new environs is time well spent. International medical graduates can explore opportunities to combine the foreign and U.S. experience to broaden the scope of emergency medicine both clinically and topographically.

Notes

1. Freida Online Specialty Training Statistics. Available at http://www.ama-assn.org/vapp/freida/spcindx/0,1238,TR,00.html.

2. The Fifth Pathway is "an avenue by which students who have attended four years at a foreign medical school may complete their supervised clinical work at a U.S. medical school, become eligible for entry to U.S. residency training, and ultimately obtain a license to practice in the U.S." More information is available at http://www.ama-assn.org/ama/pub/category/9306.html.

3. NRMP Match Data, available at http://www.nrmp.org/data/programresults 2003-2007.pdf accessed August 1, 2007.

4. Visit http://www.ama-assn.org/vapp/freida/srch/ to locate the URLs for home pages.

chapter 27

Changing Residencies:
The Applicant with Prior Training

Matthew O'Neill, MD

Resident Physician, Emergency Medicine Residency, The New York-Presbyterian Hospital

I've had great luck with residents who have previous training.
— An emergency medicine program director

First, do not worry! Many emergency physicians have prior training in different fields. You will be stunned to learn of the exciting lives your attendings and colleagues have previously had. If you have a prior experience, the bottom line is that most emergency medicine program directors will welcome your interest very enthusiastically. However, when reviewing an applicant with prior training, there will be a number of considerations a program director may have. Most of these are the very same concerns a program director will have for any candidate, yet, an applicant with previous training may encounter additional scrutiny.

You are in this profession as a calling...which extracts from you at every turn self-sacrifice, devotion, love and tenderness to your fellow man.
— William Osler, Physician

Being a professional physician requires maturity. As a working professional (regardless of the field you trained or worked in previously), you have had responsibilities to employers, patients, and colleagues—you have had real work experience. Many program directors in emergency medicine are enthusiastic about people who have had prior experience because, first, they bring unique experience and expertise to the program, and, second, the candidate has accomplished something by the mere fact of having worked a year of residency responsibly. When you go on interviews, you will meet a number of doe-eyed youngsters in their fourth year of medical school who have nothing like the experience you have. The fact is, some program directors are more inclined to hire someone who has had prior professional experience rather than hire an applicant who progressed from high school to college to medical school without having ever been employed.

The obvious advice is, if you have prior experience in any field, and it does not matter what field, you must play that experience up as a great asset to your professionalism. Prior training in residency, business, the arts, emergency medical services, the sciences—it's all good! As an emergency physician you will do it all and you will need to get the job done: you will manage a large number of people and data, budget resources, supervise students, teach and lecture, you will have great craftsmanship and manual dexterity, you will stay cool under pressure, and you will have better "people skills" than any other field because you will constantly be managing crises. Anything you have done previously is an asset.

The power to do good is also the power to do harm.
— Milton Friedman, Economist

For the applicant with prior residency training, financial considerations are perhaps the most confusing. The fact is, training residents is a business, and that business relies on federal training grants from which residents and medical centers are paid. For each resident, and for each year of training, a large amount of funding is awarded to the medical center (upwards of six figures per year, per resident) to pay the resident's salary and benefits and to pay the faculty for teaching that trainee.

That fact noted, the complexity of how residents consume this funding is well beyond the scope of this chapter. Not only is the subject fraught with ineffably confusing minutia, it is extremely boring reading. Suffice to say, for a given resident who seeks to switch into emergency medicine, every medical center may pose a unique set of financial concerns. The federal funding the applicant may or may not be associated with may be relevant, as well as the degree to which any given medical center is dependent or independent on those federal funds. Your own circumstance is a subject best discussed with the program directors at your own medical center and at the residencies you are interested in. Look at it as a way of expressing an interest in emergency medicine.

Me, I want more.

—Mike Muir, Singer and Songwriter

For the applicant with prior residency training, logistical matters may be the most important. Specific concerns such as, "Does the type of program I am switching into emergency medicine from matter?" or "Can I get advanced standing due to my previous experience?" may be at the forefront of your mind.

An emergency physician does not perform craniotomy or cardiac catheterization (typically), but they do perform a very broad range of services and evaluations. Accordingly, almost any previous residency experience is advantageous; however, prior experience in certain fields may be more or less "attractive" to program directors. For example, an applicant with prior training in internal medicine or orthopedics may be more attractive to a program director than prior training in dermatology, psychiatry, or rehabilitation. It may be an unfortunate prejudice, but emergency physicians tend to evaluate more of certain types of problems than others, and acquiring a resident who has experience in those areas makes the residency stronger as a whole. Nonetheless, for applicants seeking to switch into emergency medicine from "low-acuity" fields, certain program directors may find your desire to practice more "high-yield" medicine a very admirable quality. Those program directors may be very interested in you, so test the waters accordingly.

A further consideration you might have as you endeavor your switch is, Will I receive advanced placement in the program due to my prior training? Unfortunately, the answer is often no. The positions filled through the NRMP match, with rare exception, are first-year, or "EM1," positions. If a candidate with prior experience were to be advanced out of the EM1 class into the EM2 class, it would reduce the size of the EM1 class and thus shift a burden of the work onto the remaining EM1 class, and it would do so for the duration of the residency. The same dilemma exists with respect to early graduation.

On the brighter side, however, a candidate with prior experience may not be required to rotate through services he or she has already fulfilled. For example, a candidate who completed an internal medicine residency may not be required to rotate through the internal medicine wards again as an intern (mercy!). Because each applicant provides a unique set of circumstances, discuss the matter with program directors as is fitting. However, do so carefully. Is it more important to have an easy ride than to have a career in emergency medicine? Most residents who switch residencies are prepared to take what they can get, no questions asked.

Alternately, PGY2-4 programs (the ones that require a preliminary year of medicine or surgery) occasionally lose residents at the tail end of the preliminary year. If you have completed or are completing an internship, you generally may be able to fill such a "vacancy" at the end of your own internship without having to take a step backward. However, emergency medicine is getting more competitive, so one can not count on those positions opening up. As a side note, rare circumstances may exist in which an open second-year emergency medicine spot may be filled by a candidate with 2 years of previous experience, usually in primary care. (See www.saem.org for a list of vacancies around the country.)

Perhaps the worst logistical quandary, however, is what to do if you are a resident who has decided to switch residencies late in the academic year. Most programs stop accepting ERAS applications in December; thus, if it is too late to submit an ERAS application, or worse, you have decided to switch after the match itself has occurred, you are now in a very difficult position. The first thing to do is to build an alliance with the program director at your current medical center, or the program director at your former medical school. Discuss your decision and your current dilemma. Because emergency medicine has become increasingly competitive, it is very unlikely that he or she will be able to offer you a residency position for the coming July. Nonetheless, a program director is your best resource for advice and for news regarding open positions around the country. Second, peruse daily the Society for Academic Emergency Medicine Web site for a list of positions that may open up after the match. If a position does open up, apply immediately—it will be filled in a matter of hours and days, not weeks.

Third, begin to contemplate the merits and faults of continuing in your current residency program for another year, versus spending the next year outside of a residency. It may be an awful and awkward position to be in, but it very well may be a decision you have to make. Discuss the question with a program director as they might give you perspective as to whether your application will be strengthened by another year of your current field, or whether it may be wiser to preserve the federal training funding you are associated with by taking the year off. Also, if you do take the year off, try to do something that strengthens your application. If you are interested in international emergency medicine, try to find a clinic to work in. If you are interested in research, try to find a lab, and so forth. Stay in touch with the emergency medicine program directors or emergency medicine attending you feel most positive about, and ask openly for help or advice when you need it. They know you are in a tough spot and generally they want to help.

Finally, an important note on propriety. Regardless of the field or type of program, program directors hate to lose residents. It makes a program look bad, and it causes an incredible nightmare of bureaucracy to replace a resident. Nonetheless, people do switch, and they do so because they need to. The moment you really know in your own heart that you are going to switch, you need to tell your current program director. They will need as much time as they can to find a replacement for you, and it is the decent thing to do. Let your current program director know that you are doing the right thing by informing he or she as early as possible. Do all this, because you will almost certainly need a letter or recommendation from your current program director as you endeavor your switch into emergency medicine. Your current program director knows you will need this letter, so it may be wise to get the subject on the table sooner than later. Also, until you decide to switch, it is usually best to discuss the matter with no one. Some residents or faculty, when they hear a rumor that one of their interns is leaving, can turn on that resident rather severely. Discuss your possible switch with people whose confidence you can trust exclusively.

Coffee is for closers.

—David Mamet, Author

Regarding residents who are switching residencies, it is important to note, and it cannot be emphasized enough, that "tourists" or "drifters" are not desired. Again, nothing creates more of a headache for a program director than when a resident leaves a program. The more you drift or bounce around residencies, the more it appears you will exit another program prematurely, and the more "red flags" you have created. Be ready to address the issue of your conviction and commitment to emergency medicine in both in your application materials, and in person. Be ready to explain very clearly how you came to realize your need to be an emergency physician.

Accordingly, matters of character are the most relevant. The match is, to some degree, a gamble, and program directors are often unsure of how a fourth year medical student will work out as an EM1. Thus, the most important part of any application is reputation and character. All candidates must demonstrate commitment and conviction to emergency medicine via some means: performance on a subinternship, letters of recommendation, personal communications, visits, or persistence alone. If you can, rotate through your current medical center's emergency department and try to establish contacts, try to obtain letters of recommendation from emergency department faculty. Emergency medicine is a small world, and every emergency physician trained somewhere, and usually knows somebody in academic emergency medicine or maybe even a program director. Find your niche, if you can, and develop it. Are you interested in outdoor medicine? International medicine? Disaster medicine? Toxicology? Emergency gerontology? Visit emergency departments and program directors when you travel, if you can, and make second visits after interviewing. Establish a reputation and work hard to maintain it.

In closing, remember: many emergency physicians have prior training in different fields or switched into emergency medicine from another field. As an applicant with prior training, you have a very distinct and a great advantage.

chapter 28

American Board of Emergency Medicine

Rita K. Cydulka, MD, MS, FACEP
Vice-Chair and Associate Professor, Department of Emergency Medicine
MetroHealth Medical at Case Western Reserve University

The concept of board certification in a medical specialty began in the United States with the establishment of the American Board of Ophthalmic Examinations in 1917. For the first time, a single standardized nationwide examination was administered to graduates of all training programs in ophthalmology and individuals who obtained a passing score received certificates that could be used to assure their patients, other physicians, and insurance organizations that they were knowledgeable in their chosen field. The specialties of otolaryngology, dermatology, and obstetrics/gynecology soon followed suit.

In 1933, representatives from these four specialty boards, along with the representatives from the American Hospital Association, the Association of American Medical Colleges, the Federation of State Medical Boards, the American Medical Association Council of Medical Education, and the National Board of Medical Examiner, founded the American Board of Medical Specialties (ABMS). The mission of the newly formed ABMS was to "maintain and improve the quality of medical care by assisting member boards in their efforts to develop and utilize professional and educational standards for the evaluation and certification of physician specialists." By 1949, all existing medical specialties were represented within the ABMS.

American Board of Emergency Medicine

With the support of the American College of Emergency Physicians, the University Association for Emergency Medicine (now the Society for Academic Emergency Medicine), and the American Medical Association, the American Board of Emergency Medicine (ABEM) became the 23rd member board of the ABMS in 1979. Emergency medicine was finally recognized as a specialty. The mission of ABEM is "to protect the public by providing and sustaining the integrity, quality and standards of training in and practice of emergency medicine." To accomplish its mission, ABEM participates in the following activities:

- The development and administration of certification (qualifying exam and oral, continuing certification, and residency in-training examinations)
- The ongoing development of a continuous certification program (emergency medicine continuous certification [EMCC]), which includes assessment of professional standing, lifelong learning and self assessment, assessment of cognitive expertise (ConCert examination) and assessment of practice performance
- The conduct of research to assess and improve the reliability and validity of its examinations
- The performance of an ongoing longitudinal study of emergency physicians to

determine those factors that promote, and detract from, a successful and satisfying career in emergency medicine
- The annual publication of demographic information regarding emergency medicine residency programs
- The review of proposed changes and the special requirements of emergency medicine that are used by the Emergency Medicine Residency Review Committee to accredit training programs
- The analysis of proposals to develop combined training programs and subspecialties within the field of emergency medicine. Emergency medicine has combined training programs with both pediatrics and internal medicine. Current emergency medicine subspecialties include pediatric emergency medicine, toxicology, sports medicine, and undersea and hyperbaric medicine.
- The participation in joint endeavors with other organizations to benefit the field of emergency medicine. Recent examples include the Emergency Medicine Core Contents Task Force, which developed the model of clinical practice of emergency medicine and active participation in the ABMS governing structure.

Current Emergency Medicine Certification Process

Emergency medicine residency graduates undertake a two-part certification examination. The qualifying examination is administered at approximately 200 professional computer-based testing centers throughout the United States and includes multiple choice and pictorial multiple choice items. Each examination appointment is approximately 8 hours in length, with approximately 6.5 hours devoted to actual testing time. Candidates who successfully complete the written examination are scheduled for an oral examination. The half-day oral certification examination includes seven simulated patient encounters (five with single patients and two with multiple patients). Successful completion of both the qualifying and oral certification examinations results in diplomat status.

Emergency Medicine Continuous Certification Process

All ABMS boards, including ABEM, have evolved from a system of "certification followed by periodic recertification," which promotes periodic study for retesting, to one of "maintenance of certification" in order to promote lifelong learning and the ongoing provision of up-to-date high-quality medical care. The four components of the emergency medicine continuous certification process (EMCC) are as follows:
- *Professional standing:* Diplomats are required to possess licenses that are active, current, valid, unrestricted, and unencumbered to practice medicine in all states where they hold licenses.
- *Lifelong learning and self-assessment:* Diplomats must successfully complete at least eight online annual self-assessment tests over the 10-year certification cycle. The readings associated with the tests are related to the model of the clinical practice of emergency medicine.
- *Cognitive expertise:* Diplomats must take and pass the comprehensive, secure examination that is administered at computer testing centers nationwide. This test is typically taken in the 10th year of the EMCC cycle, but it may be taken earlier.
- *Assessment of Practice Performance:* Diplomats will attest to participation in an acceptable national, regional or local practice improvement (PI) program. The current expectation is that diplomats will attest to patient care-based PI activity twice and communication skills/professionalism PI activity once during each 10-year certification cycle.

A Final Thought

There are many opportunities for diplomats to become involved with ABEM (as oral examiners, item writers, case reviewers, exam team leaders, and directors) as well as with other emergency medicine organizations. This involvement not only helps those organizations in their efforts to develop and advance the specialty but also benefits the diplomats themselves by creating a sense of accomplishment within an environment that promotes the development of strong personal and professional relationships, many of which are lifelong and sustaining.

chapter *29*

American Osteopathic Board of Emergency Medicine

Beth A. Longenecker, DO, FACEP, FACOEP
Examiner, American Osteopathic Board of Emergency Medicine

Bryan Staffin, DO, FACOEP
Secretary, American Osteopathic Board of Emergency Medicine

The American Osteopathic Board of Emergency Medicine (AOBEM) is responsible for the process of certification in emergency medicine and its subspecialties for osteopathic physicians. Members of the American College of Osteopathic Emergency Physicians founded the AOBEM at the same time that they established residency training in emergency medicine. Residency approval came from the American Osteopathic Association (AOA) Committee on Post-Doctoral Training, while certification came from the AOA's then Advisory Board for Osteopathic Specialists (currently known as the Bureau of Osteopathic Specialists). The final approval of both residency and certification occurred at the AOA Board of Trustees meeting in 1980.

The first certification examination was given in 1980. Beginning with the second certification exam, the process became the current three-part process. Part I consists of the written exam, Part II consists of the oral and practical exam, and Part III consists of a submission of clinical charts and a peer review process of chart review. To be eligible for certification by the AOBEM, one must be a graduate of an osteopathic medical school who has completed a 4-year postgraduate program in emergency medicine. To date, this has meant completion of an internship year that meets AOA approval as well as a PGY2-PGY4 residency accredited by either the AOA or the ACGME. In July 2008, all osteopathic residency programs will transition into a PGY1-4 format. The AOBEM is currently revising standards to accommodate this change. As part of this revision of bylaws, residents will become eligible to sit for Part I (written) board examinations in the spring of their senior year of residency. Parts II and III are completed after satisfactorily completing residency training and begin independently practicing emergency medicine.

An additional change to the format of the AOBEM written board examination is the implementation of a computerized testing system. This is currently undergoing a trial period. The first computerized examination will be administered on March 26, 2008. The format allows individuals to test at a local learning center rather than flying to Chicago to sit for the written examination. Part II will continue to be given in Chicago, and Part III does not require travel or on-site evaluation.

In the early 1990s, the AOA and health care organizations were clearly moving to the arena of "recertification." Following suit, AOBEM established in 1994 the recertification examination. This resulted in "time-dated" certification that required renewal every 10 years. Both ABEM and AOBEM entered the arena of continuous recertification in 2003. The osteopathic equivalent to the allopathic LLSA is the COLA (Continuous Osteopathic Learning Assessment). Each year, a different subset of the core curriculum of emergency medicine is reviewed and updated through use of selected articles of recent interest. In order to maintain board certification, one must review these articles and take an online examination. In addition, a formal recertification examination (FRCE) must be taken every 10 years. This examination consists of an abbreviated written and oral examination.

AOBEM has established other areas of certification. In 1995, the AOBEM became a member of the conjoint board in sports medicine and was given sole jurisdiction in the "certification of added qualifications" (CAQ) in emergency medical services. In 1997, the AOBEM was granted jurisdiction in medical toxicology (a CAQ that will allow diplomats of any AOA board who meet the eligibility requirements to sit for the AOBEM exam). Examinations in sports medicine are offered yearly, while examinations in EMS and medical toxicology are offered every other year. A CAQ in pediatric emergency medicine is in development.

For more information about the AOBEM, including downloadable examination applications, deadlines for applications, and contact information, visit our Web site. The deadline for beginning the process of certification through AOBEM is September 1, each year. If you have any questions about the process of certification, please feel free to contact us at AOBEM.org.

chapter 30

Residency Review Committee for Emergency Medicine

David T. Overton, MD, MBA, FACEP
Residency Review Committee for Emergency Medicine

Organized medicine is replete with confusing acronyms, and one for you to be familiar with is the RRC, or Residency Review Committee. There are RRCs for all the specialties; this discussion deals with the RRC-Emergency Medicine, or the RRC for Emergency Medicine. The RRC-Emergency Medicine only accredits allopathic residency programs. Osteopathic programs are accredited by the American Osteopathic Association (AOA).

The RRCs all function under the auspices and direction of the Accreditation Council for Graduate Medical Education (ACGME). The RRC-Emergency Medicine is composed of representatives from the American College of Emergency Physicians, the American Board of Emergency Medicine, and the American Medical Association. These individuals are senior educators in emergency medicine, usually current or former program directors and chairs.

Additionally, the RRC-Emergency Medicine has an elected resident representative from EMRA. The EMRA representative is more than simply symbolic; he or she is a full, functioning, voting member of the committee, with a workload comparable to that of other committee members.

The RRC's main responsibilities are to (1) establish program requirements with which all emergency medicine residencies must comply and (2) accredit residencies by assessing their compliance with the program requirements. The program requirements for emergency medicine residencies can be found on the ACGME Web site (www.acgme.org). These are revised and updated every few years. The RRC also develops guidelines for emergency medicine residencies, which can also be found on the ACGME Web page.

Program accreditation is the most important function of the RRC. Without accreditation, residency programs cannot exist. There are different levels of "accreditation," each with associated nomenclature. The specific accreditation that each program holds is given on the ACGME Web page and outlined as follows:

- New programs are granted "provisional" accreditation for 3 years. There is no negative stigma associated with the term "provisional;" it just means that it is a new program.
- Established programs typically hold "full accreditation," sometimes termed "continued accreditation," "continued full accreditation," or simply "accreditation." This can range from 1 to 5 years, although the vast majority of established programs are accredited for 4 to 5 years. In most cases, 3 or fewer years of accreditation for a well-established program should be considered a red flag.
- Programs judged by the RRC to have substantive problems may be placed on "probation." Probation is a huge red flag, although not always a fatal flaw. Probation can sometimes jolt a program or institution into making the necessary changes to substantially improve the residency. Still, be very careful.

- Finally, some newer programs are placed on "continued provisional" status after their initial 3 years of provisional. This, too, should be considered a red flag, as provisional programs are normally expected to advance to full accreditation after their 3 years at the provisional level.

For established programs, the accreditation cycle typically goes something like this:

- When a program is due for reaccreditation, the program will prepare a written application thoroughly describing the program, called the program information forms (the "PIF"). This is a rather lengthy and detailed document (some have been close to 1,000 pages) that is mailed to the RRC.
- Next, a site visit is scheduled. This is a 1-day, on-site visit where a representative of the RRC (but NOT an actual RRC member) meets with the program director, faculty, staff, and residents and inspects the facilities. His or her job will be to confirm the information contained in the application that the program submitted.
- After the site visit, the site visitor prepares a written report that is submitted to the RRC.
- The site visitor's report, together with the PIF and other materials, are reviewed by two members of the RRC. These two RRC members, in turn, prepare their own written reports and recommendations.
- The full RRC meets twice a year for several days. The two reviewing RRC members present their findings and recommendations to the entire committee, which will decide and vote on (1) any citations for the program, (2) its new accreditation status, and (3) the length of its accreditation cycle.

The word "citation" sounds bad but is not necessarily bad. Virtually all emergency medicine programs receive citations (my anecdotal impression is that the average number of citations per program is about six). So, the mere fact that a program received some citations is not necessarily a big deal. It is the nature of the citations that matters. Some are minor paperwork issues, while others are more serious.

- Several weeks after the RRC meets, the program director receives a letter outlining the program's new accreditation status, its citations, and its number of years of accreditation.

Not surprisingly, residency program directors have somewhat of a love-hate relationship with the RRC. On one hand, they appreciate and understand the need for residency standards and share the goal of maximizing residency quality. On the other hand, they sometimes chafe at an outside bureaucracy sitting in judgment of them and telling them what to do, and often lament (usually loudly) individual requirements that they disagree with (or simply find it hard to comply with).

What is really important to the medical student interested in emergency medicine?

- Remember that the RRC-Emergency Medicine maintains and enforces very high educational standards for its residencies. This gives you some assurance that virtually all accredited residencies will contain the tools needed to make you an excellent emergency physician.
- Remember that the RRC and the ACGME are made up of exceedingly dedicated individuals who have resident education and welfare as their number one priority.
- Use the ACGME Web page as one of your tools to evaluate programs, by determining programs' accreditation status and their length of accreditation. Remember that probation, continued provisional, and short accreditation cycle lengths are red flags.

Last, during your residency, you may have the opportunity to participate in an RRC site visit first hand, as the visitors routinely interview a group of program residents. Although this may sound intimidating, it should not be. Rest assured that any resident comments to the site visitor are strictly confidential. However, remember that your comments may be quoted (anonymously) and your voiced opinions may well affect accreditation decisions. Thus, it is important to reasonably measured and thoughtful in your behavior. On one hand, residents should be honest, open, and forthcoming regarding pros and cons of the program. On the other hand, this is probably not a good time to give someone a piece of your mind, just because you are still in a bad mood over the recent lousy midnight shift.

In conclusion, the RRC-Emergency Medicine is another of the many organizations that make up the House of Emergency Medicine. Although its activities are largely invisible to the individual resident and student, it has a tremendous impact on the quality of your residency education and your day-to-day life in residency.

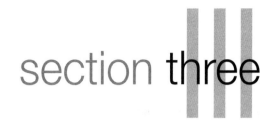

section three

Emergency Medicine
The Research

chapter 31

Emergency Medicine Research: An Overview

Judd E. Hollander, MD, FACEP
Professor, Clinical Research Director, Department of Emergency Medicine, University of Pennsylvania
President Elect–Society of Academic Emergency Medicine

Emergency medicine spans virtually all disciplines in an undifferentiated manner and has a unique perspective focusing on the acute and emergency care of time-sensitive and life-threatening diseases. Emergency medicine has made great strides in the past decade but still lags behind other specialties with respect to federal funding. Your generation of physicians will help solidify our place on the map, through growth in research interests, enhanced research training, and success in answering the research questions important to our specialty.

What Is Emergency Medicine Research?

Emergency medicine research questions are prompted by the recognition of new illnesses or injuries (or complications thereof), by the development of new potential treatments, or by the realization that some time-honored diagnostic or therapeutic maneuvers are unsupported or even refuted by the literature. "Hot topics" in emergency medicine research include the accurate diagnosis and early, aggressive management of acute coronary syndrome and stroke; the identification, tracking, and treatment of emerging infectious diseases; responses to social and public health issues; disaster preparedness; the application of new technologies in the emergency department; and health care resource utilization and policy development. The next generation of emergency medicine research appears focused on multidisciplinary collaborative research through the development of trial networks. At present, there are several federally funded research networks that focus on specific patient groups (NETT [neurological emergencies], PERC [pulmonary embolism], ROC [resuscitation], MARC [asthma], PECARN [children], EMERGIDNET [infectious disease]). Organized emergency medicine would like to see the formation of a large trans-National Institutes of Health (NIH) network that would allow investigators from all disciplines and all institutes to conduct translational and clinical trials in acute illness to improve the care of patients.

How Can You Get Involved in Emergency Medicine Research?

Opportunities for interested students to pursue emergency medicine research are diverse. Students should seek such opportunities by contacting the research director of their local emergency department. Before you do so, you should decide which questions interest you. Don't just go to a faculty mentor and say, "I want to do research." Think about issues that you have identified or observed in your clinical practice. Peruse some emergency medicine journals. Find something that you want to work hard to address. Research is tedious if you are not interested in the question you ask. Just working on someone else's project, if you are not interested (at least somewhat) in the area, can be brutal.

Once you determine where your interest lies, review the literature in that area. Use MEDLINE and/or department Web sites to look through the research interests, recent publications, and current projects done by the faculty. See what is already known about the topic. Think about what knowledge gaps can be filled. Discuss this with some of your fellow students, residents, and faculty on a clinical shift. Other clinicians will give you insights into the scope of the problem and whether or not you have a sufficient number of patients with that issue at your institution.

You will then need to identify a specific mentor. Remember the mentor is someone to help you conduct research (or maybe someone you help conduct research) but not someone to be your best friend (although you may develop a nice relationship). Treat the mentor with respect and show that are interested in the topic and well read in the area. A mentor without a strong research track record might be able to help you frame the clinical question, but there is a reason they do not conduct research. Mentors with a strong research track record are generally focused and busy. Successful researchers will always want to train new people, especially in their area of interest. If your idea is unrelated to the mentor's focus, he or she may still be willing to help, but you really want a mentor who can teach research skills and has an interest in your area. Sometimes, you need two mentors— one to help design the research and one with a knowledge and interest in the specific area.

Make sure your mentor is available to meet on a regular basis. Obviously, the mentor must have the time to do the project with you and be fairly accessible. This is rarely an issue for those students joining an ongoing project but can be problematic when working on an independent study. In addition to testing your hypothesis and publishing your work, you also want to know if the mentor will help you network and meet colleagues. Will he work with you to submit your work to a research meeting? Will she support you (both academically and financially) if you have an opportunity to present your work? If you are joining your mentor on his or her own project, make sure that your mentor will make you an author on the project that you work on. It is also worth your while to speak with upperclassmen and recent graduates who matched in emergency medicine about potential mentors. Your emergency medicine interest group might also have classmates who can speak to their experiences.

Funding Options

Your school's administrative offices frequently provide information about grants and available funding. Contact the director of your combined degree office or research office and ask for school or institutional packets and/or Web sites that list known sources of external funding. Frequently, you will be directed toward competitive grants from large research organizations like the American Heart Association or American Cancer Society. The Doris Duke Foundation, American Heart Association, and some other foundations offer "year out" training grants for students seriously interested in research. These grants come with criteria for acceptable projects, but the terms are often broad, thus allowing many different areas of study to fall under their umbrella. Additionally, some medical schools offer funding for research, especially the summer between the first and second years.

Start-up support for medical student research projects and funds for training researchers in emergency medicine has generally been through the specialty's organizations, the Society for Academic Emergency Medicine (SAEM) and the Emergency Medicine Foundation (EMF) associated with the American College of Emergency Physicians (ACEP). Both organizations emphasize training and fellowship grants, although EMF also supports specific projects without a training emphasis. They award as much as $800/month for 3 months to medical students and/or residents to encourage research in emergency medicine. The deadline is typically in late February or March, with awards made for the following academic year, July through June. On the application, they are most interested in what you are going to do, what you will gain from the experience, and, very important, that you have selected a qualified mentor who will have the time and research experience to ensure the project is completed. Information can be found on the EMRA, ACEP, and SAEM Web sites.

Your Research Future

If you really want to conduct research for your career, you need to get formal training. In most other specialties, the federal government (NIH) is the primary source of medical research funding. For emergency medicine investigators, federal research support has played a small role. In the four major emergency medicine journals in 1994, only 37% of studies were funded, and among the funded research, only 24% received support from the federal government.[1] Furthermore, only 0.05% of NIH training grant dollars awarded to medical schools go to departments of emergency medicine, resulting in only $50.66 per resident.[2] This is dramatically lower than that of virtually all other medical specialties.

After two decades in which federal grants to emergency medicine researchers were extraordinarily rare, the mid-1990s marked a turning point for federal funding of emergency medicine-based investigators. Recently, residency-trained emergency physicians have been competitive for first-time NIH grants, including Mentored Clinical Scientist Investigator Awards (K awards). In 2004, the ACEP Scientific Review Committee surveyed emergency medicine academic chairs regarding the success of first-time NIH submissions. Data were collected on 38 first-time NIH submissions. Of the grants that had been reviewed, 31% were funded on the initial submission. These numbers compare favorably for physicians from other specialties submitting NIH proposals.[3]

One reason that NIH R01 and NIH T32 training grants are difficult to obtain stems from the undifferentiated nature of emergency care, which does not fit very well with the highly discipline specific focus of individual NIH institutes. The recent introduction of the NIH Clinical and Translational Science Awards (CTSAs) may serve as the vehicle for emergency medicine training grants. The NIH recently awarded CTSAs to 12 academic health centers. These grants have training grants within them that are not discipline specific and span the whole range of training from medical student through junior faculty, thereby opening the doors for future emergency physicians to pursue formal training in clinical and translational research. The decision on who receives these grants rests with the institution. Tapping into CTSA grants represents the best opportunity for emergency medicine to receive training grants from the NIH and pursue the standard training process to become a researcher—fellowship training.

The Best-Kept Secret

One of the most enjoyable aspects of a productive research career is getting the opportunity to network and socialize with colleagues from around the world at national meetings. While a resident, I was amazed that some faculty members could remember the name of authors on publications. As my research career grew, I met many of the leading investigators and discussed their research directly with them. Now I understand how my mentors could remember the authors of many papers. Getting to know people across the country, see them regularly, and know about advances in medical care long before they are published is one of the greatest pleasures and benefits of being a researcher. If things go well for you, you may also get the opportunity to make your own contribution to improve the care of patients that may affect practice literally around the world.

References

1. Ernst AA, Houry D, Weiss SJ. Research funding in the four major emergency medicine journals. *Am J Emerg Med.* 1997;15:268-270.
2. Institute of Medicine Committee of the Future of Emergency Care in the United States Health System Board on Health Care Services. Hospital-based emergency care. At the breaking point. Table 8-1, p 228. Available at www.iom.edu.
3. Kotchen TA, Lindquist T, Malik K, Ehrenfeld E. NIH peer review of grant applications for clinical research. *JAMA.* 2004;291(7):836-843.

chapter 32

Medical Student Research and Resident Scholarly Projects

Sunday Clark, MPH, ScD
Research Director, Department of Emergency Medicine
New York-Presbyterian Hospital

Jonathan Fisher, MD, MPH
Instructor, Medicine, Harvard Medical School
Beth Israel Deaconess Medical Center

"**Because I said so!**" How many times did we hear that phrase uttered when we were growing up. The phrase was not very satisfying then, and it is even less now that we are adults. Medical education was traditionally a process where pearls were handed down from senior physicians to young physicians in training. These pearls often became dogma and took on a life of their own. The days of anecdotal medicine are gone. Emergency departments are becoming overcrowded. The population as a whole is getting older. As more care is being shifted to the ambulatory setting, the acuity of patients is increasing. The Institute of Medicine reports that anywhere from 44,000 to 98,000 deaths a year are due to medical errors.[1] Health care costs are skyrocketing.

How are emergency physicians going to provide cost-effective, evidence-based, high-quality medicine in this challenging environment? This is where research comes into focus. It is through research and understanding the research process that emergency medicine will be able to improve patient care and grow as a specialty.

As a medical student, you may not yet grasp the importance of research and its affect on the practice of medicine. You may hear physicians talking about this study or that journal article and may not appreciate why these contributions are so important to medicine. You may think that research is something one does to pad their CV. But eventually you come to realize that research is about answering questions to improve patient care and quality of life. As you go through residency training, you will find yourself constantly asking senior residents and attendings questions about patient care. Should you get test X? Should you give drug Y? Many of the answers to your questions come from empirical evidence derived from research. Ultimately, it will be research that will help you decide how to best care for your patients.

Research can help us advance the care of patients by finding new diagnostic and therapeutic modalities. Even if you are not a researcher yourself, you need to understand the research process so that you can critically evaluate the evidence and decide whether research findings are applicable to your patients. One has to understand how a study is designed and carried out in order to evaluate whether its conclusions are sound and should be incorporated into clinical practice.

There are three basics types of research: basic science, clinical, and epidemiological research. Basic science research is also known as bench or laboratory research. It is the area that medical students may be the most familiar with during their first 2 years of medical school. It focuses on cellular and animal models of the disease process. It also is the area that is the least developed in emergency medicine. Clinical research is at the patient level. Questions often focus on how we diagnose and treat patients. Epidemiological research looks at questions on a population level. Who comes to the emergency department and why? Areas such as injury prevention and access to care are just some examples. Clinical epidemiology is a melding of clinical and epidemiological research.

As a medical student, there are many reasons to become involved with emergency medicine research. It may be to learn about research, to find out more about the specialty, to get to know the faculty, or to answer a specific question. While you may not have a specific topic of interest, it is important to have a desire to learn about research methodology and participate in designing and implementing research studies. The exposure to both emergency medicine and the research process you get by taking part in emergency medicine research projects will be invaluable. As a resident, performing research will expand your understanding of the research process and contribute to your growth as physician clinically.

Undertaking a research project requires a dedicated time commitment. While most resident schedules allow for a dedicated month-long block of time that is often used for research purposes, it is unrealistic to expect to take most research projects from conception to completed project during a single month block. Even relatively small projects, such as simple retrospective studies, will require several months to a year to finish. The process is often periods of intense work separated by down time. In today's research environment, it also is important to factor in regulatory requirements, such as institutional review board review. If you have a month block that you are planning to use for research, you should have most of the groundwork done before the month starts or plan on using the month to get your project up and running with the expectation that it will continue after your dedicated research month has ended. Having a plan in place well before your research month will allow you to use your time efficiently for designing your study, collecting and analyzing the data, and writing your abstracts and manuscripts. Residents interested in research should think about getting involved with faculty on a project by the end of the first year or at the beginning of the second year so that he or she will have time to develop and complete projects on their own as a senior resident.

Residency Review Committee (RRC) requires that all residents be involved in scholarly activity as part of training. How each program meets this requirement varies greatly. Some programs require residents to produce a publishable quality case report, review, or chapter, while others expect a research abstract presentation or even an original publication. No matter which program you choose, there will always be academic and research opportunities. Residency programs come in all type and flavors; some programs will have a more focus on research than others.

As an emergency medicine applicant evaluates various residency programs, it is important to take a look at a department's research infrastructure. One quick and easy way to look at program is to look at the productivity of the department. How many abstracts are presented at national meetings? How many publications? However, these benchmarks only scratch the surface. What kind of support exists for research? Are there people to help with data collection and biostatistical analysis? Some programs have people, such as research coordinators and research assistants, who spend time in the emergency department enrolling patients in various studies. Are there research facilities for those interested in basic science? What kinds of funding are available? While funding for emergency medicine research is often limited and sometimes comes from industry sources, some programs may have large research budgets. If a department has a large amount of NIH funding, it can be a sign of a strong research department. There are mechanisms for inexperienced researchers to obtain funding when starting out. The Emergency Medicine Foundation is a good place to start to find funding for projects. Overall, the important thing to look for in a program is the availability of strong research mentors. Are there faculty and senior residents who have successful research careers? Collaborating with an experienced mentor is one of the best ways to get started on a productive research career.

In general, programs with a 4-year format tend to provide more time for research and have a more academic focus. There are also many 3-year residency programs with strong academic and research track records. If you are considering a career in academic emergency medicine or a research fellowship after residency, the amount of research experience you gain during residency will help you be competitive for jobs at academic centers after you finish residency. Graduating with experience presenting original research at national conferences and having several publications will make it easier to get an academic position because you have already demonstrated your ability to produce research.

Pursuing a research fellowship may also be a good idea for those interested in an academic career in emergency medicine. There are several research fellowships in emergency medicine and many other opportunities in other specialties too. Research fellowships vary in length from 1 to 2 years and often include a Masters of Public Health. The SAEM Web site contains a listing of emergency medicine fellowships in addition to residency programs. Research fellowships will help teach young investigators the intricacies of research methodology and strategies to successfully obtain grant funding. After formal training is completed, a fellow will ideally have developed an area of expertise and obtained grant funding to continue research in that area. Fellowship training and the resulting research will help you obtain a research faculty position in a major academic center.

Because the RRC requires that training take place in an environment of inquiry and scholarship, no matter which residency you choose, you will be exposed to research. It will be up to you to shape the experience so that it is most beneficial to you and your career goals. As part of any emergency medicine residency, you must acquire a solid foundation in research so that you can critically evaluate the literature regardless of whether you go on to a career in research. Remember, we are all researchers every time we see a patient and ask a question.

Reference

1. Kohn LT, et al. *To err is human: building a safer health system.* Washington, DC: National Academy Press; 2000. Available at http://www.nap.edu/catalog/9728.html.

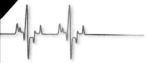

chapter 33

Evidence-Based Medicine in Emergency Medicine: An Introduction

Peter C. Wyer, MD, FACEP
Columbia University College of Physicians & Surgeons

Evidence-Based Medicine: What Is It, Fruitfully?

No doubt you have heard the term "evidence-based medicine" (EBM) and may even have formed an opinion about its merits and usefulness. Most negative opinions about EBM reflect misconceptions regardinsg what it is and how it is conceptualized by the individuals who first advanced the term.[1] Let's start by describing the attributes of their vision.

EBM is best defined in two stages. First, what is evidence-based clinical practice? Second, what special expertise is required to practice in this way? Evidence-based clinical practice is most succinctly defined as a patient-centered model of clinical decision making in which clinical research is routinely considered in tandem with the social and clinical circumstances and also the values and preferences of the patient.[2,3] All three components are implied whenever a clinical decision is made. To maximize the validity of a decision for an individual patient, the strength and applicability of the available research evidence must be properly assessed, the patient's circumstances, including the nature of her disease process or processes and social and living circumstances must be accurately characterized, and her values and preferences carefully considered. The challenge to the evidence-based practitioner is to facilitate the process of bringing these three domains accurately and saliently to bear on those important health care decisions for a particular patient that lie within the physician's scope of practice. Figure 1 represents this model.[3]

The Haynes construct coheres closely with the definition of competency in "patient care" provided by the Accreditation Council on Graduate Medical Education (ACGME), which includes the requirement that learners be assessed on their ability to "make informed decisions about diagnostic and therapeutic interventions based on patient information and preferences, up-to-date scientific evidence, and clinical judgment."[4]

Hence, practicing EBM is not only about the evidence. However, to do it competently requires the development of some specialized skills pertaining to finding and evaluating clinical evidence relevant to specific questions. This is where the instructional literature on EBM comes in.

The required EBM skills are embodied in an oft-cited definition, advanced in 1996: "Evidence based medicine is the conscientious, explicit, and judicious use of current best evidence in making decisions about the care of individual patients."[5]

This definition highlights the need to be able to bring the best and most relevant evidence to the decision table routinely (*conscientious*), and with consideration of its validity and applicability to the problem at hand (*judicious*). It recognizes that not all evidence is equally strong nor is it equally applicable to specific circumstances.

The skills required to manage the evidentiary side of evidence-based practice are commonly described with reference to four domains: "ask," "acquire," "appraise," and

A Model for Clinical Decisions

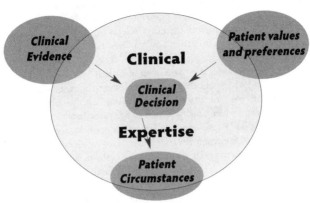

Adapted from Haynes 2002

Figure 1. Model of evidence-based practice in which clinical expertise is defined as the ability to coordinate decision making on behalf of individual patients with explicit reference to three independent but overlapping domains. Adapted from Haynes 2002.[3]

"apply."[6,7] The mastery of these skill domains entails knowledge regarding how to ask appropriate questions, choose appropriate online resources, assess the quality of studies and structured reviews, and understand the potential impact on patient outcomes of various categories of results. An understanding of different study designs and of how they relate to specific types of questions are included elements of such mastery. A multiplicity of sources, including full textbooks, are devoted to elaborating these skill sets and how best to learn and teach them.[8-10]

Summarizing, if there are two fundamental principles of EBM, they are to (1) understand the hierarchy of evidence and (2) understand that evidence from research is never a sufficient basis for a clinical decision to be made.

Evidence-Based Medicine: What Isn't It, Fruitfully?

Now that we have defined evidence-based practice and EBM as understood by its advocates, we can, from the standpoint of a "survival guide," quickly dispense with some of the commonly encountered misconceptions.

EBM, fruitfully, is *not:*
— Finding literature that agrees with your preconceptions
— A sexy marketing label to be placed on anything you want to promote
— A negative epithet to be attached to anything you want to reject
— A rejection of clinical experience and patient values in favor of evidence from randomized trials
— Something that anyone has already been doing for the past 30 years

A comment on the last exclusion is in order. When EBM was introduced in 1992 as a paradigm for learning and teaching clinical practice,[11] it was still not quite possible to practice it in a truly "conscientious" way. The World Wide Web had not yet made the Internet widely available to patients and their physicians. Conscientious practice of EBM ultimately requires the development of advanced resources and information systems that have only begun to emerge in the past 15 years. Such resources and systems largely remain to be developed within emergency medicine to address the special needs of evidence-based practice in our specialty.

What Am I Expected to Know and Learn About EBM?

Objectively, EBM skills constitute mandated competencies for both undergraduate and graduate medical learners throughout North America. The Medical School Objectives Project of the Association of American Medical Colleges lists EBM skills as required elements within the undergraduate curriculum.[12,13] These include "the ability to translate current clinical research into lay language for patients." The ACGME competency framework governs U.S. residency programs in all specialties.[4] As noted above, the "patient care" competency includes language that coheres with the published model of evidence-based practice. The skills pertaining to the EBM domains "ask," "acquire," "appraise," and "apply" constitute elements of another ACGME competency, "practice-based learning and improvement (PBLI)." PBLI frames these skills within a performance-based, or behavioral, model, frequently termed "improvement learning."[14] Within this construct, residents are expected to ask questions, perform literature searches, evaluate evidence relevant to their patients' problems, and formulate plans for revision of practice as a result of such inquiries.

Finally, the principal guideline for residency training in emergency medicine, the Model for the Clinical Practice of Emergency Medicine,[15] lists "evidence-based medicine" and "interpretation of the medical literature" as required curricular elements.

EBM is relatively new. Commitment to and understanding of it may vary from school to school, program to program, and even faculty member to faculty member. However, the values and premises that it represents go to the heart of current efforts at curriculum reform on both undergraduate and graduate levels and are consistent with the goal of life-long learning. The ACGME is expected to begin rigorous evaluation of competency achievement within specific residency programs within another 5 years of this writing. Interim evaluation modalities for the ACGME competencies include the use of portfolios, in which students or residents document activities pertinent to PBLI.[16] Such instruments are particularly compelling insofar as they constitute vehicles for student and resident learning as well as for evaluation of both learners and programs.

What Would It Look Like to Learn and Use Evidence-Based Medicine in an Emergency Department?

A common objection to EBM is that "it takes too much time."[1] This might particularly appear to be the case in the time-pressed setting of emergency care. Efficient use of online resources, including customized resources, constitutes one component of the answer. A strategic approach to researching questions, prioritizing those that come up most often and that pertain to a disproportionate number of patients is another. Most important, for EBM skills to be learned and used in practice, their relevance must be integrated into the elements of clinical reasoning. An emergency medicine resident's eye view of the process of encountering and acquiring EBM skills over a 3- to 4-year training cycle, which also elucidates their relationship to logic and critical reasoning, was recently authored by a visionary emergency medicine resident with the help of this writer.[10]

Research Opportunities

As extensive as is the literature on EBM system development, methodology, and education, this area remains a frontier zone for new ideas and research. Particularly relevant to emergency medicine are the development of specialty specific electronic resources, including preappraised, synthesized resource, education research initiatives, and innovative approaches to prediction rule and guideline implementation. Clinical knowledge translation is closely related to EBM and constitutes an area of development that offers a multiplicity of research opportunities to students, residents and young investigators within our specialty.[17]

References

1. Straus SE, McAlister FA. Evidence-based medicine: a commentary on common criticisms. *CMAJ.* 2000;163:837-841.

2. Guyatt G, Montori V, Devereaux PJ, Schunemann H, Bhandari M. Patients at the center: in our practice, and in our use of language. *ACP J Club.* 2004;140:A11-A12.

3. Haynes RB, Devereaux PJ, Guyatt GH. Physicians' and patients choices in evidence based practice: evidence does not make decisions, people do. *BMJ.* 2002;324:1350.

4. ACGME. Outcome Project: General Competencies. Available at: http://www.acgme.org/outcome/comp/compFull.asp#3. Accessed September 6, 2005.

5. Sacket DL, Rosenberg WMC, Gray JAM, Haynes RB, Richardson WS. Evidence based medicine: what it is and what it isn't. *BMJ.* 1996;312:71-72.

6. Shaneyfelt T, Baum KD, Bell D, et al. Instruments for evaluating education in evidence-based practice: a systematic review. *JAMA.* 2006;296:1116-1127.

7. Straus SE, Green ML, Bell DS, et al. Evaluating the teaching of evidence based medicine: conceptual framework. *BMJ.* 2004;329:1029-1032.

8. Guyatt G, Rennie D. *Users' guides to the medical literature: a manual for evidence-based clinical practice.* Chicago: AMA Press; 2002.

9. Straus SE, Richardson WS, Glasziou P, Haynes RB. *Evidence-based medicine: how to practice and teach EBM.* 3rd ed. Edinburgh: Elsevier Churchill Livingstone; 2005.

10. Weingart S, Wyer P. *Emergency medicine decision making: critical choices in chaotic environments.* New York: McGraw-Hill Companies; 2006.

11. Evidence-Based Medicine Working Group. Evidence-based medicine: a new approach to teaching the practice of medicine. *JAMA.* 1992;268:2420-2425.

12. Medical Informatics Advisory Panel. *Contemporary issues in medicine: medical informatics and population health: report II of the Medical Schools Objective Project.* AAMC; 1999.

13. Clinical Research Advisory Panel. *Contemporary issues in medicine: basic science and clinical research: report IV of the Medical Schools Objective Project.* AAMC; 2001.

14. Headrick LA, Richardson A, Priebe GP. Continuous improvement learning for residents. *Pediatrics.* 1998;101:768-774.

15. 2005 Emergency Medicine Model Review Task Force. The 2003 model of the clinical practice of emergency medicine: the 2005 update. *Ann Emerg Med.* 2006;48:e1-e17.

16. O'Sullivan PS, Cogbill KK, McClain T, Reckase MD, Clardy JA. Portfolios as a novel approach for residency evaluation. *Acad Psych.* 2002;26:173-179.

17. Lang ES, Wyer PC, Haynes RB. Knowledge translation: closing the evidence-to-practice gap. *Ann Emerg Med.* 2007;49:355-363.

Emergency Medicine
The Fellowships and Subspecialties

chapter 34

Emergency Medicine Fellowship Training: An Overview

Jeremy T. Cushman, MD, MS
Past President, EMRA
Director, EMS Fellowship, Division of EMS and Office of Prehospital Care
Department of Emergency Medicine, University of Rochester School of Medicine and Dentistry

By its very nature, the specialty of emergency medicine covers a broad and diverse body of knowledge. Whereas the specialties of medicine and surgery have multiple defined subspecialties, emergency medicine is just beginning to grow out of its specialization to meet a clinical need and into a diverse specialty with numerous unique subspecialties. The number of fellowship training programs has nearly quadrupled in the past 20 years, reflective of the continuing evolution of emergency medicine practice. This may be the result of emergency physician's increased appreciation for additional training or perhaps it is out of emergency medicine's "adoption" of so many diverse niches in which medical care can be provided (air medicine, disaster medicine, international medicine, etc.).

The reasons for pursing fellowship training are as varied as the fellowships available. Unlike other specialties where fellowship training usually results in that person practicing the subspecialty full-time (for example, few gastroenterologists practice general internal medicine), nearly all emergency medicine subspecialties involve the continued practice of emergency medicine. There are varied reasons for this, but as you look at the list of emergency medicine fellowship opportunities (see table page 133), it is hard to imagine any of them not providing some type of clinical care in one way or another. Further, many of the subspecialties explore emergency medicine's unique role in public health (environmental health and injury control), our ability improvise and provide care in austere or otherwise uncontrolled environments (air medicine, disaster medicine, emergency medical services, international medicine, and wilderness medicine), our background in caring for severely injured or ill patients (critical care, palliative care, toxicology), or our interest in leadership, research, and education (administration, research, and medical education and simulation).

Similar to other specialties, pursuing a fellowship allows an individual to know more about a subject or an area that is of particular interest to them. Unlike many other medical specialties, however, fellowship training in emergency medicine typically leads to a smaller salary. The SAEM 2004-2005 Salary and Benefit Survey found that fellowship-trained faculty made approximately $9,000 less per year, although this is likely accounted for by the fewer number of clinical hours that fellowship-trained faculty work.[1] This is particularly important for the candidate to consider as pursuing a fellowship will limit his or her earning potential for the duration of the fellowship, further compounding the years spent living off student loans and lean budgets. Fortunately, many emergency medicine fellowships include clinical work in the emergency department, further augmenting the salary support offered to the fellow.

With this said, the economics of emergency medicine subspecialization become apparent. Pursuing fellowship training and subspecialization in emergency medicine is not met with the same financial rewards witnessed in other specialties. The medical community and lay public do not yet recognize the importance of fellowship-trained emergency medicine subspecialists and therefore are not willing to provide them with the salary support to practice only that subspecialty. In short, it is rare to find an emergency medicine subspecialist who does not need to work clinically in the emergency department to provide them with sufficient salary support.

Although fellowship training may not result in a larger salary, it may secondarily improve job opportunities, job satisfaction, and career longevity. For those interested in an academic career, completing a fellowship will establish your niche to fill in the department, perhaps placing you in a better position to compete for resources for your specific area of interest (research, pediatrics, ultrasound, etc.). A graduate of a fellowship program may also be more attractive to an academic department because of specific training and demonstrated experience. In the end, academic departments look to what you will be able to contribute to the program and fellowship training will clearly establish that potential contribution.

Most complete fellowship training immediately after residency. However, there is nothing that should prevent an individual from completing a fellowship after working in the community for a few years. In fact, the level of clinical maturity that comes with an applicant who has been "in the trenches" for a period of time may be particularly beneficial and allow them to have greater focus and application of their fellowship training. The other extreme may be the medical student who chooses the field of emergency medicine because of a specific desire to pursue subspecialty training in toxicology, disaster medicine, or hyperbarics, for example. With the option of either a 3- or 4-year emergency medicine residency, one may tend to gravitate to the 3-year residency with plans to pursue subspecialty training. The increase in time and financial stresses associated with the 4-year training programs when combined with a 1- to 3-year fellowship may be a difficult stress to bear depending on individual circumstances.

Unlike residency, the majority of fellowship programs do not use a common application such as Electronic Residency Application System (ERAS), nor do they often require the same application materials or have common deadlines. The decision to pursue a fellowship should be made in the second year of residency (third year in 1,2,3,4 or 2,3,4 programs). Because many programs operate on a rotating admission schedule, it is important to begin to inquire about fellowship programs during your second year to be sure that you have every opportunity to pursue the program of interest. Professional associations (both emergency medicine and subspecialty specific) are often the best sources for discovering fellowship training programs. The SAEM fellowship catalog is another fantastic resource listing the various fellowship programs available.

The majority of emergency medicine fellowships do not have standard curricula like residency programs, which follow the requirements set forth by the Residency Review Committee for Emergency Medicine. Those fellowships that result in board certification through ABEM or ABHPM are the exception, and tend to have similar, although not identical, curricula in order to meet certification requirements. This is extremely important to recognize as there are a large number of fellowships available to emergency medicine graduates, and should you choose, for example, a geriatric emergency medicine fellowship, the didactic and experiential curricula may be significantly different from one site to another. Careful evaluation of a program prior to application is vital to ensure that the fellowship program meets your specific needs and career interests.

The application process, as suggested, is quite variable. Many programs require a curriculum vitae and letters of recommendation, while others use a formal application. It is imperative to inquire about the application process when finding out about the programs. An on-site interview is a must and is just as important as the residency interview to determine whether you fit the program and the program fits you. The decision as to which programs to pursue is a personal one. There is much less pressure than the mystique and suspense of the match, but you cannot blame the computer on where you end up. Careful research and preparation will ensure you make the choice that is right for you. Important questions to consider when evaluating a fellowship program include the following:

- What is the fellowship curriculum? What portion of it is experiential, and where and how does it occur? What portion of it is didactic, and where and when does it occur?
- Will you complete formal coursework toward an advanced degree/certification? What is the degree/certification, and is it reimbursed?
- Who will be your mentor? What are their qualifications?
- What other key faculty will you interact with during the fellowship, and how will they contribute to your subspecialty education?
- What financial support will you receive (continuing medical education, reimbursement for presentations, research funding, salary)?
- What ancillary support will you receive (secretarial staff, research staff)?
- Will you have office space, a computer, copying capabilities, library resources?
- What will be your clinical requirement, and what setting will it be in (academic versus community)?
- Are there any publishing or presentation expectations?
- Are there any required teaching or educational responsibilities?
- Who are the current and former fellows and what is their contact information? Just like residency interviews, often the best sources of information are those that have recently participated in the program.

As Table 1 demonstrates, there is a broad array of fellowship training opportunities available. Many programs do not result in board certification with a few notable exceptions: hyperbaric medicine, pediatric emergency medicine, sportsmedicine, and toxicology fellowships result in board certification by the American Board of Emergency Medicine in conjunction with other sponsoring boards. Each of these specialties is discussed in detail in subsequent chapters. The most recent addition to subspecialty certification is that of palliative care medicine, and Dr. Susan Stone provides us with more information in a subsequent chapter.

The American Board of Physician Specialists (ABPS), a non-American Board of Medical Specialties certification body, recently announced the availability of board certification for disaster medicine. Important to note is that although fellowships in disaster medicine exist (as discussed by Dr. Kristi Koenig in a later chapter), there are no national standard curricula and certification through ABPS is based on experience and participation in disaster management and education. This will likely change in future years as this new subspecialty continues to grow and evolve.

Critical care is a subspecialty that receives significant interest from emergency medicine residency graduates, and although numerous training opportunities exist, the barriers to subspecialty board certification by emergency medicine residency graduates remain. Further detailed description of the opportunities and certification challenges within the subspecialty of critical care are detailed by Drs. Farcy, Chiu, and Scalea in a later chapter.

The lack of subspecialty certification in some areas of emergency medicine should not minimize the importance and opportunities provided by these fellowship programs. Many programs offer advanced course work in the form of a master's of business administration (MBA), master's in public health (MPH), or a master's of science (MS) in clinical research, education, or even emergency medical services. Others still may offer certificates of advanced training, such as ultrasound fellowships offering certification as a registered diagnostic medical sonographer (RDMS).

Obtaining an advanced degree from a training program is likely to be as powerful as attaining board certification. Further, when board certification becomes available in these

content areas, persons having undergone previous fellowship training will likely be eligible to take a new certifying exam. For those programs where both subspecialty board certification and an advanced degree are not available, all is not lost. When looking at other specialties, we see the importance of advance training without the tangible certificates of a degree or board certification. Surgery, orthopedics, and anesthesia provide examples of advanced training without formal certification. The intensive knowledge and experience you gain from a fellowship program will be a recognized asset for your future career, regardless of whether you become board certified.

The following table highlights the 24 known types of fellowship programs available to emergency medicine graduates. Subsequent chapters provide greater details regarding the more common fellowships available and will be an excellent guide to the types of curricula associated with any fellowship program. As the specialty of emergency matures, so will the formalization of many of the subspecialties into programs with standardized curricula and board certification. The ability to subspecialize offers the interested physician tremendous potential to further examine a specific aspect of emergency medicine, with the personal and professional benefits of such training.

Fellowships Available to Emergency Medicine Graduates		
Fellowship	**Length**	**Certification**
Administration	1 year	No
Air medicine	1 year	No
Cardiovascular emergency medicine	1 or 2 years	No
Clinical forensic medicine	1 or 2 years	No
Critical care	1 or 2 years	No*
Disaster medicine	1 or 2 years	Yes, ABPS
Prehospital (EMS)	1 or 2 years	No
Environmental health	2 years	No
Geriatric emergency medicine	1 year	No
Government EMS	1 year	No
Hyperbaric medicine	1 year	Yes, ABEM
Injury control	1 year	No
International emergency medicine	1 or 2 years	No
Medical education	1 year	No
Medical informatics	1 year	No
Medical simulation	1 year	No
Neurology/neurovascular	1 or 2 years	No
Palliative care	1 year	Yes, ABHPM
Pediatric emergency medicine	2 or 3 years	Yes, ABEM
Research	1 to 3 years	No
Sports medicine	1 year	Yes, ABEM
Toxicology	2 years	Yes, ABEM
Ultrasound	1 year	No
Wilderness emergency medicine	1 year	No

ABEM, American Board of Emergency Medicine; ABHPM, American Board of Hospice and Palliative Care Medicine; ABPS, American Board of Physician Specialists.
*Certification is available through the European Society of Intensive Care Medicine.

Reference

1. Kristal SL, Randall-Kristal KA, Thompson BM. The Society for Academic Emergency Medicine's 2004–2005 Emergency Medicine Faculty Salary and Benefit Survey. *Acad Emerg Med.* 2006;13:548-558.

chapter 35

Pediatric Emergency Medicine

Ramon W. Johnson, MD, FACEP, FAAP
ACEP Board of Directors 2006-2007
Mission Hospital Regional Medical Center and Children's Hospital of Orange County

Robert W. Schafermeyer, MD, FACEP, FAAP
President, ACEP, 2000-2001, Chair, Pediatric Emergency Medicine Sub Board 1995-1996
Emergency Physician, Carolinas Medical Center

Pediatric emergency medicine—a joy, a challenge, an opportunity for any physician who enjoys acute care medicine and interacting with children and their families. The unique aspects of care of the pediatric patient led to a subspecialty, pediatric emergency medicine. Pediatric emergency medicine practices have existed since at least 1976, with many of these early practices predominantly at children's hospitals in the United States. Many early practitioners came from the field of pediatrics and some came from the field of emergency medicine.

While the emergency physician is trained to care for critically ill and injured children and provides the majority of health care services to children, some physicians want to devote a significant amount of their clinical, administrative, teaching, and research time to enhancing emergency care of children. In March 1991, the American Board of Medical Specialties approved the subspecialty of pediatric emergency medicine for the American Board of Pediatrics (ABP) and for the American Board of Emergency Medicine (ABEM). The first exam was administered in 1992 and is given every 2 years. There are approximately 50 subspecialty programs in the United States and 5 in Canada.

Requirements

To enter this subspecialty training of pediatric emergency medicine, you must first complete a residency in emergency medicine or in pediatrics. You apply to the pediatric emergency medicine subspecialty programs, and then participate in the National Resident and Fellowship Match Program, which occurs in December.

The goals and objectives for the training program are to produce an individual who is not only clinically proficient in the practice of pediatric emergency medicine, especially in the management of the acutely ill and injured child in the setting of an emergency department, but also capable of teaching, performing research, and defining a standard of care for their department, institution, and community. Such individuals become content experts to assist hospitals, local EMS agencies, and regional and statewide medical organizations to improve the care of children.

The core content for this subspecialty includes resuscitation, trauma, medical and surgical emergencies, toxicology, environmental emergencies, psychosocial emergencies, EMS, epidemiology, administration, ethics, legal issues, procedures, and the care of physically and sexually abused children. The majority of your clinical experience will occur in the emergency department, where you will have the opportunity to provide emergency

care for children and treat the full spectrum of illnesses and injuries.

You will develop special competence in resuscitation including cardiopulmonary, trauma, disaster and environmental medicine, airway management, procedural sedation, transport, and triage. You must master a range of technical and procedural skills in children of all ages beyond those acquired in the primary residency program.

Fellowship training has the additional benefit of teaching and promoting research in the field of pediatric emergency medicine. This skill set becomes extremely valuable for those individuals seeking positions in academic emergency medicine.

The two boards have a few different requirements in order to take the certifying exam for pediatric emergency medicine. The graduate of a pediatric residency must complete a 3-year training program with the first 2 years based mostly in a clinical setting and the third year devoted more to a research project. The ABP requires 3 years of fellowship training as a minimum for all of their subspecialty programs. At least 4 months of the clinical time during the 3 years must be spent in an adult emergency department, where the subspecialty resident should receive education and experience in community EMS, adult trauma, and toxicology.

A graduate of an emergency medicine residency training program must complete at least 2 years of clinical training with at least 4 months of this time spent on pediatric rotations in ambulatory clinics, inpatient units, neonatal services, and critical care. A research year may be optional or a third year may be required by the program director. You should inquire if a third year is required before you apply as this may influence which programs you choose.

Why Subspecialize?

There are many reasons why you might choose to pursue a subspecialty. While you may enjoy the practice of pediatrics or emergency medicine, you may wish to have an area of special expertise where you are viewed as an expert. It gives you an area of expertise and allows you to develop additional educational and research skills. Most importantly, you choose a subspecialty because you enjoy caring for and advocating for children.

Other reasons to subspecialize include the opportunity to work in a clinical setting where you might otherwise be excluded. For example, if you completed an emergency medicine training program, you may be less likely to work in a children's hospital emergency department. However, if you complete the subspecialty training in pediatric emergency medicine, you have a wider choice of emergency departments in which to work. As with any subspecialty, your personal curiosity, desire for in-depth knowledge in a particular content area of emergency medicine, and professional satisfaction are the key reasons to choose pediatric emergency medicine as your subspecialty.

Professional Opportunities

The variety of job opportunities has grown tremendously over the past 5 years. Many academic, children's, and general acute care hospitals are seeking pediatric emergency medicine specialists.

In addition, the unique knowledge obtained from fellowship training opens up a wide variety of opportunities outside of the practice of medicine. These include not only teaching opportunities both nationally and internationally but also consulting opportunities for hospital systems desiring to expand their pediatric capabilities, medicolegal opportunities, and advisory roles with state, national, and federal agencies.

Caring for children requires meticulous attention to detail, but their ability to recover from serious illness and injury makes it worthwhile. By saving a child's life or restoring his/her health, you appreciate the rewards of the practice of pediatric emergency medicine.

chapter 36

Geriatric Emergency Medicine

Michael Stern, MD
Instructor of Medicine, Cornell University Weill Medical College, New York-Presbyterian Hospital

Neal Flomenbaum, MD, FACP, FACEP
Emergency Physician-in-Chief, Professor of Clinical Medicine
Cornell University Weill Medical College, New York-Presbyterian Hospital

What Is Geriatric Emergency Medicine, and Why Is It Important?

According to the most recent U.S. Census Bureau data, there are currently more than 35 million people aged 65 and over, or 13% of the population, living in the United States. By 2030, this percentage will increase to approximately 21% of the population, or 76 million people. Moreover, the fastest growing segment of the population is the age group of 85 years and older.

Compared with previous generations, older people today are living longer and healthier lives, with lower rates of disability and poverty and remaining independent and highly functional well past retirement. Advances in health education, technology, and medicine have enabled the elderly to survive longer and better with chronic medical conditions such as heart disease, diabetes, depression, and arthritis. At the same time, many of the elderly still suffer from functional impairment, chronic underlying illness, and acute exacerbations of chronic illnesses that cause them to seek emergency care in ever-increasing numbers.

The elderly currently account for 18% of emergency department visits nationwide. The complexity of their clinical presentation and evaluation, their consumption of emergency department resources, their length of stay in the emergency department, and their rates of inpatient admission to the hospital are all significantly higher for the elderly than for younger patients. And it is expected that in the future, older patients will increasingly rely on the emergency department for both their acute and subacute health care needs.

The emergency physician of the 21st century will require an enhanced skills set and innovative strategies to provide the emergency care necessary for geriatric patients to overcome what some have characterized as a *sentinel event*—a potentially catastrophic illness or occurrence that may be life-threatening and ultimately jeopardizes their ability to return to their former lifestyle. After an emergency department visit, geriatric patients can experience a functional decline and a reduction in their health-related quality of life. Approximately 25% of elderly patients will return to the emergency department within 90 days of their initial visit. And based on several studies, an emergency department visit by a geriatric patient confers an increase in 1-year mortality. Clearly, this population of elderly emergency patients is particularly vulnerable and requires focused expert care.

Postresidency training in geriatric emergency medicine represents a new attempt to deal with these increasingly frequent issues. Geriatric emergency medicine training focuses

on the unique characteristics of the geriatric emergency patient—the effects of the physiology of aging, the particular pathophysiology of older patients as manifested by special geriatric syndromes and atypical presentations of classic disease states, specific toxicologic emergencies associated with polypharmacy, the problem of oligoanalgesia (the undertreatment of pain) in the emergency department, the impact of comorbidities on both clinical care and outcome, end-of-life issues in the acute care setting, and the complexities of the interface between community, nursing home, and inpatient settings. The emergency physician who develops expertise in these areas will also be in a better position to apply this expertise to similar needs in younger patients as well.

Opportunities in Geriatric Emergency Medicine: A Geriatric Emergency Medicine Fellowship

The primary goals of a currently non-ACGME-accredited geriatric emergency medicine fellowship are (1) to provide recent emergency medicine residency graduates with an understanding of the unique and often complex needs of the large geriatric population who require emergency care and (2) to provide residency-trained emergency medicine physicians with the fundamental skills required to build an academic research career in geriatric emergency medicine through collaboration with nationally respected researchers in divisions of geriatric medicine.

Through a multidisciplinary approach, the geriatric emergency medicine fellow can receive extensive experience in both primary care and consultative care for geriatric patients in numerous health care settings, including emergency departments, inpatient units, nursing homes, clinics, and the patients' homes.

Clinical Component

The geriatric emergency medicine fellow should participate fully in clinical, educational, and research activities in the emergency department. A particular focus in the emergency department is the early recognition and management of the most common geriatric syndromes: falls, dizziness, loss-of-consciousness, delirium, depression, dementia, hip fracture, infection (particularly urinary tract infection and pneumonia), and polypharmacy. The appropriate selection and utilization of assessment tools for the rapid detection of clinically significant cognitive impairment are stressed. Paramount to the fellow's training is the development of an understanding of the impact of comorbidities on the acute event, the atypical clinical presentations, and the tendency of elderly patients to present to the emergency department later in the course of their clinical syndromes or disease states. Another objective is the ability to effectively risk-stratify geriatric patients in terms of disposition (avoiding both the premature discharge from the emergency department and the potential pitfalls and the dangers of an unnecessary hospital admission). Understanding the importance of the psychosocial factors impacting on the treatment and discharge of these patients from the emergency department is a key component of successful management of this segment of the emergency department population.

The geriatric emergency medicine fellow must participate as an active member of the health care team on rounds led by attending geriatric physicians on any inpatient unit dedicated to geriatric patients. Because most of these geriatric inpatients are admitted through the emergency department, effectively dealing with case-specific and general issues at the intersection between emergency treatment and inpatient management is a goal of this rotation. Specific clinical objectives are learning how to most effectively manage such common geriatric inpatient problems as hip fractures (preoperative and postoperative care), rehabilitation, infection, congestive heart failure, atrial fibrillation, coronary artery disease, anticoagulation, pneumonia, chronic obstructive pulmonary disease, acute and chronic renal failure, stroke, deep venous thrombosis and pulmonary embolism, and oncologic care. In addition, gaining a firm knowledge of the ethical and legal issues related to the care of geriatric patients (e.g., do-not-resuscitate orders, advanced directives, and health care proxies) is essential, as is a focus on understanding and utilizing the multidisciplinary team approach to patient care.

Another goal of geriatric emergency medicine training is the improved understanding and practice of palliative care and pain management. The geriatric emergency medicine fellow participates with the Palliative Care Consult Service throughout the hospital for patients at the end-of-life and those suffering from chronic pain syndromes. In addition, the fellow participates with the Geriatric Consult Service to gain experience in the interface between geriatric medicine and the other medical and surgical services to which the emergency department admits elderly patients.

The geriatric emergency medicine fellow also helps provide clinical care to elderly patients in several intensive care units (ICUs), such as the surgical intensive care unit (SICU), medical intensive care unit (MICU), coronary care unit (CCU), and burn unit. On these units, the geriatric emergency medicine fellow focuses on the ICU management of critically ill elderly patients newly admitted from the emergency department. Particular objectives are an understanding of the physiologic reserves of the elderly, pathophysiologic disease states and comorbidities, and their combined effects on clinical care and outcomes. In addition, goals include learning the appropriate utilization of critical care pharmacologic agents and choosing among several alternatives the ones that best address the needs of the elderly. Vasoactive medications and pharmacologic agents for procedural sedation and analgesia, as well as medical instrumentation, hemodynamic monitoring, and mechanical ventilator parameters, should be emphasized. Issues regarding quality of life, end-of-life decisions, withdrawal of care, and effects on and reactions of surviving family members, particularly elderly spouses, are dealt with, as well as the psychosocial aspects of discharged, ill elderly patients returning to the community.

The geriatric emergency medicine fellow should also participate in providing clinical care in state-of-the-art nursing homes and long-term care facilities. There, the fellow can gain clinical experience on in-patient floors, taking "call" at night with the on-call physician responsible for managing emergencies in nursing home patients, and gain a better understanding of the criteria for transferring nursing home residents to the emergency department. At times, the geriatric emergency medicine fellow can help obviate the need for emergency department transfers. The geriatric emergency medicine fellow can also help evaluate new inpatient nursing home clients for elder abuse and participate in the care of patients at the numerous specialty clinics available to their residents. The geriatric emergency medicine fellow should also spend time at a state-of-the-art community-based outpatient care center.

With an increasing number of elderly patients with chronic medical conditions living longer at home, home-based clinical care is steadily gaining ground in the United States. To that end, the geriatric emergency medicine fellow should participate in a house call program that provides health care to older, homebound individuals. In this way, the fellow will better understand the multiple issues that elderly, community-dwelling individuals face in terms of health care access, medication administration, adverse effects and polypharmacy, self-neglect, and environmental considerations (i.e., what constitutes a safe home environment for an elderly person with or without comorbidities).

Educational Component

The geriatric emergency medicine fellow can play a pivotal role as educational liaison between the departments of emergency medicine and geriatrics. Working closely with both the emergency medicine residency program director and the geriatric faculty, the fellow can help develop a geriatric curriculum for the emergency medicine residency that will include a comprehensive written curriculum and detailed bibliography, and a required

residency reading list, as well as a 36-month geriatric emergency medicine lecture cycle. Throughout the year, the geriatric emergency medicine fellow should participate in and help implement a formal emergency medicine didactic curriculum and should present those core content lectures requested by the program director.

Research Component

Early in the fellowship year, a geriatric emergency medicine fellow should be provided with all of the basic tools required for research. The training may begin with a 6- to 8-week intensive didactic program in clinical epidemiology and health sciences research that will provide an introduction and overview to research methodology, biostatistics, databases, decision analysis, qualitative research, and behavioral science and health services research. The geriatric emergency medicine fellow should be required to develop a significant research question, as well as the appropriate methodology, form of statistical analysis, and protocol design to study it, with the goal of obtaining extramural funding. Extending this grounding in clinical research for the geriatric emergency medicine fellow, the physician leaders of the geriatric and emergency medicine departments should supervise the grant application process. All geriatric emergency medicine fellows should be required to prepare an abstract describing the research project and present the findings at a national scientific conference. Upon completion of the project, the fellow is expected to prepare a manuscript for publication in a peer-reviewed journal.

The Future

Geriatric emergency medicine fellowship training at present is still in its infancy, with only one or two programs offering the full range of activities described here. Yet, as a concept, geriatric emergency medicine training has been germinating for several years. The demographics of our aging population, the complex structure of our current health care delivery system, the ever-rapid advancements in biotechnology, pharmaceuticals, and medical knowledge, and the specific utilization patterns of emergency departments by older adults for both acute and chronic problems have all contributed to a sharpening focus on the unique but important characteristics that govern the care of geriatric patients in the emergency setting. Attention is now being paid as never before by health care professionals/experts and politicians on both the local and national stage. Geriatric emergency medicine interest groups convene at hospitals and medical colleges as well as at national medical conferences. The U.S. Department of Health and Human Services has sponsored *Healthy People 2010* to improve the nation's delivery of medical care to the elderly, and both public and private research organizations are funding aging research to an unprecedented extent.

The comprehensive clinical, research, and educational experience that a geriatric emergency medicine fellow obtains from 1 or 2 years of postresidency training will enable the geriatric emergency medicine fellow to become a leader in this exciting new academic discipline. As interest continues to increase, more programs will be started at academic medical institutions across the country, and the likelihood that geriatric emergency medicine fellowship training will become an official ACGME-accredited fellowship will increase. As more emergency physicians are trained in geriatric emergency medicine, elder emergency care will improve. Education regarding this unique population will begin to trickle down to both emergency medicine residents and those training in other medical and surgical specialties. There is currently a huge discrepancy between the percentage of elderly patients seen in the emergency department and the percentage of didactic lectures mandated by residency programs to address geriatric emergency medicine topics. This same glaring gap characterizes the questions on the written board exam given by the American Board of Emergency Medicine (ABEM), where officially only 4% of the total questions address the subject of geriatric patients. In the future, these gaps will narrow in order to ensure the provision of improved care to older patients.

The future of geriatric emergency medicine will also rely heavily on clinical research, as data are necessary not only to elucidate specific characteristics of this population but also eventually to guide evidence-based care. The opportunities in geriatric emergency medicine research are almost limitless. And the potential pool of elderly study subjects is expanding with the population. Historically, geriatric patients have been poorly studied. Few prospective, randomized trials, regardless of the topic, have focused on elderly patients as a specific cohort. The majority existing data are in the form of subgroup analyses of older patients within more-inclusive cohorts. Well-designed studies investigating pertinent diagnostic and treatment questions will surely raise the standard of care for geriatric emergency medicine patients. Not only will the elderly benefit, but our society as a whole will begin to reap the rewards of a healthier, older population.

Geriatric emergency medicine fellowship training may not suit every emergency medicine resident's goals and plans at present, but for a few clear thinking and far-sighted pioneering emergency physicians, the career benefits will be limitless.

chapter 37

Critical Care/Trauma

William C. Chiu, MD
Program Director of Emergency Medicine Critical Care Fellowship,
R Adams Cowley Shock Trauma Center, Baltimore, Maryland

David A. Farcy, MD
Director of Emergency Department Critical Care, Mount Sinai Medical Center, Miami, Florida

Thomas Scalea, MD
Physician-in-Chief, R Adams Cowley Shock Trauma Center, Baltimore, Maryland

Ideally, critically ill patients should receive initial evaluation and stabilization in the emergency department. Soon thereafter, patients should be transferred to an intensive care unit (ICU) to receive further stabilization and definitive care. The emergency department phase of care should be limited to the necessary diagnostic tests, treatment, and initial stabilization. Unfortunately, this is not a reality in many hospitals in the United States. Critically ill patients can remain in the emergency department for many hours or days.

Critical illness is a time-related disease. Over 30 years ago, R. Adams Cowley coined the term "the golden hour" to describe the time-sensitive nature of critical injury.[1] Emanuel Rivers et al.[2] clearly demonstrated that early goal-directed therapy in the emergency department improved long-term survival in patients with septic shock. Although we often segment patient care into phases such as emergency department or ICU treatment, optimal patient management is a continuum of care that should begin at the time of patient presentation.

It is unlikely that the challenge of emergency department crowding of critically ill patients will improve in the near future. Many hospitals designate approximate 10% of inpatient beds as ICUs and an additional 15% as intermediate-care or step-down beds. However, approximately 40% of patients require high-dependency beds and an additional 20% require ICU beds. Critically ill patients consume approximately 33% of the average hospital's resources.[3,4] Some of this demand can be met by the use of dedicated intensivists, who can decrease patient costs, streamline ICU care, decrease morbidity and mortality, and improve patient outcome.[5,6] However, there is a nationwide shortage of critical care physicians. Two-thirds of critically ill patients currently do not receive care from a trained intensivist at any time during their ICU stay.[7] This deficit is predicted to increase with only approximately one-fourth of the demand being met by 2020.[8]

Emergency medicine residency has superb initial triage and stabilization training but is lacking in sufficient longitudinal critical care experience to allow emergency physicians to provide full service critical care in the emergency department or ICU. Training in critical care for emergency physicians has the potential to improve care in critically ill patients presenting to the emergency department and can help solve the current shortage of intensivists.

Critical care is not currently recognized as a board-certified specialty program for emergency physicians in the United States. Boards such as internal medicine, pediatrics, anesthesia, and surgery all have a certification processes allowing trainees in any of these specialties to become certified in critical care, with each specialty administering its own exam. Recently, the American Board of Internal Medicine and the American Board of Pediatrics chose to no longer allow emergency physicians to sit for their critical care certification exam. While there are no current pathways through the American Board of Medical Specialties (ABMS) for an emergency physician to become certified in critical care, an alternative pathway exits through the European Society of Intensive Care Medicine (ESICM). The European exam is a two-part examination. A written multiple-choice examination is taken after 12 months of critical care training, and an oral exam is taken after completion of 24 months of critical care training.

Critical care training is available for emergency physicians. Currently, there are 35 critical care fellowship programs that accept emergency physicians (http://www.acep.org). In 2005, the American Board of Internal Medicine instituted a 6-year residency program that combines emergency medicine, internal medicine, and critical care. This has recently been approved by the ACGME. Currently, only Long Island Jewish Medical Center, Albert Einstein College of Medicine, Henry Ford Hospital, and the University of Maryland Medical Center offer this program.

The fellowship application process is not centralized and there is no fellowship match, so the application process may vary considerably between institutions. Generally, an interested applicant should begin the process when they start their last year of training. However, some programs strongly encourage early application, so individual programs should be contacted to specify application details.

The curriculum varies from institution to institution. Approximately three quarters of the time is typically spent in the various ICUs within the program such as the burn, medical, or neurologic ICU. Electives are offered in related subjects such as radiology, and there is a research requirement at nearly every program.

Job opportunities for the emergency physician trained in critical care are clearly growing. It is likely there will be increased pressure placed on the credentialing process based on the strong recommendation in the Institute of Medicine recent report on emergency care in the United States.[9] The Institute of Medicine recommended that board certification in critical care be made available to any physician who has successfully completed fellowship training.

Emergency physicians trained in critical care are able to find employment in a variety of practice settings. The emergency physician trained in critical care may choose to work exclusively in the emergency department or ICU but may also have a combined practice. Individual hospital bylaws should be examined to determine if board certification is required for staff privileges, and some hospitals may accept the European board certification as a substitute for American medical specialty certification.

Emergency medicine residency training is insufficient on its own to effectively practice in an ICU. However, critical care training for emergency physicians is a natural extension of emergency medicine training and clearly represents the wave of the future.[10-12] The field of critical care medicine will continue to grow in importance as well as in popularity and will almost certainly become an integral part of our health care system.

Resources

EMRA Critical Care Committee: www.emra.org
ACEP Critical Care Section: www.acep.org/webportal/membercenter/sections/ccmed
Coalition for Critical Care Medicine in the Emergency Department (C$_3$MED):
   http://health.groups.yahoo.com/group/C3MED/

References

1. Cowley RA. The resuscitation and stabilization of major multiple trauma patients in a trauma center environment. *Clin Med.* 1976:83:14-22.
2. Rivers E, Nguyen B, Havstad S, et al: Efficacy and safety of recombinant human activated protein C for severe sepsis: the Recombinant Human Protein C Worldwide Evaluation in Severe Sepsis (PROWESS) Study Group. *N Engl J Med.* 2001;344:599-709.
3. Berenson RA. *Intensive care units (ICUs): clinical outcomes, costs, and decision-making (Health Technology Case Study 28).* Prepared for the Office of Technology Assessment, US Congress, OTA-HCS-28. Washington, DC: US Government Printing Office; 1984.
4. Coursin D, Macciloi G, Murray M. Critical care and peri-operative medicine: how goes the flow? *Anesthesiol Clin North Am.* 2000:18:527-538.
5. Reynolds HN, Haupt MT, Thill-Baharozian MC, et al. Impact of critical care physician staffing on patients with septic shock in a university hospital medical intensive care unit. *JAMA.* 1988;206:3446-3450.
6. Hanson CW, Deutschman CS, Anderson HL, et al. Effects of an organized critical care service on outcomes and resource utilization: a cohort study. *Crit Care Med.* 1999;27:270-274.
7. Pingleton SK. Committee on Manpower of Pulmonary and Critical Care Societies: a report to membership. *Chest.* 2001;120:327-328.
8. Angus DC, Kelley MA, Schmitz RJ, et al. Current and projected workforce requirements for care of the critically ill patients with pulmonary disease: can we meet the requirements of an aging population? *JAMA.* 2000;284:2762-2770.
9. Institute of Medicine. *Hospital-based emergency care: at the breaking point.* Washington, DC: Institute of Medicine; 2000.
10. Huang DT, Osborn TM, et al. Critical care medicine training and certification for emergency physicians. *Crit Care Med.* 2005;33:2104-2109 and . *Ann Emerg Med.* 2005;46:217-221.
11. Osborn T, Scalea TM. A call for critical care training of emergency physician. *Ann Emerg Med.* 2002;39:562-565.
12. Bozeman WP, Gaasch WR, Barish RA, et al. Trauma resuscitation/critical care fellowship for emergency physicians: a necessary step for the future of academic emergency medicine. *Acad Emerg Med.* 1999;6:331-333.

chapter 38

Emergency Ultrasound

Jill Corbo, MD, RDMS
Director, Emergency Ultrasound Fellowship, Jacobi Medical Center
Associate Professor of Emergency Medicine, Albert Einstein College of Medicine

Michael J. Lambert, MD, RDMS, FACEP
Fellowship Director, Emergency Ultrasound, Resurrection Medical Center, Chicago, Illinois

Joseph P. Wood, MD, JD, RDMS, FACEP
Mayo Clinic, Arizona

Emergency medicine was formally recognized as a distinct specialty in September 1979. As a specialty, we are devoted to the swift recognition and prompt and appropriate care of medical and surgical problems. By its nature, the scope of our practice has always overlapped with that of other specialties. For example, while we do not provide the full panoply of services offered by cardiologists, we are skilled in ECG analysis and the clinical evaluation of patients presenting with acute chest pain. In the same vein, while we do not provide the same spectrum of diagnostic ultrasound found in radiology departments, emergency physicians have demonstrated they can perform skillful screening ultrasound exams at the bedside. The literature has demonstrated that where emergency departments are equipped with a portable ultrasound unit, and the physicians possess the necessary skills to perform and interpret bedside studies, patient care is enhanced in the following ways:

- Time to definitive diagnoses of life-threatening conditions (e.g., hemopericardium or abdominal aortic aneurysm) is greatly reduced.
- Emergency department length of stay is significantly reduced for pregnant patients with first-trimester pain or bleeding and patients experiencing abdominal pain secondary to cholelithiasis or cholecystitis.
- Patient satisfaction is improved because of the reduction in waiting times for diagnostic imaging, a better understanding of their disease process, and the increased time spent with the emergency physician performing the ultrasound study.

The key to performing safe and effective ultrasound studies in the emergency department is to limit the scope of the examination by answering simple questions in a focused study. The time constraints of a busy emergency department preclude us from performing comprehensive diagnostic imaging studies. However, it has been demonstrated that emergency physicians can use bedside ultrasound swiftly and accurately to determine the following:

- Is there an intrauterine pregnancy?
- Are gallstones present?
- Is hydronephrosis present?

- Does the patient have an abdominal aortic aneurysm?
- Is there fluid in the pericardial sac?
- Is there evidence of a deep vein thrombosis?
- Is there vascular compromise to an ovary or a teste?
- Is there fluid in the peritoneal cavity?

Emergency physicians who limit themselves to answering a focused question with one of three answers ("yes," "no," "indeterminate") will find bedside ultrasound enormously helpful in clinical decision-making and rarely will make mistakes. Because there is more potential harm in making a misdiagnosis than an indeterminate conclusion, emergency physicians should seek confirmatory studies when the results of the bedside exam are indeterminate. This approach of "picking the bottom fruit" is no different than one employed by many community hospitals in which emergency physicians interpret extremity radiographs, but consult with a staff radiologist via teleradiography on head CT scans.

While there have been inevitable "turf battles" between radiologists and emergency physicians, these boundaries have been resolved effectively by AMA Resolution 802, which states diagnostic ultrasound belongs to no single specialty. This position requires each specialty to promulgate policies addressing the training and credentialing standards to match the scope of ultrasound practice within the specialty. Since then, the clinical application of ultrasound by the emergency physician has greatly expanded. Ultrasound is now considered a part of the core content of emergency medicine, and virtually every emergency medicine residency program offers some training. Programs that have a faculty member with appropriate protected time devoted to ultrasound education and research will be in the best position to ensure its residents receive appropriate training and experience prior to commencement.

There is no set national training standard at this time; however, guidelines have been suggested by each of the governing bodies of emergency medicine. The American College of Emergency Physicians (ACEP) recommends that residency include both training in acquisition and image interpretation. Credentialing consists of 25 to 50 documented and reviewed ultrasound examinations per primary application and 150 examinations for general privileges. The Society for Academic Emergency Medicine has a policy stating a board-certified emergency physician who has completed 40 hours of didactic training and performed 150 exams should be eligible for hospital credentialing in emergency department ultrasonography.

Postgraduating training in emergency ultrasonography usually entails a 1-year fellowship following the completion of an emergency medicine residency. Over the past decade, over 18 new fellowship programs in the United States have been created. Because emergency ultrasonography is not an ACGME-recognized subspecialty, components of each training program will vary. Most fellowships include performing and interpreting ultrasounds, quality assurance and review, education, and research. In 2005, ACEP established guidelines for emergency ultrasound fellowships that include a minimum of 800 ultrasound examinations, at least one research project with submission to a national meeting such as ACEP or SAEM, one interdepartmental quality assurance work/project, and three separate lectures on emergency ultrasound to their department (available at: http://www.acep.org/webportal/PracticeResources/PolicyStatements/pracmgt/UseofUlt rasoundImagingbyEmergencyPhysicians.htm). Many fellowship programs also require certification by the American Registry for Diagnostic Medical Sonography examination (ARDMS). (See Web site for more information: http:/www.ardms.org).

Emergency screening ultrasound is now a nationally accepted tool for the rapid assessment of the emergency patient. Emergency ultrasound has been incorporated in residency training and numerous fellowship programs have been created. Emergency medicine focuses on diagnosis and treatment of acute illnesses and injuries that require immediate medical attention. Emergency ultrasound affords emergency physicians the tool with which to provide this service.

chapter 39

Palliative Medicine

Susan C. Stone, MD, MPH
Associate Professor of Clinical Emergency Medicine, Director of Palliative Care
Los Angeles County Medical Center and Keck School of Medicine of the University of Southern California

Palliative medicine is the discipline of medicine that specializes in care of patients with incurable and end-stage illness. The patients for whom a palliative care physician cares are often seen in emergency departments. For example, patients with advanced congestive heart failure, cancer, chronic obstructive pulmonary disease, or dementia may initially come to the emergency department, and during evaluation, a palliative care consult may be called to provide pain and symptom management recommendations and to help guide discussions about advance directives or further care. Additionally, the consultant can determine hospice eligibility or may even be on staff at a hospice.

As of June 2006, there are a total of 49 active programs with 119 fellowship positions. Fellowships are typically 1 year in length, and for applicants intending to stay in an academic setting, a 2-year fellowship may be completed. The second year provides an opportunity to participate in research but is not a requirement for board certification. The fellowship programs offer a year of experience in the key competencies required to be a specialist in hospice and palliative care. Overall, time will be spent on inpatient consult services, in outpatient settings, and with hospice programs in the community. While covering the inpatient service, consults may involve care for patients in the emergency department. The outpatient experience may involve a clinic or office setting, and the hospice experience will include home visits to patients who have chosen to receive comfort care in the home. Many programs will offer experience working with the pain service. The American Academy of Hospice and Palliative Medicine Fellowship Program Directory is available at http://www.aahpm.org/fellowship/directory.html.

The American Board of Hospice and Palliative Medicine (ABHPM) was formed in 1995 to establish and implement standards for the certification of physicians practicing hospice and palliative medicine. ABHPM creates and administers the certifying examination, works to implement high standards for training, and contributes to setting the standards for excellence in palliative medicine. In 2006, the American Board of Medical Specialties (ABMS) accepted the hospice and palliative medicine examination for certification. Currently, there are 10 ABMS boards, including emergency medicine, that serve as a prerequisite to fellowship training. After completion of a fellowship, the examination is administered annually. The Society for Academic Emergency Medicine currently has a Palliative Care Interest Group, which is a source of education and for meeting other emergency physicians interested in this growing specialty. Additionally, there is research being conducted by several emergency physicians on integrating palliative care education into the current practice of all emergency providers.

Regarding career options, palliative care can be practiced alongside emergency medicine or as a full-time career. Some emergency physicians work on consult services in the hospital or in outpatient clinics. Another option is to work as a medical director of a hospice. The training in emergency medicine dovetails into the palliative care practice, because rapid assessment and treatment of complex symptoms are core to emergency medicine.

Additionally, training in the critical care aspects of emergency medicine is very useful when providing consultation to the ICU teams or even in the emergency department. Think of the intubated patient with a severe head injury who is not improving and the many issues regarding pain assessment and management, family dynamics, and other difficult topics that may arise, such as code status. Clearly, there is tremendous overlap.

chapter 40

Emergency Medical Services

Jeremy T. Cushman, MD, MS
Past President, EMRA
Director, EMS Fellowship, Division of EMS and Office of Prehospital Care
Department of Emergency Medicine, University of Rochester School of Medicine and Dentistry

Joshua Moskovitz, MD, MPH
University at Maryland

Emergency medical services (EMS) is an important component of the specialty of emergency medicine. It encompasses numerous areas of prehospital and interhospital care, and in many ways is an extension of the emergency department. Seen by many as the subspecialty nestled at the crossroads of emergency medical care, public safety, and public health, EMS has many unique opportunities for physician involvement.

EMS Systems and Medical Direction

The structure of EMS systems varies widely across the United States as there are no federal statutes dictating system composition; however, their operation is generally consistent from locale to locale. There are multiple levels of providers within each system, from certified first responder (CFR) to emergency medical technician (EMT) and paramedic with progressive increases in skills and abilities to render out-of-hospital care. Systems provide varying levels of care, from basic life support (BLS) to advanced life support (ALS) and may be configured as commercial, volunteer, fire-based, municipal, or public utility services.

Each EMS system has a medical director, but their role within the specific agency can vary from minimal to intricate involvement in daily activities. EMS medical direction has historically been a volunteer role; however, the quality of an EMS system is often directly related to the involvement of the EMS medical director in system operations. As a result, more and more agencies are compensating medical directors for their professional services and increasing their oversight and role within the EMS system.

The medical director provides guidance in two forms: online and offline medical direction. On-line medical direction is the form of directing patient care to prehospital providers via real-time voice communications using radio or telephone. Off-line medical control is the process of deriving preestablished policies, protocols, and procedures for the provision of medical care. This includes both "standing orders" and criteria delineating when to call on-line medical control for authorization to perform certain procedures or administer certain medications. With medical direction comes the important responsibility of continuous quality improvement, whereby the medical director in concert with the agency use a review process to identify concerns in patient care, system improvement, and training needs.

In addition to providing medical direction, EMS physicians may be involved in disaster planning, preparedness, and response for their local /regional agency; are involved in fire and rescue operations; respond to certain scenes and mass casualty incidents to

render out of hospital care; provide direct patient care in both ground and air ambulances; are involved with area hospitals and organizations to determine alternative sources of care; work with the 911 system to refine emergency medical dispatch protocols and procedures for dispatching the appropriate prehospital resources; and work with interfacility transport services and specialty transport teams. EMS physicians are also integral in prehospital provider training and system quality improvement.

EMS Fellowships

EMS physicians and medical directors provide more than just clinical care. A thorough understanding of prehospital operations, disaster preparedness and response, oversight and training responsibilities, medicolegal implications of prehospital care, protocol development, and local, state, and federal guidelines applicable to prehospital care are required. As a result, the last decade has noted a proliferation of EMS fellowships for emergency medicine residency-trained graduates.

There is currently no subspecialty certification for prehospital or disaster medicine, and completion of a fellowship in EMS, prehospital care, or disaster medicine is considered a certificate of added qualification. Fellowship training is particularly useful for individuals seeking to become medical director of a large agency or system or interested in academic pursuits as an EMS physician.

EMS fellowships are sponsored by one or more institutions and may be 1 or 2 years in length. Two-year programs often require coursework leading to a master's degree in public health, business administration, research, or emergency health services. There is no accreditation body for EMS fellowships, although SAEM sponsors the Medtronic/PhysioControl EMS Fellowship program and fellowships approved as an SAEM-approved training site have completed a detailed application and peer-review process ensuring a diverse and comprehensive fellowship curriculum. It is thus extremely important for the potential applicant to carefully evaluate the fellowship program to ensure that it meets one's individual training needs.

The fellowship curriculum typically includes the following content areas: history of EMS; legislation and legal issues specific to prehospital care; EMS system design; air medical transport; personnel/human resources; financial aspects of prehospital and interhospital care; equipment familiarization; training requirements of providers and how to become an effective EMS educator; communications technologies, equipment, and procedures; disaster management; role of EMS in public health; on-line and off-line medical direction including quality assurance, emergency medical dispatch, and agency operations; EMS research; participation in EMS field operations including mass casualty incidents, mass gathering events, and disasters; and familiarization with hazardous materials and fire ground operations. It is important that the fellowship have not only didactic instruction on these core content areas but also extensive hands-on experience and participation in all of these activities during the fellowship. Further, the program should foster the fellow''s leadership development through involvement in local, regional, state, and national organizations.

The EMS fellow typically works 10 to 12 hours per week clinically as an attending physician in the emergency department, which is necessary to maintain one's clinical skills. Additional opportunities for training through the fellowship may include tactical operations, urban search and rescue, high angle/specialty rescue, disaster medical assistance teams, and other unique subspecialties of prehospital and disaster medicine.

Emergency medicine is inextricably tied to EMS and provides a unique area of subspecialization for interested physicians. The diversity of fellowship training is reflective of the many areas of expertise required to provide medical direction and oversight of prehospital and interhospital care. Whether it is disaster planning or quality assurance reviews, scene response, or mass gathering medical care, the variety and intensity of experience are unparalleled and offer a unique opportunity to provide medical care at the crossroads of public health and safety.

chapter 41

Disaster Medicine

Christopher A. Kahn, MD
Fellow, Emergency Medical Services and Disaster Medical Sciences
Department of Emergency Medicine, University of California, Irvine

Kristi L. Koenig, MD, FACEP
Professor of Clinical Emergency Medicine, Director of Public Health Preparedness
Co-Director, EMS and Disaster Medical Sciences Fellowship
Department of Emergency Medicine, University of California, Irvine

Hurricane Katrina, the terrorist attacks of 9/11, or the Southeast Asia tsunami—each of these events requires expertise in the field of disaster medicine, one of the newest emerging subspecialties of emergency medicine. Emergency physicians have clinical training to manage a wide spectrum of emergencies and also nonemergent patients without access to regular medical care. In addition, emergency medicine teaches physicians how to think in systems and deal with populations of patients as well as individuals. These features make emergency physicians uniquely qualified to train in disaster medicine. Although currently less than a dozen exist nationwide, postresidency fellowships in disaster medicine are becoming increasingly common, sometimes in combination with EMS or other training (such as international emergency medicine). Disaster medicine is a multidisciplinary specialty; management of disasters extends beyond the traditional field of emergency medicine and involves public health, community emergency management, law enforcement, and cooperation with a wide array of stakeholders. Disaster fellows are trained in both research and operational aspects of disaster management to include mitigating, preparing for, responding to, and recovering from a disaster. In addition, an understanding of administration and legislative authorities at all levels (local, state, and federal) is a key component of disaster fellowship education. Fellows work with several distinct groups of people, each with an interest in protecting the community from the effects of disasters.

Although clinical skills during a disaster have some unique aspects, disaster medicine fellowships spend little time on imparting a clinical skills set, and much more time on teaching a methodology for planning, advocacy, education, and research. The disaster medicine physician is a useful resource for helping communities develop disaster response plans, research better ways to respond to disasters, and assist government officials with setting funding priorities which affect future policies and legislation. Accordingly, some fellowships include master's-level training in public health or public administration.

Research is an important aspect of a disaster medicine fellowship. The subspecialty is still in its infancy and little science underlies many of the assumptions currently made in disaster management worldwide. It is generally not feasible to perform a prospective, randomized controlled study of a disaster, so appropriate research methodologies are being developed to form an academic foundation for the science of disaster medicine. Many disaster plans are based on "lessons learned" from observing prior disasters, rather than on

scientifically derived and tested hypotheses. Unfortunately, the "lessons learned" often are the same from one disaster to another, suggesting that this terminology is outdated because lessons may not be learned at all. A major focus of current disaster medicine fellowships is to build a scientific basis for disaster medicine.

Response to disasters is also a common feature of disaster medicine fellowships, whether as part of a formal government resource such as a disaster medical assistance team or urban search and rescue task force, or as part of local and regional groups. Although these responses are, by their nature, sporadic and unpredictable, most fellowships will attempt to allow the fellows to respond to disasters as part of their education.

After completing a fellowship, many disaster medicine physicians choose academic careers, combining clinical work with research, education, advocacy, and disaster response. However, it is also possible to be an important local community resource for disaster planning while working in a nonacademic setting. Given their unpredictability, very few physicians focus solely on clinical response to disasters.

At this time, no central resource describing disaster medicine fellowships exists. The Society for Academic Emergency Medicine maintains a list of fellowships. However, given the rapid changes in the field of disaster medicine, this list is likely to be incomplete when you are considering your fellowship training. You may wish to discuss your fellowship plans with a mentor at your institution who is familiar with disaster medicine and who may be able to help you find a fellowship program that suits your needs. Also, interest groups for disaster medicine can be found within the major emergency medicine organizations and are likely to prove a valuable resource for residents contemplating a career in disaster medicine.

chapter 42

Air Medical Transport

Kenneth Robinson, MD, FACEP
Medical Director, Program Director, LIFE STAR, Hartford Hospital, Hartford, CT
Associate Professor, Department of Traumatology and Emergency Medicine
University of Connecticut School of Medicine; Past President, AMPA

James C. Suozzi, DO, NREMT-P
Emergency Medicine Resident
Integrated Residency in Emergency Medicine at the University of Connecticut

Kenneth A Williams, MD, FACEP
Medical Director, Lifeguard EMS Rhode Island Hospital, Providence, RI; Associate Professor
Emergency Medicine, The Warren Alpert Medical School of Brown University; Past President, AMPA

History of Air Medical Transport

Air medical transport can be traced to World War I, when Serbian patients were evacuated in a French fighter plane. By World War II, air medical transport became an integral part of military medicine when the allies evacuated large numbers of casualties by fixed wing aircraft. The first documented helicopter evacuation occurred during the latter stages of World War II in Burma. By the time of the Korean and Vietnam conflicts, helicopter transport of wounded soldiers became an essential part of the military's trauma system. The successful use of helicopter air medical transport in the Vietnam conflict led to the development of civilian helicopter EMS programs. In 1969, the Maryland State Police in conjunction with the University of Maryland began the first air medical transport program in the United States. Currently, there are approximately 251 air medical transport programs in the United States, transporting about 450,000 patients annually.

Description of Air Medical Transport

Air medical transport is the use of aircraft, both helicopters and fixed-wing airplanes, to move and care for patients. It is a growing and evolving field for which there are progressively more indications for utilization. There are four subcategories of air medical transport:

1. *Helicopter EMS* (HEMS) response to the incident scene, occasionally including hoist rescue or similar operations, with patient transport typically to tertiary care/trauma center emergency departments

2. *Helicopter interfacility* transportation, where a patient is cared for during transport between hospitals, typically to receive higher-level care at a tertiary receiving hospital

3. *Fixed wing* transports, where a patient is flown (typically over longer distances and/or through more challenging weather than with helicopter transport) between airports near sending and receiving hospitals. Typically, ground

ambulances or helicopters are used to transport the patient from hospital to airport.

4. *Commercial fixed wing* transports, where a patient is accompanied by medical personnel during flight on a scheduled commercial aircraft. These patients are typically transported for long distances and are less ill than are patients flown in a dedicated fixed-wing aircraft.

Most types of EMS helicopters have a range of about 150 nautical miles. In rural areas, when the weather precludes helicopter flight or when the most appropriate tertiary care is a significant distance from the referring facility, airplanes (fixed-wing) are used. Commercial airlines are also used to transport patients; this practice is more common elsewhere in the world than in the United States and involves a designated section of the airplane configured to accommodate a patient and medical crew in some cases. In other cases, the patient is well enough to be accompanied in regular seating.

Ground critical care transportation (GCCT) is also commonly thought of as part of air medical transport because many of the GCCT systems developed out of existing air medical transport programs as a means to provide the same high level of care in a ground ambulance. GCCT is useful for shorter transport distances, urban transport, and certain complex cases and when weather precludes helicopter flight.

Air medical transport and GCCT offer the highest level of out-of-hospital patient care. In the case of air medical transport, this mode is also the fastest way to move a patient between two facilities or from the scene to a hospital when distance and landing zone parameters are optimal. GCCT is often more rapid over shorter distances and when landing zones are inconvenient. Critical care transport crews are highly trained and in most systems are prepared to care for a wide range of patients, including all ages from neonatal through adult and with most critical illnesses and injuries and including acute stroke, myocardial infarction, sepsis, shock, trauma, intracranial hemorrhage, and the high-risk obstetrical patient. The air medical helicopter or fixed wing is internally configured to duplicate the medical care and monitoring capabilities of an intensive care unit, as are dedicated ground critical care ambulances.

The indications for air medical transport continue to expand as new, time-dependent interventions are developed and as health care systems become increasingly specialized and regionalized. Patients qualifying for air medical transport have a need for either the aircraft (due to a remote or island location, congested or weather-impaired roads, time-critical condition), the crew (need for highest level of out-of-hospital care), or both. In most cases, the patient is critically ill or injured and therefore requires rapid transportation and the highest level of out-of-hospital care available.

Role of Physicians in Air Medical Transport

All physicians should have a basic understanding of air medical transport system capabilities and availability. This knowledge is important for the safe and effective air medical referral of patients or receipt of patients from air medical transfer. In addition to basic system history and operations, flight physicians must be knowledgeable about safe aircraft operations, clinical care in the aviation environment, altitude physiology, and a variety of other topics. The Air Medical Physician Association and the National Association of EMS Physicians have collaborated on developing this core curriculum for flight physicians.

Medical direction of an air medical program requires even more training and experience, including management, legal issues, quality improvement systems, billing and finance, and other topics needed to safely and properly lead a program.

The role of the physician in air medical transport varies widely. Some participate only as the referring physician, while others partake in direct patient care as the flight physician or system supervision as the program medical director. Air medical transport systems are present throughout the country, and all emergency physicians will have frequent interactions with the system and flight crews as the referring or receiving physician. All emergency physicians should have at least a fundamental understanding of the structure of the local air medical transport system, the indications for appropriate utilization, and the capabilities of the local flight crews.

Aside from the referring or receiving physician, physicians can serve as a flight physician, medical director, program director, or administrator of a transport system or state EMS system. A number of studies have shown that medical crews consisting of a nurse, paramedic, or respiratory therapist can be trained to provide care equivalent to that of a physician in the out-of-hospital setting so long as there is committed physician medical direction. Most systems in the United States use nurses, paramedics, or respiratory therapists for their flight crew. There are a few programs that use physicians, either residents or attendings, as part of the regular flight crew. In this role, the flight physician provides and directs patient care during transport.

Every air medical transport program requires a medical director. This physician is ultimately responsible for all care provided by the medical crew. The medical director determines the standards of care or medical protocols used by the flight crew. In addition, he or she provides initial and recurrent training. This person also retrospectively reviews all activity of the medical crew to determine appropriate utilization and opportunities for further education. In many flight programs, the program director is also a physician, but this role does not necessarily have to be filled by a physician. The program director is responsible for all operations of the transport program, including business management, hiring and coaching/mentoring, marketing, and strategic planning. Last, some physicians involved in air medical transport have become medical directors of larger systems or of state EMS systems.

Requirements for a Physician in Air Medical Transport

The training necessary for a physician involved in air medical transport is dependent on the role the physician plays in the transport system. The referring or receiving physician must have knowledge of the indications for air medical transport as well as the capabilities of the flight crew and aircraft. The flight physician role requires competency in a wide range of medical conditions and emergency procedures. In addition, this physician must have significant training in safety issues and have a strong understanding of issues related to the role of air medical transport in the local EMS/health care system as well as a working knowledge of altitude physiology. A prerequisite for a medical director is the knowledge base and skills of the flight physician. Additionally, the medical director must have training in educating medical professionals and in mentoring and coaching and must be very collaborative. Because air medical transport systems have matured and are so complex, the knowledge base and skills necessary for the medical director are mostly commonly gained in postresidency fellowship in air medical transport or EMS.

Air Medical Experience in Emergency Medicine Residencies

Emergency medicine residency programs differ widely with respect to the exposure to air medical transport that they provide for the residents. Some training programs have no exposure to air medical transport other than the occasional transport of patients into or out of their institution. Residencies based at hospitals with flight programs often offer more significant exposure to air medical transport. This participation may be flying with the team as an observer or in a program of graded responsibility of the resident on the flight crew. Residents in programs with close relationships with an air medical transport program may serve as an integral member of the flight crew. At these programs, there is a resident on every flight and the resident is often the team leader.

The medical student or resident interested in pursuing a career in air medical transport should seek a residency that provides a significant exposure to air medicine. A program in which the resident flies as an integral member of the flight team is optimal. The 2 to 3 years of experience as a flight physician will provide a solid understanding of the role of air medicine in a health care system and will be invaluable throughout his or her career. A fellowship in air medical transport or EMS is also recommended in order to fully learn and experience the administrative and leadership responsibilities of the medical director of an air medical transport program.

Air Medical Fellowships

A fellowship in air medical transport or EMS provides not only the education but also the initial credibility necessary for beginning a career in air medical transport. Air medical transport fellowships and EMS fellowships often have unique curricula. Each training site will have expertise in different educational opportunities; therefore, the educational experience will differ. The prospective fellow should determine which aspects of air medical transport or EMS are most interesting and find a fellowship that emphasizes those aspects of the specialty. The length of such a fellowship varies from 1 to 2 years. A fellowship focusing solely on air medical transport may be 1 year, whereas a combined air and ground fellowship or a fellowship that includes an MPH in the curriculum may be 2 years. The curricula for air medical transport and EMS fellowships vary widely and may include any or all of the following educational opportunities: experience as the medical crew leader on a helicopter or fixed wing or ground ambulance; instruction and experience with administrating the local EMS or air medical transport service; interaction with local, state, and federal regulatory agencies; and experience with other local municipal agencies, military operations such as the Coast Guard, and tactical EMS teams. Another goal of fellowships is to teach the basics of research and most fellowships require participation in research activities. Last, most fellowships include opportunities for teaching local medical students, residents, and EMS providers.

chapter 43

Wilderness Medicine

Paul Auerbach, MD, FACEP
Clinical Professor of Surgery, Division of Emergency Medicine, Stanford University School of Medicine

Jay Lemery, MD
Director, Wilderness and Environmental Medicine Division
New York Presbyterian –Weill Cornell Medical Center

Over the past few decades, the field of wilderness medicine has become increasingly recognized as a medical subspecialty. Professional societies have formed with the goal of promotion of the field and collaboration among its practitioners. Commercial groups have been successful in marketing wilderness medicine training courses to health care practitioners from first responders to physicians.

Many of these changes have been due to shifts in our society and, thus, our patient demographics. There has been a tremendous increase in environmental recreation. Visits are increasing at the national parks and recreation areas, more people are participating in "extreme" and "ecochallenge" sports, and there has been a proliferation and success of groups offering outdoor experiences (National Outdoor Leadership School [NOLS] and Outward Bound). The demographics of people venturing into the backcountry are evolving. With the graying of America and the Baby Boomer generation, the complexity of wilderness medicine-related injuries has increased. Simple orthopedic injuries on the trail now are more likely to present along with diabetes, osteoporosis, and coronary artery disease. With the geriatrification of patients comes the increase in the mobility of our society. Patients are frequently seeking care for injuries and illnesses sustained thousands of miles away in remote and exotic locations. Not only do many wilderness medicine maladies have delayed sequelae, but also patients will seek follow-up care at their home institutions. In a sense, patients are increasingly bringing the wilderness to you, whether you work in Montana or in New York City.

What does all this mean for the graduating emergency physician? Commensurate with these changes, there have never been more opportunities for physicians to practice wilderness medicine.

The Wilderness Medical Society (WMS) began in 1983 with the goal of promoting wilderness medicine education to health care providers in all areas. Its motto is "combining your profession with your passion," and that perhaps best represents the myriad of opportunities for new physicians. One of the most significant considerations regarding a career in wilderness medicine will be dictated by your financial profile. Many opportunities in remote and exotic locales will offer innumerable rewards, although substantial remuneration will not be one of them. Recent graduates with debt may not have the schedule flexibility to work outside an emergency medicine practice, although opportunities do exist to work in practices proximal to rugged and rural environments, and agencies such as the Indian Health Service will arrange for debt repayment for physicians who commit to practicing in these areas for a set time period.

The following is a discussion of other strategies to incorporate wilderness medicine into your emergency medicine career.

Academic Wilderness Medicine

Many academic medical centers are active centers of wilderness medicine education and research. There are dozens or courses around the United States where medical faculty teach residents and/or medical students the basics of wilderness medicine. Most of these courses are active in outdoor, hands-on, scenario-based education. The preponderance of these courses last from 1 to four weeks, and the longer ones will change geographic locales to stress the different environmental challenges of alpine versus desert versus coastal areas. Two excellent resources for course offerings are the WMS Web site (www.wms.org) and a recent detailed review by Morton and Marshall.[1] There are likewise many institutions active in wilderness medicine research from all over the United States, Canada, and Europe. The most relevant papers can be found in the peer-reviewed journals *Wilderness & Environmental Medicine* and *High Altitude Medicine* or at national wilderness medicine conferences (most prominently run by the Wilderness Medical Society or California ACEP).

There are currently two 1-year academic fellowships in wilderness medicine, at Stanford University and the University of Utah, which both stress an emphasis on original research, clinical experience, and wilderness medicine education. There are many other wilderness medicine-related fellowships that emergency medicine graduates have pursued, including hyperbaric and undersea medicine, space medicine, international emergency medicine, aviation medicine, and EMS/prehospital care. Two programs in aerospace medicine are presently available at the University of Texas Medical Branch/NASA and Wright State University School of Medicine.

Disaster Preparedness and Wilderness Medicine

Although this topic is still virgin territory, the potential for explosive growth in this field is so vast that it should be considered a separate career path. How is wilderness medicine related to disaster preparedness? The recent national disasters of an unprecedented scale (the attacks of September 11 and Hurricane Katrina) have had tremendous impacts on our government priorities, and disaster response planning has become a national mandate at the federal, state, and local levels. In 2007 alone, the Department of Homeland Security will award more than $1.6 billion in grants to encourage such initiatives, and planners have realized that knowledge of wilderness medicine skills—and its emphasis on medical improvisation and treatment in austere conditions—is an integral part of a disaster response strategy.[2] Many EMS systems are now incorporating wilderness medicine skills as part of their disaster training. Opportunities abound through federal grants and thought medical advisory roles for physicians with an interest in wilderness medicine to create research and/or training programs for disaster response teams.

Advisory Positions

Although lucrative jobs in wilderness medicine may be difficult to come by, the demand for advisory roles is not, and this is an excellent and readily available way for career emergency physicians to partake in wilderness medicine and diversify their careers beyond the hospital setting. Almost every community in the United States must deal with extreme weather conditions and natural disasters specific to that area. Community lectures on heat and/or cold stress is a simple place to start that can foster goodwill for you and your profession, as well as provide a valuable educational service. Advisory roles to local authorities, be they urban parks or larger state parks, are always appreciated, and lectures to EMS, fire crews, or rangers are an excellent way to practice wilderness medicine on a local level. Larger municipalities on the county and state level will need medical advisement for search and rescue, backcountry evacuation, and air transport protocols.

There are a plethora of outdoor groups on a local, regional, or national level, such as local summer camps, YMCA, Adirondack Mountain Club, US Lifeguard Association, National Ski Patrol, National Association for Search & Rescue, and thousands others, that serve millions of outdoor enthusiasts, and these are ideal places for an emergency physician to offer consultation. The networking potential and benefits to interaction with such groups can provide many returns to one's career. For those with a more flexible schedule, international groups such as the Himalayan Rescue Association offer a chance to provide care to an underserved population of Nepal and to foreign climbers in one of the most majestic areas of the world.

Commercial Opportunities

There are ways to turn your knowledge of wilderness medicine into a profit. Private organizations that teach wilderness medicine courses to all comers have been quite successful over the past few decades. Groups such as SOLO, WMA (Wilderness Medicine Associates), and NOLS have made commercial success in their educational courses. Through continuing medical education (CME) courses via an academic institution (ACEP) or through a private travel company, many physicians have created a profitable niche for themselves (or subsidized their vacations) through guest lecturing and/or running these courses. Beyond the CME opportunities, there is a smaller market of expedition groups looking for medical support on their trips. Whether in the form of a commercial expedition (providing medical care for paid customers), a research or extreme recreation team (e.g., climbing uncharted Antarctic peaks), or a private group adventure, physicians are valuable and sought-after members of these organizations. One word of caution: the medical liability of treating people in these settings can be as dubious as the settings themselves, and a thorough contractualization of legal consequences should be undertaken by all parties prior to the trip.

Another potential commercial opportunity can be in the form of authorship of wilderness medicine-related topics to the daily press, periodicals, or even the televised media. Wilderness medicine topics are often dramatic and sexy to the general public. A physician with developed writing skills combined with the medical understanding may easily market his or her skills toward journalism. On a lesser scale, news crews and journalists are often looking for commentary on topical wilderness events. Stories of the latest heat wave or that lost hiker in the mountains will often include "expert" testimony from a wilderness medicine practitioner.

Military

Perhaps the largest and most consistent place where wilderness medicine is practiced on a daily basis is in the military. It is here that some of the most important research on wilderness medicine originates. Although the military services actively teach wilderness medicine courses, many preclude civilian participation.

Summary

Wilderness medicine is a field as varied as the diverse planet we inhabit and offers career opportunities on many levels. As you finish residency and are newly formulating your practice path, seek a niche that will sustain you professionally and philosophically. Not only will you find personal fulfillment, but your patients will reap the benefit from a physician in balance between his or her work and life.

References

1. Morton PM, Marshall JP. Wilderness medicine education for the physician. *Emerg Med Clin North Am.* 2004;22:539-559.
2. US Department of Homeland Security Web site: http://www.ojp.usdoj.gov/odp/.

chapter 44

Hyperbaric Medicine

Stephen R. Thom, MD, PhD, FACEP
Professor of Emergency Medicine and Chief, Hyperbaric Medicine
University of Pennsylvania Medical Center

Undersea and hyperbaric medicine is one of the newest subspecialties in emergency medicine. Currently, there are six institutions that offer fellowships in hyperbaric medicine, three of which are Accreditation Council for Graduate Medical Education (ACGME) certified. Our experience has been that approximately two thirds of fellowship-trained physicians go into private practice and the rest remain in academics. The academic pathway provides a rewarding clinical practice with extremely broad opportunities for basic and clinical research. Many of the community-based hyperbaric medicine programs in the country are operated by emergency physician groups. Specialty training in undersea and hyperbaric medicine allows physicians to modify their professional activity to include a gratifying practice with less moment-to-moment stress than in a typical emergency department.

The only admission requirement for the 1-year fellowship training programs is board eligibility in any of the disciplines approved by the American Board of Medical Specialties. Therefore, this opportunity is open to all residents who have graduated from an emergency medicine residency. There are now in excess of 400 medical centers in the United States and Canada that operate clinical hyperbaric chambers. Credentialing of physicians to operate these facilities is becoming stricter because board-certified physicians are sought.

Overwhelmingly, the largest aspect of hyperbaric medicine practice is hyperbaric oxygen (HBO) therapy. The specialty also involves evaluation of individuals exposed to alterations in ambient pressure, such as scuba divers. HBO therapy is a patient treatment modality in which a person breathes 100% O_2 while exposed in a treatment chamber to increased atmospheric pressure. Treatments are typically conducted at pressures two to three times higher than normal atmospheric pressure (14.7 psi), or 2 to 3 atmospheres absolute. The hyperbaric chamber per se is not the therapeutic agent. Oxygen is the therapeutic drug and the chamber serves as a dosing device. The mechanisms of action for HBO are based on both elevated pressure and increased oxygen tension in the patient's tissues. Elevated pressure is typically viewed as the predominant treatment goal in bubble-related disorders such as air embolism and decompression sickness. Elevated oxygen partial pressures trigger several effects that are helpful when treating carbon monoxide poisoning, diabetic and other refractory wounds, anaerobic or mixed necrotizing infections, compromised skin grafts and flaps, osteoradionecrosis, some thermal burns, and several types of peripheral ischemia. Mechanisms of action include mobilization of bone marrow stem cells and modification of adhesion molecule function on circulating leukocytes.

A number of disorders treated with HBO are diagnosed in the emergency department and many of these cases require critical care support. These issues make hyperbaric medicine a natural progression following training in emergency medicine. Because of the variety of conditions that are treated, hyperbaric medicine also offers the opportunity for close clinical collaborations with all other types of medical and surgical specialists.

chapter 45

Sports Medicine

Thom Mayer, MD, FACEP, FAAP
Medical Director, NFL Players Association

Peter Paganussi, MD, FACEP
Team Physician, The Potomac School

What Is Sports Medicine?

On the surface, the answer would appear to be simple—the care and treatment of athletes. However, practicing the increasing popular specialty of sports medicine has become far more complex—and satisfying—as the specialty has broadened its horizons. Certainly, all emergency physicians evaluate and treat sports medicine patients, ranging from musculoskeletal injuries to concussions to heat illnesses. However, the practice of sports medicine has come to involve much more than the episodic care of illnesses and injuries in athletes.

Sports medicine was previously largely an avocation in that emergency physicians, orthopedists, family medicine physicians, pediatricians, and internists often volunteered for "sideline coverage" for teams in order to evaluate and treat ill and injured players. However, during the 1980s, there was an explosive growth in knowledge, research studies, and the evidence-based practice of both musculoskeletal and nonmusculoskeletal illnesses and injuries in athletes. This culminated in 1991 with the certifying boards for emergency medicine (ABEM), family medicine (formerly ABFP, now ABFM), pediatrics (ABP), and internal medicine (AMIM), seeking and gaining approval from the American Board of Medical Specialties (ABMS) to offer subspecialty certification in sports medicine. This was approved in March 1992 and the ABFM has administered the examination since it was first offered in 1993.

Sports medicine has come to comprise two distinct yet related subgroups of physicians. First, operative sports medicine is practiced primarily by orthopedists with a deep and abiding interest in the care and treatment of athletic injuries. For the first time in 2007, the American Board of Orthopaedic Surgery (ABOS) will offer a subspecialty examination, which is open to all ABOS diplomats with 2 years of experience in sports medicine. After 2012, fellowship training will be required to sit for the subspecialty examination. Some orthopedists currently do postgraduate fellowship training in academic medical centers to improve their knowledge of orthopedic sports medicine. The primary society for the practice of orthopedic sports medicine is the American Orthopaedic Society for Sports Medicine (AOSSM; http://www.aossm.org); comprising orthopedists with a deep interest in and commitment to operative sports medicine.

Practicing sports medicine also encompasses the nonoperative medical treatment of athletes, which includes but is far broader than the treatment of musculoskeletal conditions. The modern sports medicine physician must be capable of treating nonoperative musculoskeletal conditions, blunt-force traumatic injuries, laceration repair, heat illnesses, reactive airway disease, nutrition issues (including eating disorders), overuse injuries, amenorrhea, and any chronic medical problems of athletes and handles, in certain settings, drug testing. This level of service was previously offered only to elite (NCAA Division I college and professional) athletes; however, the growth of sports medicine is such that virtually all high school and many junior high school/intermediate school teams have some level of sports medicine coverage, particularly in urban and suburban areas.

Why Sports Medicine?

The primary attraction to sports medicine is the same for emergency medicine and all other physician careers—the satisfaction of offering a high level of medical care to a deserving and appreciative patient population. That said, the specialty is rapidly growing, with reams of research being generated on how best to handle a protean list of issues facing athletes on a daily basis. While sports medicine has previously referred to a generally young population of athletes, the importance in popularity of regular exercise has expanded the specialty to include middle-aged and even geriatric athletes as well. Perhaps one of the reasons that emergency physicians are drawn to sports medicine is their natural proclivity toward a broad range of generally treatable illnesses and injuries. In that respect, it is an absolutely natural extension for an emergency physician to be interested in the subspecialty of sports medicine. The vast majority of nonoperative sports medicine physicians continue to practice their primary specialty, in addition to their sports medicine career.

What Are the Career Opportunities in Sports Medicine?

While there is certainly allure and attraction to the elite level practice of sports medicine with professional teams, players associations, and college athletics, there are far more opportunities than just these available. For example, there are over 3,000 colleges and universities participating in NCAA athletics and over 20,000 high schools offering varsity athletics across the country (with many more high schools being built each year). Thus, there are literally dozens of sports medicine opportunities for physicians interested in this specialty in all but the most remote rural areas. To be sure, reimbursement for team physician coverage is generally either limited or on a voluntary basis, except in those academic medical centers where team physicians are employed through the university. Even in professional athletics, the direct compensation for team physician coverage is far more meager than generally appreciated. However, the satisfaction and enthusiasm enjoyed by sports medicine physicians are generally extremely high—and the primary reason for practicing the specialty. While many operative and nonoperative sports medicine physicians are former college or professional athletes, this is certainly not a prerequisite.

What Is Postgraduate Training in Primary Care Sports Medicine?

There are over 90 Accreditation Council for Graduate Medical Education (ACGME)-accredited nonoperative sports medicine fellowship training programs in the United States, which entail 1 to 2 years of fellowship. Entry into the training programs generally requires successful completion of residency training in emergency medicine, pediatrics, family medicine, or internal medicine. In addition to training in the broadest possible aspects of musculoskeletal examinations, illnesses, and injuries, training programs include as a part of the curriculum training issues, return to play criteria, drug testing, banned substances, heat illnesses, altitude-related performance issues, performance-enhancing supplements, strength and flexibility training, reactive airway disease management in athletes, special issues for female athletes, and both exercise stress testing and exercise-induced asthma testing. Coverage of specific teams is a requirement in all fellowships, and most require fellows to cover year-round sports of a diverse nature.

ACGME guidelines require that fellows spend one-half day per week refining their skills in their primary specialty, as well as 1 day per week for a minimum of 10 months in sports medicine clinic activities. In general, the difference between 1- and 2-year fellowships is dedicated and required time for research in the latter. Clinical activities account for a minimum of 50% of the time in the program, with the remainder spent in teaching, research, didactic training, and maintenance of the primary specialty skill. In selecting a training program in sports medicine, it is essential that the applicant contact graduates of the program (particularly recent graduates) to discuss with them their thoughts on the training experience. For a list of questions for potential applicants, the following question adapted from Dr. James Jaggers, Team Physician, DePauw University (www.saem.org/saemdnn/Home/ViewByRole/Fellowship/SportsMedicine), cannot be improved on:

Questions to Investigate in Selecting a Fellowship in Sports Medicine
1. What will be the extent of your experience with sports teams? Which sports? How much autonomy will you have?
2. Does the program provide you with the opportunity to work with Division I or elite athletes?
3. What are the structure and quality of the relationship between the PCSM faculty and fellowship training program and the orthopedic surgeons?
4. Who will be your mentors and faculty? What is their level of involvement in team sports and organizations at the national level?
5. How many fellows have graduated, where have they gone, and how can I contact them regarding their experience as a fellow, and how it has prepared them for their practice?
6. Is the program "emergency medicine friendly," and can I contact the emergency medicine group to assess their support of the fellows?
7. Does the program have an adequate didactic and research focus?
8. Will you have protected time for research, study time, and development of lectures and other tools?
9. How is the fellowship funded?
10. Is the fellowship accredited? How have the graduates performed on the certifying examination?

Following completion of the sports medicine fellowship and certification in the sponsoring board, candidates are offered the opportunity to take a written exam administered by ABFM, which is given once per year and consists of questions submitted by representatives of the sponsoring boards. Additional requirements include maintenance of an active medical license and the usual requirements for any certification examination.

What Are the Sports Medicine Societies, and Who Do They Represent?

The American Orthopaedic Society for Sports Medicine has previously been described as a professional society of orthopedists dedicated to the operative care and treatment of athletes. It offers a variety of training programs, generally of extremely high quality (http://www.aossm.org).

The American Medical Society for Sports Medicine (AMSSN; www.AMSSN.org) represents primarily nonoperative sports medicine physicians, comprising emergency physicians, internists, family medicine physicians, pediatricians, and physical medicine and rehabilitation physicians. AMSSN has a rich and active Web site, including a site for current sports medicine opportunities, a listing of both accredited and nonaccredited sports medicine fellowships, and provides training courses in clinical sports medicine topics.

The American College of Sports Medicine (ACSM; http://www.ACSM.org) represents physicians from all specialties involved in the care and the treatment of athletes, as well as athletic trainers and other allied health care professionals. ACSM provides a national conference annually, including basic science and clinical research, as well as sponsoring the "Team Physician Course Series."

What Are the Sports Medicine Journals or Newsletters?

In addition to some articles in the referred subspecialty journals for the parent board, the following (generally nonrefereed) journals and newsletters are available:

The Physician and Sports Medicine
International Journal of Sports Medicine
Medicine and Science and Sports and Exercise
Clinical Sports Medicine
Sports Medicine Alert
Sports Medicine Digest

Our experience in sports medicine has been, without exception, positive, stimulating, and gratifying in the extreme. We highly recommend it as a subspecialty, particularly for physicians who maintain exercise and athletic pursuits throughout their lifetime—as, indeed, all of us should! Please feel free to contact us if we can be of help.

chapter 46

Medical Toxicology

Lewis R. Goldfrank, MD, FACEP, FACMT
Medical Director, New York Poison Center
Professor and Chairman of Emergency Medicine, New York University

Louis J. Ling, MD, FACEP, FACMT
Senior Associate Medical Director, Hennepin Regional Poison Center
Associate Medical Director for Medical Education, Hennepin County Medical Center
Professor of Emergency Medicine and Associate Dean for GME, University of Minnesota

Although pediatricians, internists, intensivists, and laboratory medicine, forensic medicine, and preventive medicine physicians participate with emergency physicians in the care of patients with poisonings and overdoses, most toxicologists have an emergency medicine background. While most incidents involve acute and chronic drug overdoses and chemical exposures, medical toxicology also includes drug abuse, reptile, arachnid and marine envenomations, poisoning from plants and natural products, drug interactions, and hazards in the workplace. For emergency physicians who subspecialize in medical toxicology, there are many diverse challenges and opportunities available, particularly in regard to the interface with public health and public policy.

In the academic world, medical schools and emergency medicine residency programs need medical toxicology faculty members to teach medical students and residents, clinical pharmacists, and nurses, among others. Toxicology research involves basic, clinical, and health-services research. Recent advances have been made in the understanding of new poisonings, antidotes, diagnostic abilities, prognostic skills, and treatment. Toxicologists investigate workplace hazards and long-term exposure with regard to illness as well as new xenobiotics. Medical toxicologists are individuals devoted to a career of continuous learning.

There are 58 regional poison centers accredited by the American Association of Poison Control Centers. Each of these must have a medical director and medical consultants responsible for the medical standards, protocols, and quality assurance established by the poison center. The medical toxicology staff provide telephone consultation to many physicians on challenging cases and develop an expertise because of their concentrated exposure to patients with poisonings. Poison centers recently have received increased federal recognition and support to expand their roles and capabilities. Much of the history and a description of the concerns of society can be found in the Institute of Medicine Report, *Forging a Poison Prevention and Control System* (available at http://www.iom.edu/CMS/3793/5931/19901.aspx, released April 21, 2004).

Emergency physicians play a critical role because patients with life-threatening poisoning present initially to the emergency department. Many medical toxicologists also have admitting or consulting privileges to treat patients with poisonings and overdoses in the hospital because they have more interest, expertise, and experience than do other physicians. Patients with severe poisonings are referred to some hospitals that serve as regional poison treatment centers, similar to trauma centers. In these centers, medical toxicologists with the necessary laboratory and critical care support provide care for these patients.

Medical toxicologists see outpatients who are potentially exposed to workplace toxins, work with industrial hygienists to improve workplace safety, and help interpret drug testing results. Medical toxicologists provide their medical expertise to employers, insurance companies, and the legal system as well as patients in sorting out complex exposures and potential drug effects and interactions.

The danger of hazardous materials incidents has created a demand for emergency physicians to prepare prehospital workers and the hospital itself for victims exposed to hazardous materials. These medical toxicologists work closely with their counterparts in EMS and disaster management to maintain society's preparedness for these incidents. The 1995 sarin gas release in the Tokyo subway increased the national concern about chemical and biological terrorism. Ricin, anthrax, botulism, and other agents in the news media have raised our awareness of these potential dangers. Medical toxicologists are on the forefront of improving the country's readiness for these potential disasters. They frequently serve as advisors or medical directors for local and state health departments and the federal government in planning and making public policy.

Poisoning and toxicology date back to ancient days, but the subspecialty of medical toxicology was officially recognized by the American Board of Medical Specialties in 1992. It is jointly sponsored by the American Board of Emergency Medicine, the American Board of Preventive Medicine, and the American Board of Pediatrics, but emergency physicians represent the majority of medical toxicologists. In 2006, there were 255 board-certified medical toxicologists, of which 208 are emergency physicians. Twenty-three fellowships are primarily affiliated with emergency medicine residency programs, and another four with occupational medicine residencies. These 2-year fellowships include a variety of experiences with inpatients, outpatients, and poison center consultation as well as learning skills in epidemiology, research, and public health. In addition to patient care conferences, didactic experience may include formal course work. Fellowships are reviewed by the Residency Review Committee and must meet the criteria published by the Accreditation Council for Graduate Medical Education (ACGME) for educational standards and quality. These requirements and the locations of these fellowships are available at www.acgme.org. Fellowships graduate up to 20 new medical toxicologists annually. The certification examination is given every 2 years in November of even years.

The American College of Medical Toxicology (ACMT) is the professional society for medical toxicologists, and it provides a forum for peer discussion, education, and interchange. The American Academy of Clinical Toxicology (AACT) includes physicians, pharmacists, nurses, and those with doctorates. It serves as an umbrella organization for many professionals who care for poisoned patients. The American Association of Poison Control Centers (AAPCC) advocates and supports the activities of poison centers and their staffs. For further information, the respective Web sites are www.acmt.net, www.aactox.org, and www.aapcc.org. These organizations sponsor the North American Congress of Clinical Toxicology (NACCT), with a meeting held every fall for didactic sessions and new research presentations. International organizations and meetings provide an outlet to network widely with counterparts throughout the world. Toxicology research is published in journals for emergency medicine, internal medicine, pediatrics, public health, and occupational medicine. In addition, there are journals devoted specifically to toxicology, which include the *Journal of Toxicology/Clinical Toxicology*. Several excellent textbooks provide an overview of common toxicologic problems.

Medical toxicology offers the emergency physician the opportunity to achieve an in-depth understanding of one area. Many toxicologists will continue to practice general emergency medicine, but increasingly some are devoting their full-time careers just to medical toxicology. Medical toxicology has attracted and will continue to attract some of the most talented residents to solve emergency medicine and society's most complex and interesting problems. The diverse roles of patient care, consultation for industry, education, public health, and government at the Centers for Disease Control and Prevention (CDC), Agency for Toxic Substances and Drug Research (ATSDR), and the Food and Drug Administration (FDA) provide a wide scope for medical toxicology practice.

chapter 47

Clinical Forensic Medicine

Nathan Berger, MD
University of Louisville, Department of Emergency Medicine

Jennie Jones, BS
University of Louisville School of Medicine

William S. Smock, MD, MS, FACEP, FAAEM
Professor, Division of Protective Medicine, Department of Emergency Medicine
University of Louisville School of Medicine

Forensic emergency medicine, also termed clinical forensic medicine, is the application of forensic medical knowledge and appropriate techniques to living patients in the emergency department. In 1991, the University of Louisville Department of Emergency Medicine and the Kentucky Medical Examiner's Office instituted the first formal clinical forensic medical training program in the United States. In 1993, the first fellowship in Clinical Forensic Medicine was established in the University of Louisville's Department of Emergency Medicine.1

The emergency physician, by design and default, evaluates and treats on a daily basis victims of gun violence, physical and sexual assault, domestic violence, child abuse, and motor vehicle-related trauma. All of these patients have injuries or conditions that have criminal or civil forensic implications. The need for the emergency physician to be trained in clinical forensic medicine in the emergency department was necessitated by the need for the physician to make accurate diagnoses and avoid forensic errors. Examples included the failure to fully document the nature of the patient's injuries at the time of presentation, inaccurate interpretation of the wounds, and failure to preserve short-lived evidence (including clothing, blood samples, projectiles, etc.).

Comprehensive documentation ideally contains three components: narrative, diagrammatic, and photographic. Accurate interpretation and documentation are invaluable to investigators and can be a resource for the physician in the event courtroom testimony is necessary. Failure to provide your patient with the highest level of forensic care is not only a disservice to your patient but also may compromise the criminal justice's system ability to find the "truth." Appropriate forensic training will also promote a collegial working relationship with the coroner and medical examiner.

Gunshot Wounds

Accurate wound descriptions, devoid of opinions as to causation or conclusions, are more helpful than are statements, which prove to be inaccurate or misleading in ensuing investigations. The most common forensic errors in the emergency department involve the interpretation of gunshot wounds, specifically, the distinction between entrance and exit wounds. The errors are invariably based on the fallacious assumption that an exit wound will always be larger than its corresponding entrance wound. In a landmark study at a Level

1 trauma center, physicians (trauma and neurosurgery, emergency medicine) were asked to assess gunshot wounds in the clinical setting and the findings were compared with autopsy results.[2] These physicians incorrectly interpreted 53% of the exit or entrance wounds in patients with multiple wounds.

Appropriate knowledge of forensics will help physicians avoid rendering forensic opinions without adequate forensic training. In the case of firearm injuries, there are five factors that determine the size of gunshot wounds, both entrance and exit: the size, shape, configuration, and velocity of the bullet as it contacts tissue and the physical characteristics of the impacted tissue itself.

Range of fire is the distance between the muzzle and the victim. There are four categories of range of fire. Each has an entrance wound whose characteristics are unique to it. The entrance wounds bear the name of the range of fire from which they are inflicted: contact (tight and loose), close (0 to 6 inches), intermediate (up to 48 inches), and long range or indeterminate.

"Tight contact" is where the barrel is pushed hard against the skin. In these wounds, all materials—bullet, gases, soot, incompletely burned pieces of gunpowder, and metal fragments—are forced into the wound. Contact wounds can very large due to the injection of gases into nonelastic tissue.

Close range is defined as the maximum range at which soot is deposited on the wound or clothing. This muzzle-to-target distance is usually less than 6 inches.

An immediate-range wound (up to 48 inches) is one that is sufficiently close to cause "tattooing or stippling." Tattooing is caused by contact with partially burned and wholly unburned pieces of gunpowder.

The long-range or distant wound (beyond 48 inches) is inflicted from a range sufficiently far that only the bullet makes contact with the clothing and skin, leaving only an abrasion collar.

Blunt Force Pattern Injuries

A pattern injury is one that is recognized by imprint left on the skin by offending object. Blunt traumatic pattern injuries include pattern abrasions, pattern lacerations, and, most commonly, pattern contusions. Pattern injuries are reproducible and are mirror images of the weapon, whether hand, gun muzzle tip, baseball bat, belt, or a golf club that inflicted them.

The pattern contusion is produced by blunt force. Blood is the tissue underlying the striking object is forcibly displaced to the sides, resulting in an epithelial print that essentially traces the outline of the weapon used.

Sharp Force Injuries Patterns

There are two types of sharp force injuries: incised and stabbed. The incised wound is one generated by a drawing motion and is therefore longer than it is deep. The stab wound is a puncture-type wound and is, as a result, deeper than it is wide. The wound margins of sharp force injuries are clean and lack the abraded edges of injures generated by blunt force trauma.

Summary

Physician misinterpretation of the nature or cause of injuries or wounds can have devastating consequences and should be no more tolerated than the misdiagnosis of an acute coronary syndrome. Forensic medicine belongs in the emergency department now out of necessity and out of the ethical obligation to fulfill a critical role in safeguarding patients.[3] Clinical forensic medicine will continue to evolve and we encourage medical students and residents interested in this subspecialty of emergency medicine to further explore educational opportunities in this field.

Fellowship Opportunities

In the United States, there are currently no formal fellowships in clinical forensic medicine. Several emergency residency programs (University of Louisville and University of North Carolina) have added clinical forensic medicine to their training. Medical students and residents interested in clinical forensic medicine should contact their local medical examiner to determine what clinical forensic training opportunities are available within their medical school or residency program.

References

1. Smock WS. Clinical forensic medicine. In *Rosen's Emergency Medicine: Concepts and Clinical Practice,* 6th ed. St Louis: Mosby/Elsevier; 2006.
2. Collins KA, Lantz PE. Interpretation of fatal, multiple and exiting gunshot wounds by trauma specialists. *J Forensic Sci.* 1994;39:94-99.
3. Olshaker JS, Jackson MC, Smock WS. *Forensic emergency medicine,* 2nd ed. Philadelphia: Lippincott, Williams, & Wilkins; 2007.

Internet

www.louisville.edu/medschool/emermed/interactive.htm
American Academy of Forensic Sciences: www.aafs.org
American College of Emergency Physicians-Clinical Forensic Medicine Section: www.acep.org

chapter 48

Administration

Eric T. Carter, MD, FACEP
Assistant Medical Director, Department of Emergency Medicine, Southlake Hospital

Philip A. Giordano, MD, FACEP
Vice-Chairman, Department of Emergency Medicine, Orlando Regional Medical Center

Kurt D. Weber, MD, FACEP
Assistant Director, Department of Clinical Trials, Orlando Regional Medical Center

An administrative fellowship in emergency medicine provides the recent emergency medicine residency graduate with a unique perspective of the operations and management of the emergency department. An effective administrative fellowship is a flexible training module that encompasses many of the aspects of emergency medicine that are not covered traditionally during residency. The goal of these programs is to provide training, insight, and understanding of the day-to-day inner-workings and management of the emergency department and how it functions within the larger hospital environment. Areas of focus can include but are not limited to three main areas: (1) business and financial aspects of emergency medicine, (2) emergency department administration including quality assurance and improvement (QA/QI), and (3) medical informatics. Because of the extensive nature of these topics, the fellowship year should be personally tailored to the interests of the fellow and can be focused in one of the aforementioned areas. The skills gained in these areas prepare the recently graduated fellow for several possible job opportunities depending on their area of choice.

The business and financial aspects of emergency medicine are very complex, and the emergency medicine resident often has little to no formal training in this area during residency. The language of *Common Procedural Terminology (CPT)* as it applies to the various procedures and evaluations in our specialty provides the basis for billing for the professional fees for emergency physicians. While this "coding" is often done by third-party billing companies, it is imperative and required for any emergency medicine group to monitor compliance with current government guidelines and laws. For this reason, the appointment of a compliance officer has become commonplace. The percentage of emergency physicians who understand the nuances of billing and coding is very small, and the job candidate who has spent his or her fellowship focused on learning these business aspects will have a considerable advantage where groups are looking to fill this need. A stipended position of managing partner in a group is often separate from the medical director or chairman position and is filled by the rare emergency physician with skills and knowledge in this area.

The administration of an emergency department has become more and more complex over the past 10 years. Overcrowding, increased acuity, and access to care are only a few of the many issues that have presented an increased challenge to managing an emergency department. The complexities of the interactions between physician groups, nursing leadership and administration make it very difficult to tackle these problems on a day-today basis without an array of committees and working groups that are present in all large hospitals. During residency, it is difficult to learn and participate at a level that allows one to understand this complex interplay. As an administrative fellow, there is a possibility to serve on all or most of these committees. A proactive fellow can cultivate professional relationships at all levels of management and become an influential member of these committees. The insight gained during this year is invaluable and inevitably leads to administrative involvement much earlier in an emergency physician's career and is often followed by an early administrative position as a director or assistant director.

Quality assurance and improvement is currently at the core of emergency department management. In the "pay-for-performance" era, this focus will only intensify further. The administrative fellow can participate in programs to measure the various benchmarks required by government and hospital initiatives and play an integral role in the design of strategies to improve these benchmarks.

An administrative fellowship can also focus solely on medical informatics. One of the biggest changes in emergency medicine has been the explosion of computerized data available to emergency department directors. Armed with these data, the ability to measure and improve throughput and efficiency has increased markedly. For this reason, advanced computer and database software skills have become a commodity. In emergency departments across the country, electronic charts and records are replacing paper. Electronic order entry and data acquisition is becoming routine for physicians. All large emergency departments need a leader in this field to serve on medical informatics committees. Chief of medical informatics for the entire hospital is often a paid position that is filled by physicians who have received supplemental training in this area.

As stated earlier, good administrative fellowships are flexible and can be focused in the area of candidate interest. For the fellow to gain truly valuable skills and insight in a 1-year period, it is very important to focus on one of the three main areas mentioned or even on a specific project within that area. Some fellowship programs offer a second year of fellowship to the current fellow before considering applications from new candidates. This second year can be very valuable to finish projects that were started and often to cement relationships within the fellowship hospital. Ultimately, this can lead to immediate administrative jobs for fellows within their current faculty or private group. Administrative fellows may also consider pursuing an advanced degree such as an MBA or MPH using their fellowship as a framework to better understand the concepts of these curricula.

For those considering an administrative fellowship, more information can be found at the Society for Academic Emergency Medicine's Web site (www.saem.org), in the resident community section. Currently, four programs are listed as offering administrative fellowships. Administrative fellowships are also offered intermittently by some of the larger emergency medicine management groups like Team Health or Kaiser. Information about their fellowships can be found on their respective Web sites. The interested resident is encouraged to research each program individually as core focus and requirements can vary from year to year. Candidates are encouraged also to speak to recent graduates of each program to gain further insight. Finding the right "fit" for the fellow to cultivate his/her administrative interests is essential to a productive fellowship, and with the wide variety of fellowship opportunities available, candidates should be able to find what they are looking for.

chapter49

Public Health

Jon Mark Hirshon, MD, MPH, FACEP
Associate Professor, Departments of Emergency Medicine and Epidemiology & Preventive Medicine
University of Maryland School of Medicine

Joshua Moskovitz, MD, MPH
University of Maryland

In many ways, public health is an ideal complement to emergency medicine. These two specialties can be viewed as the Ying and Yang of health. For example, after treating countless children with head injuries from bicycle accidents, the necessity of preventing injuries through public health interventions such as helmets emerge. Emergency medicine, a field crafted on providing care to all comers, whether acute, destitute, or critically ill, feels the effects of societal problems often long before the primary care specialties or the coffers of Medicare and Medicaid are affected. Public health transforms experts in the management of acute illness and injury into far-sighted interventionists.

There are many different degrees that focus on increasing the general health awareness of the physician, while teaching public health perspectives, policy intervention strategies, and management techniques. Public health-related master's degrees include the fields of health administration (MHA), health science (MHS), and public health (MPH). All three degrees have some levels of overlap. While the MHA student may take public health courses like biostatistics, epidemiology, and environmental health, their focus is on the structure and effectiveness of health service organizations. The MHA also includes business management skills that are necessary for health administration leaders. It is an excellent degree for someone with an interest in health care administration.

The MHS degree is broad in scope and similar to the MPH but may not require prior health experience or training for matriculation. Areas of specialization range from health policy and management, to the epidemiology of parasitic diseases. Each public health school that offers an MHS should be researched thoroughly, as they all have different opportunities for specialization and investigation.

The MPH has historically been the most popular degree for physicians. It begins with a core sequence of courses in biostatics, epidemiology, environmental health, public health biology, and social/behavioral science. Afterward, specialization and focus depends on the school. Areas of emphasis could include: biostatistics and epidemiology, health policy and management, emergency management and disaster preparedness, child and adolescent health, women's and reproductive health, public health nutrition, infectious diseases, immigrant and urban health, international health, and law and public health. The MPH is specifically directed toward those with prior health care experience and training and can be an excellent complement to a medical degree.

An MPH can be attained at different times during the medical education process. While many students are entering medical school with such advanced degrees, some are taking a year's sabbatical before completing their medical studies. It is common to find students who take a year to study between second and third year or between the third and fourth year of medical school. Each time frame offers unique advantages. A sabbatical between the second and third year allows one to complete their last 2 clinical years of medical school uninterrupted and is the traditional approach, as witnessed by PhD and MBA students. Advocates of studying between the third and fourth year argue that one has a better clinical base to understand the communication and implementation difficulties faced by public health officials in trying to impact the health of populations. Third year is also seen by some as the most difficult portion of medical school, and this hiatus is viewed as a welcome change of pace. It should be noted that some medical schools offer combined MD/MPH degrees in 4 or, more commonly, 5 years.

Taking a sabbatical during medical school allows a student to pursue the degree at an independent university. Several public health schools allow completion of the MPH in as little as 9 to 11 months, while others offer online coursework. This flexibility may allow the student to choose a public health school based on reputation and program specialization and complete their course of study in the available time.

One can also wait until residency or fellowship to pursue an MPH. Many fellowships, especially those in emergency medical services, tend to have an MPH or other Masters component attached to the 2-year specialization. An advantage of such a program includes tuition remission through the fellowship sponsor, while disadvantages include completing the MPH in a public health school at the training site and potentially missing opportunities based on the school's breadth of courses.

The utility of your new MPH degree is vast. It is a wonderful complement to a medical degree, because it adds a broader view of health to the traditional clinical perspective learned in medical school. Physicians with this degree have many opportunities both domestically and abroad. Internationally, this degree indicates that the individual is familiar with treating populations and not just individuals, and thus knowledgeable about developing or improving health care systems. There are a number of other significant topic areas at the interface between emergency medicine and public health, such as injury prevention, interpersonal violence, substance abuse, and emerging infectious diseases.

Domestic applications of the MPH are as diverse as the international opportunities, and include medical direction of an EMS system, creation of a hospital's disaster preparedness program including exercises and drills, or possibly working directly in public health. Health departments at the local, state, and federal level tend to have physicians in charge, some of which are emergency medicine trained. Collaboration between the health department and the emergency department is critical, especially because emergency departments are often at the center of many of societies' major health care issues, such as difficulties with access to health care, drug abuse, and responses to disasters both biological (avian influenza) and physical (explosions and earthquakes). Other opportunities exist for physicians with public health training, including working on the frontiers of knowledge through innovative research, especially in the application of clinical medicine. The statistical and epidemiological coursework taken through an MPH can aid in study design, data collection, data analysis, and presentation of research results. For academicians, the knowledge gained from such an advanced degree can be a critical step during the early phases of an academic career.

No matter how you pursue a public health-related master's degree, the training that you receive will be invaluable. Public health professionals can be found changing the face of medicine through the delivery of health care services, studying innovative interventions, applying medical care, and more. They are routinely sought after to manage and improve topic areas that impact the population's health. A MPH can set you on the right path to make a difference, more than one patient at a time.

chapter50

International Emergency Medicine

Stephanie Rosborough, MD, MPH
Director, International Emergency Medicine Fellowship, Department of Emergency Medicine
Brigham and Women's Hospital, Harvard Medical School

More emergency physicians than ever are becoming interested in international work. While some are content to participate in a brief medical mission or relief project, others decide to make international emergency medicine the focus of their careers. International emergency medicine is a dynamic, research-driven subspecialty that seeks to improve health care around the world.

What Do International Emergency Medicine Specialists Do?

Develop emergency medicine overseas. In most countries, emergency medicine is either not a recognized medical specialty or still in the infant stages of development. Even in nations with highly sophisticated health systems, emergency departments (or "rooms") are often staffed by providers with no specialized training in emergency medicine—interns, moonlighters, or even just a nurse. Where there are full-time emergency physicians, their scope of practice is sometimes limited to the most obviously sick patients—trauma, stroke, cardiac arrest—while other patients are triaged to on-call specialists. In the least-developed health systems, there is no emergency care at all.

International emergency physicians help our colleagues in other countries build the specialty of emergency medicine. This includes developing residency training programs, supporting the growth of national societies for emergency medicine, conducting exchange programs and training sessions, and advising health systems on the need for quality emergency care. Sharing the lessons learned from more than 30 years of U.S. emergency medicine development is a large part of this work.

Respond to international disasters and humanitarian crises. Large-scale public health emergencies due to natural disasters and conflicts are a growing problem worldwide. In 2005, there were more than 600 natural disasters, an 18% increase from the year before. In 2006, almost 20 million people worldwide had been driven from their homes by conflict and disaster. And more than 90% of today's war victims are civilians. Providing medical care to the survivors of disasters and humanitarian crises can be a daunting task.

Flexibility, broad medical training, and the ability to work well with a team under stress make emergency physicians ideal aid workers. But cool nerves and a will to help are not enough. Effective international emergency physicians also train to provide survivors of humanitarian crises with clean water, emergency shelter, proper sanitation, and personal security. They learn about international humanitarian law and human rights—the basis of international relief work. Some international emergency physicians also conduct research to improve disaster response methods or to document crimes against humanity.

Promote international health. The lack of emergency care is only one of many health disparities between rich and poor countries. Poverty, malnutrition, epidemics, and the lack of drugs and medical staff are just a few of the problems that contribute to poor health in the world's populations.

There are many ways that international emergency physicians help improve health care in underdeveloped countries. Some build partnerships with particular clinics or hospitals to provide equipment, training, and medical care. Others take an interest in specific diseases, such as malaria or HIV/AIDS. Other international emergency physicians are drawn to a certain geographic area and focus on improving care in that region.

How Can You Get Involved?

First, get to know the field of international emergency medicine by joining the international sections of ACEP, SAEM, and EMRA. By talking with other physicians in these groups, you can develop a sense of the work done by international emergency physicians. Consider attending an international meeting, such as the International Conference on Emergency Medicine (ICEM) or the World Congress on Disaster and Emergency Medicine (WCDEM).

Second, stay up to date on international health issues and emergency medicine development. *The Lancet* and the *British Medical Journal* have a strong international health focus, and the *Annals of Emergency Medicine* and *Academic Emergency Medicine* publish articles on emergency medicine in other countries. Reuters AlertNet (www.alertnet.org) is a good first stop for those interested in disasters and humanitarian crises.

Last, find time during residency to gain experience in international medicine. Arranging an elective abroad can be time-consuming, but you will be rewarded with a unique opportunity to sharpen your clinical skills and immerse yourself in another culture. Start early by seeking out local physicians who participate in international health projects. Those interested in disaster response could consider joining the nearest DMAT (Disaster Medical Assistance Team).

Thinking about a career in international emergency medicine? Then check out the list of international emergency medicine fellowships on the SAEM Web site. Each fellowship focuses on a slightly different part of international medicine, so take time to find the best fit for you. You just may find yourself on the road to one of the most rewarding careers in emergency medicine.

chapter 51

Neurologic Emergencies

Andrew S. Jagoda, MD, FACEP
Treasurer, Foundation for Education and Research in Neurological Emergencies (FERNE)
Professor, Department of Emergency Medicine, Mount Sinai School of Medicine

Charrise M. O'Neill, RN, BS, CCRC
Executive Director, Foundation for Education and Research in Neurological Emergencies (FERNE)

Edward P. Sloan, MD, MPH, FACEP
Chairman and President, Foundation for Education and Research in Neurological Emergencies (FERNE)
Professor, Department of Emergency Medicine, University of Illinois at Chicago

There are many varied neurological emergencies that lead to significant morbidity and mortality for emergency department patients. Patient outcomes can be optimized by the delivery of excellent care by emergency physicians during the first hours after the onset of symptoms, including timely diagnosis, treatment, consultation, and disposition.

A variety of neurological emergency disease states are commonly treated by emergency physicians in the emergency department. These conditions include:

- Seizure and status epilepticus
- Traumatic brain injury
- Acute ischemic stroke
- Intracerebral and subarachnoid hemorrhage
- Central nervous system infection
- Headache syndromes
- Spinal injury
- Neuropsychiatric disorders

Academic Emergency Medicine published in 2005 a report describing the status of neurological education in emergency medicine residency training programs.[1] Stettler and associates conducted a survey of 126 emergency medicine residency programs to determine what methods were being used to educate residents on neurological emergencies. The group concluded that the primary method of educating residents to treat neurological emergencies is through didactic lectures and that expanding clinical rotations or electives to enhance education in neurological emergencies also warrants future attention. This chapter outlines some of the resources available for enhancing one's education and research in neurological emergencies and the various career options available to the interested student.

Education

Residency programs include the management of neurological emergencies throughout the curriculum; however, many have added rotations on neurology or stroke services to enhance the didactic curriculum. The Foundation for Education and Research in

Neurological Emergencies (FERNE) is a group of emergency physicians with an interest in optimizing the care of neurological emergency patients. FERNE leverages technology and organizational collaboration to promote excellent emergency care for patients with neurological emergencies, supports quality neurological emergencies research, and provides state-of-the-art educational programs for student, resident, faculty, and other practitioners of emergency medicine. Additional information including clinical resources may be found at their Web site (www.ferne.org).

Fellowship Training

Currently, there is only one neurovascular emergency fellowship program, at the University of Cincinnati. This fellowship provides the emergency medicine residency graduate with training in acute neurovascular emergencies in collaboration with the Greater Cincinnati/Northern Kentucky Stroke Team. This training is accomplished through clinical experience involving acute stroke intervention at The University of Cincinnati and other regional hospitals, as well as through didactic education in research methodologies, biomedical statistics, and principles of research design. Additional training is provided by the Department of Neurology and the Division of Neuroradiology in the utilization of neuroimaging, including computed tomography, magnetic resonance imaging, magnetic resonance angiography, and transcranial Doppler. The fellow also directly participates in stroke call and ongoing acute interventional trials.

This program is the only one of its kind in the United States, and two fellowship positions exist for a 2-year fellowship that combines the traditional 1-year neurovascular fellowship with an additional year of neuro-critical care training. This program provides an outstanding opportunity for the interested individual to explore the many academic and research opportunities associated with the diagnosis and management of emergent neurological conditions.

Research

There are tremendous opportunities for research in the diagnosis and management of neurological emergencies; a number of funding opportunities exist as well. The Directed Neurological Emergencies Grant Program is jointly sponsored by the Emergency Medicine Foundation (EMF) and the Foundation for Education and Research in Neurological Emergencies (FERNE). Applicants may apply for up to $25,000 of the funds. The grants are awarded to researchers in established emergency medicine research programs to support research specifically in the topic of neurological emergencies. The goal of this directed grant program is to fund clinical research in the treatment of acute disorders of the neurological system, such as the identification and treatment of diseases and injury to the brain, spinal cord and nerves.

The Emergency Neurology Clinical Trials Network (ENCTN) includes emergency physicians from U.S. research and academic centers and facilitates high priority, interdisciplinary, multi-institutional research into the diagnosis and treatment of neurological emergencies to optimize care and improve outcomes for patients who seek care in emergency departments. Further information on this research network can be found at http://nett.umich.edu/nett/welcome.

Career Opportunities

There are numerous opportunities for emergency physicians to pursue a career with a focus on the optimal treatment of patients with neurological emergencies. These include:

- Educating within an emergency medicine residency program or hospital on optimal neurological emergencies patient care
- Conducting neurological emergencies research with EMF/FERNE funding or other sources of funding

- Working with ENCTN to conduct neurological emergencies research
- Collaborating with industry in developing new products for use in managing patients with neurological emergencies
- Networking within your hospital with other providers of neurological emergency care to develop guidelines for optimal patient care
- Becoming a member of the ACEP Clinical Policies Committee in order to develop guidelines that optimize neurological emergencies patient care
- Working with the SAEM Neurological Emergencies Interest Group in promoting research and education in this area of interest
- Working with FERNE or other organizations to optimize this patient care

Summary

There are many opportunities to pursue a career in emergency medicine with a focus on the optimal care of patients with neurological emergencies. Whether it involves research, education, or the development of state-of-the-art treatment guidelines, a focus in this treatment area will enhance your career in emergency medicine and make the care of these critically ill and injured patients maximally fulfilling.

Reference

1. Stettler B, Jauch EC, Kissela B, Lindsell CJ. Neurologic education in emergency medicine training programs. *Acad Emerg Med.* 2005;12:909-911.

chapter 52

Medical Simulation

Matthew Spencer, MD, and Linda Spillane, MD
Department of Emergency Medicine, University of Rochester School of Medicine and Dentistry

Medical simulation is an exciting and rapidly expanding field for those interested in education, competency assessment, patient safety, and biomedical modeling and design.

What Is It?

Simulation is an instructional method in which a variety of "tools" are used to create a learning environment in which individuals, teams, or groups can practice a wide range of clinical skills and receive immediate feedback regarding their performance. Tools include standardized patients, screen-based computer programs, task trainers, virtual reality simulators, and computer-assisted full body patient simulators. The use of simulation allows learners to test their medical knowledge and decision-making, communication, and teamwork skills in a safe environment. Simulation applications in medical training are numerous and have become more realistic as the sophistication of computer along with mannequin-based technologies has advanced.

Medical Applications of Simulation

Training

The applications of simulation in medical training are limitless and have already become integral parts of training from medical school through residency. Standardized patients are routinely used in medical school training to teach and assess clinical and communication skills. Task trainers such as arms for intravenous line insertion and mannequins for intubation practice, are often used to teach basic procedural skills. Full body computer-assisted mannequins, such as the Laerdal SimMan and METI Human Patient Simulator, are tools used to teach and assess the care of patients with a variety of more complicated critical conditions such as respiratory failure, myocardial infarction, arrhythmias, and shock. Patient scenarios can be constructed and used as a tool to teach not only clinical skills but also communication, teamwork, professionalism, and systems management skills. Virtual reality-based laparoscopic and endoscopic simulators are also being used by many programs for residents, fellows, and attendings to practice new procedural techniques before performing them on patients.

Assessment

The use of simulation as a method of assessing competence is already here. Several specialty boards including the American Board of Emergency Medicine (ABEM) use case-based oral simulations as part of the board certification process. The National Board of Medical Examiners (NBME) and the Education Commission for Foreign Medical Graduates (ECFMG) both require students to pass a clinical skills exam (CS), which incorporates multiple standardized patient encounters, as part of the licensing process.

Also, several emergency medicine residency programs use high-fidelity mannequin-assisted simulations to provide a formative assessment of residents' clinical skills. The use of simulation techniques to credential physicians to perform high-risk procedures such as procedural sedation will most likely soon become commonplace.

Patient Safety

Patient safety initiatives involving simulation have focused on improving communication and teamwork skills through crisis resource management. In the future, simulation may also be used to test the safety of the interface between people and both new devices and the processes used to deliver health care.

Training Opportunities

Several opportunities exist for residents interested in pursuing advanced training in simulation. Although there are no opportunities for board certification in medical simulation, there are several structured fellowships available for physicians who want to develop expertise in this area. Advertised fellowship positions in medical simulation can be found at both Brown University and Yale University, and there will be many more that follow. As simulation centers spring up at major academic centers across the country, there may be an opportunity to hand-craft a fellowship combining a master's in medical education with a focus on medical simulation. Additionally, there are many courses sponsored by simulation centers designed to introduce faculty to the basics of designing a simulation center. These courses include how to obtain funding, how to design and organize the simulation space, how to write cases, how to use different instructional techniques and debriefing strategies, and how to conduct research in this new educational environment. These courses are appropriate for those interested in becoming involved in the field without pursuing a fellowship or advanced degree.

Resources

There are several valuable resources for those interested in more information regarding medical simulation.

1. The Society for Academic Emergency Medicine (SAEM) has a simulation interest group that all members may join. Information about this group can be found on the SAEM home page or the interest group Web site (http://www.emedu.org/sim/).
2. The Society for Simulation in Healthcare (SSH) is a multidisciplinary society that sponsors an annual meeting and the journal *Simulation in Healthcare*. The Web site for the organization is http://ssih.org/.

chapter 53

Advanced Alternate Degrees

Gregory P. Conners, MD, MPH, MBA, FAAP, FACEP
Professor of Emergency Medicine and Pediatrics, Vice Chair of Emergency Medicine
Chief, Division of Pediatric Emergency Medicine, University of Rochester

College, medical school, residency—with all the hard work it takes to become an emergency physician, why would you bother with yet another degree? The answer, of course, is as individual as you are. You may want to pursue an academic career and believe that you need additional research training to do it right. (That is why I decided to pursue a master's of public health [MPH] degree, even after doing a fellowship). You may want to take on a leadership position, and need to learn more about how to manage and lead others (which is why I later enrolled in a master of business administration [MBA] program). You may see a future role for yourself as an educator and want to pursue formal training in education. Emergency physicians are often interested in becoming public policy leaders; a degree in that area can help you acquire the necessary skills. Along with specific training, a graduate degree can help distinguish you as someone special among physicians; in a sense, the "letters after your name" serve as credentials that may help with getting that next grant, job, or other opportunity.

There are, of course, a wide variety of graduate degrees available. Some important factors to consider when examining programs include:

- Master's versus a doctoral degree program
- Format: Full-time, part-time, executive; traditional classroom, distance learning
- Timing
- Cost
- Personal support

Master's or Doctorate

An additional doctoral degree beyond an MD is a large undertaking. Although most such programs are research intensive, resulting in a PhD or similar degree, others may be more practice oriented. While a master's degree is, in general terms, typically a supplement to an MD, an additional doctoral degree is more often career defining. Occasionally, physicians working toward a master's degree may find themselves so drawn to the field that they extend their studies into a doctoral program. These decisions are unique to each physician and require extensive introspection and planning.

Format

Full-time graduate study is the most practical option when it is part of a greater educational experience, such as when combined with medical school. Once a physician has begun a clinical career (and taken on the other responsibilities of professional life), it can be difficult to revert to full-time student life. However, of any medical specialty, emergency medicine may be the most compatible with part-time clinical work, given its shift-based nature. More commonly, a practicing physician who is interested in a graduate degree will undertake part-time study, perhaps one or two courses at a time, taken over several years.

Although still stressful, this does allow time for a reasonable balance between the "work" and 'school" aspects of life. An emergency physician can, for example, work more night and weekend shifts than his or her colleagues, in order to make time for that Monday-Wednesday-Friday mid-day biostatistics or evening accounting course. An alternative format is the "executive" degree, still largely the realm of MBA programs. These programs are designed to meet the advanced degree needs of the practicing mid- or upper-level manager, typically meeting on alternate weekends, every Friday, or some other, regular time period. Because schedules do not change every semester, this sort of program allows long-range life and work planning. Executive MBA programs are typically more expensive than part-time programs, because, along with tuition, the program might "provide" books, meals, and other related items. Along with class time, these programs typically have extensive homework and group meeting requirements.

Graduate study need not mean classroom attendance. Distance learning (generally over the Internet) has become increasingly prevalent and accepted in recent years, and this will undoubtedly continue. Although there is typically a brief on-campus requirement as part of the degree program, the majority of the class time is spent at a computer. Depending on the structure of the program, this may be taken at whatever time is most convenient. Distance learning is especially valuable to those either without access to quality local graduate programs or who simply cannot make the time to attend traditional classes.

Timing

What is the best time in your career to pursue a graduate degree? In some ways, it makes sense to include it in while in medical school and residency. You are in "training mode," rather than enmeshed in your career and trying to carve time for school. You may not have started a family. You may be able to get accepted to a combined degree program (e.g., MD/MPH) that can reduce the additional time necessary to complete your degree. Also, you will have the additional training, and the additional credential, throughout the entirety of your professional career.

On the other hand, if you were to wait until you are into your career and really need the training you will obtain in graduate school, you will be more focused on your education. You can concentrate on meeting the specific goals of your education, and constantly think about how to apply what you are learning every day to what you are doing at work right then. Additionally, you will be prepared to use the personal and professional connections you may make.

Cost

Unless you are independently wealthy, an important factor in any decision-making regarding graduate study is the financial one. If you enroll in graduate school as a full-time student, you may be able to defer student loans. Those taking graduate courses in medical school are likely taking on additional tuition costs, as well as delaying the time until an attending physician's salary. Later in your career, you might be able to get someone else to pay your tuition bills. Some fellowship programs, for example, may include an option of an MPH or similar degree as part of the training. Faculty positions may include tuition-free or reduced cost graduate education as a standard part of a benefits package. This may, of course, limit you to study in your own local university. If tuition benefits are not standard, you may be able to negotiate such a benefit with your chief or chair as part of your specific employment package, especially if you can convince him or her that the additional cost will ultimately provide an additional benefit to the emergency department that makes it beneficial for all concerned.

Personal Factors

Being an emergency physician is a stressful job. Adding in graduate study can make life even more stressful, even as it enhances your career. Consider how additional graduate study may change your family and personal life, and whether this will work for you. You will need to weigh financial consideration, program quality versus availability, and how much time your class and homework time will take away from other obligations, including those to your family and friends. Trying out a course or two is one way to test whether the academic material and the life changes will work for you.

Specific Degree Programs

Although there is a wide variety of graduate educational opportunities available, many emergency physicians have pursued degrees either in public health or related fields or in an area of management. This section provides some details of these fields of study.

Public health. Public health training can help the emergency physician with clinical research training or with understanding the greater context of health care. Graduate public health is typically taught in one of two settings, either the school/college of public health or a department of (something like) community and preventive medicine of a medical school, college of human services, allied health, or a similar title. Either sort of program may be accredited by the Council on Education for Public Health, and it is worth spending some time on their Web site (www.ceph.org) if you are considering this option. The most common degree path is toward the master's of public health (MPH), which can be either quite general or focused in such areas as health services research, epidemiology, international health, maternal-child health, and health policy, among others. Some programs offer MS degrees allowing deeper specialization, such as the master's of science in clinical epidemiology (MSCE). Doctoral programs are also available. An interesting variation, especially for those with more of a political/community orientation, is a master's of public policy (MPP) degree, which may or may not be offered in the same setting as an MPH, depending on the organization at that university.

Management. These programs can help physicians learn the language of hospital administration, an especially valuable asset for anyone planning on taking leadership positions. The most commonly pursued graduate degree in management is the master's of business administration (MBA). An MBA may represent a general overview of business management principles or be focused on such areas as health care management, management of the nonprofit organization, or the more traditional business fields such as finance, accounting, and operations management. As graduate management training has become more popular among physicians and other health care professionals, a number of related programs have emerged. Thus, along with the growing number of health care MBA programs, master''s programs in medical management (MMM), administrative medicine, and even related programs in public administration, are now available.

Education. As educational programming in medical schools and residencies takes on greater rigor and earns more recognition, formal training in education may make sense to emergency physicians. Master's degrees in education (MEd) are widely available but vary tremendously in their quality; it is important to find a high quality program that matches your needs. Doctoral programs are also available for those with especially well-developed needs.

Law. A legal degree (typically a JD) can serve an emergency physician in a wide variety of ways. Being highly regulated, emergency medicine has such a variety of interactions with the legal system, and a consulting practice by someone with backgrounds both in emergency medicine and the law can be quite successful. An academic career could also be quite productive. Finally, a physician-attorney may be especially well trained to take on leadership positions, either in private practice, in academics, or of the professional itself.

Summary

Like any other aspect of your professional education, a graduate degree program can offer significant benefit, but it comes with significant costs, both financial and in terms of time and energy. The ability to tailor graduate study to your own personal interests makes it different from medical school and residency. The ultimate cost-benefit balance will differ for everyone, but it is worth thinking about for any ambitious budding emergency physician.

section five

Emergency Medicine
Life Issues

chapter 54

Mentoring in Emergency Medicine

Gloria Kuhn, DO, PhD, FACEP
Professor, Vice-Chair of Academic Affairs, Dept of Emergency Medicine
Wayne State University School of Medicine; Professor, Department of Internal Medicine
Section of Emergency Medicine, Michigan State University College of Osteopathic Medicine

"A mentor is a purveyor of dreams."
—Peter Rosen, MD, emergency physician

In preparation for writing this article I looked at the literature on mentoring. A systematic review on the topic found 3640 citations, demonstrating that there is a great deal of interest in the subject.1 Reading some of these papers and citing the information would certainly provide me with content for this paper. And yet, and yet … . What I remember from many years ago is Peter Rosen standing in front of a group of educators giving a talk on mentoring and telling us that a mentor is a purveyor of dreams. He was the last of four speakers on the topic. I don't remember what any of the others said. Peter was the one who had caught, for me, the true essence of the relationship.

In the rest of this paper, I will give advice on the value of being mentored, how to find a good mentor, and what to do as a mentee. And yet if that is all I write about, I have missed describing the most important things about this relationship. I do not believe that one can be successfully assigned to a mentor unless the mentor and mentee are lucky enough to have mutual interests and can establish a close and mutually satisfying relationship. I do not believe that someone can be a true mentor if the motivation is to fulfill the requirement of an institution that they serve in this capacity. I do believe that the young come to find guidance and help from those who have gone before them, and many are generous in providing help.

A true mentor is someone the mentee might wish to emulate; the mentor must be liked and trusted and have shared interests. The mentor has gone before, knows the path, and offers guidance but never imposes his or her will. The mentor is there to help the mentee reach his or her full potential. That is done by listening, asking questions, and helping to clarify thoughts and goals. Only then is advice offered. There is a richness to the relationship that transcends time and space. Mentors can be found in many ways, through telephone calls, e-mail, in structured programs, or by going to someone's office and asking for help. Many cite relatives as their best mentor. At the beginning of the relationship are shared interests, but at the end are realized dreams for both the mentee and mentor.

History and Definition

The concept of mentoring is at least 2600 years old and probably older. Homer describes the relationship in *The Iliad* when Ulysses, who must go to war, entrusts the training and intellectual and spiritual guidance of his 2-year-old son to his best friend, Mentor. In the 1970s, large private-sector corporations in the United States adopted mentoring as a method of supporting and guiding junior staff. In the 1990s, within medicine, various groups and institutions have introduced mentoring programs for medical students, residents, fellows, and academic junior faculty. Researchers have long used mentoring to train young researchers, give them access to needed laboratory facilities and resources they could not garner on their own because of inexperience and lack of reputation, and help them establish themselves in their new careers. Although it was before the concept of formal mentoring programs in medicine, figures like Sir William Osler and William Stewart Halstead, founder of the American residency training system of progressive responsibility, certainly rank among outstanding examples of mentors for countess young physicians and their influence lives on to this day.

The term *mentoring* may be defined very broadly so that a number of roles and relationships between mentors and mentees, or protégés, may be viewed as mentoring. Berk notes that since the 1970s more than 20 definitions of mentoring or mentors have appeared in the literature. A committee on mentoring at Johns Hopkins University composed the following definition, which is cited here because of its completeness: "A mentoring relationship is one that may vary along a continuum from informal/short-term to formal/long-term in which faculty with useful experience, knowledge, skills, and/or wisdom offers advice, information, guidance, support, or opportunity to another faculty member or student for that individual's professional development.[2]

The Relationship

A mentor may serve as a role model, provide information, guide career decisions, provide introductions, act as a supervisor, help mentees in achieving the necessary skills for success and career advancement, and, perhaps most important, assist the mentee in becoming inculcated into the prevailing culture he or she wishes to enter, whether it be in business, medicine, or another profession. Mentors frequently write letters of recommendation or introduction.

The relationship may be formal or informal, part of a structured program in a medical school or residency program, or begin as the result of a young student asking advice and help from a more experienced individual. Many mentoring relationships begin early on for high school, and even grade school students, as they seek to find their niche in life and choose careers. Many highly successful people cite those early relationships as having pointed them along their ultimate paths to success.

College students often seek advice from physicians, teachers, and relatives as they consider entering medicine. The prospect of facing 10 to 15 years of schooling and training is often daunting to young students, and encouragement by physicians who have gone before them and can demonstrate that not only is the task possible but immensely satisfying is extremely important. Medical students need guidance in how to succeed in their studies, manage their time, and begin to take on the roles and responsibilities, as well as the professional persona, of a physician. Residents also need guidance as they cope with the stresses and responsibilities of their specialty. The seeking of advice and guidance continues for young physicians as they face graduation, choosing practice venues, and constructing successful careers.

Types of Mentoring Relationships

Mentoring relationships may be part of a structured program or may occur (most often the case) because a potential mentor and mentee have shared interests and form the relationship to the mutual benefit and satisfaction of both. In structured programs, mentoring can be on a one-to-one basis, as a group of mentees with one or more mentors, or as peer mentoring (an example might be an entering medical student being assigned to a more senior student, who has volunteered for the position, who is aware of the "ropes").

The main goals of structured mentoring programs include helping the mentee enter the culture of the institution, assisting mentees in choosing an area of specialization in medicine, increasing the mentee's competence in research or other specialized work, assisting the mentee in gaining expertise/recognition, providing entrée to a network of valuable contacts who will welcome and provide future opportunities for collaboration, and, especially in the area of research, giving the mentee access to needed resources for conducting research. Research has shown that academic physicians who have a strong mentoring relationship are more productive as measured by the number of published manuscripts produced, grants obtained,[3] and promotions.[4] Perhaps most important, faculty with mentors are significantly more satisfied with their careers than are those without mentors.[5]

Some literature has stated that in medicine, mentoring is more important for the academic physician than physicians who enter private practice, but I disagree. For those in private practice, the mentor is frequently a respected member of their group, a hospital colleague from another specialty, or someone met as a result of engaging in activities as a result of membership in a professional society. Although the relationship is frequently informal, it is no less important and meaningful to the career and emotional well-being of both the mentee and mentor.

As noted, there are a number of models used in structured mentoring programs. One model uses an assigned relationship between the mentee and more senior individual(s). In this model, there are frequently assigned meetings with goals and objectives and an attempt to evaluate the outcomes of the mentoring program. A variation of this model is a semiformal program that uses faculty who volunteer to be mentors. In this model, there is less monitoring of outcomes and it is often left to the mentors and mentees to determine frequency and content of meetings and what the relationship will be like. There are also models that use more senior medical students as mentors for entering medical students.

Residency and fellowship programs frequently use all or any of the above models as they guide residents throughout their years of training. Some residents have asserted that their program director has been their best mentor and guide during their years of training, and many program directors see this mentoring relationship as their chief value and duty to their residents. They also describe this as the most satisfying aspect of their job. Other residents have formed close relationships to various faculty members. Whoever has the position of mentor, this person will guide, advise, and generally give support and assistance in the transition from medical student to the role of a competent attending physician, with clear goals for the start of a career. These relationships often continue for many years, in the case of medical students with those who assisted them early on in critical decision making, and in the case of residents with those they credit with having profoundly influenced their professional development.

Practical Advice

Finding a mentor may be a challenge but there are programs to assist in at least making contact with a potential mentor. Interestingly, it has been suggested that personality plays a role in the ability to find and engage in a successful mentoring relationship.[1,6]

Many medical schools have formal programs for mentoring, and the Society for Academic Emergency Medicine (SAEM) has a virtual mentoring program for medical students interested in emergency medicine. This can be accessed from the Web site http://www.saem.org/saemdnn/ and clicking on the link "students." Mentors may be found by simply calling, writing, or e-mailing a recognized individual or leader and asking for advice or help. Most physicians are generous with their time and wish to help those coming behind them. It is important that a mentor have some or all of the following characteristics: knowledge/or experience of interest to the mentee and a willingness to engage and allot time for the relationship.

Some students may be reticent in contacting someone who is not personally known to them and asking for help. Additionally, they may not want to state that they are looking for a mentor as this may imply an intense relationship that they are not yet ready to commit to or may feel that it is asking a very large commitment from someone who does not know them. A graceful way to begin the relationship is to contact the possible mentor and state that they are looking for advice on a topic. If distance is not a problem, a face-to-face meeting can be arranged. If the conversation goes well, as it usually does, it is now time for the student to ask if they can contact the person again. E-mail has made it possible to find mentors in distant locations and arrange for e-mail correspondence, telephone communication, or a possible future meeting.

Suggestions for Establishing a Successful Relationship

There are some suggestions for actions to take and others to avoid in order for the relationship of mentor and mentee to be successful. For the mentee, these actions include being punctual for a meeting, having an agenda, and following through on promised actions, accepting or at least considering accepting critique, being courteous and grateful, and accepting challenges. Some actions for mentees to avoid are overreliance on the mentor, blindly accepting advice from the mentor without thinking about the value of that advice for achieving the mentee's goals, or not determining if the advice fits with the mentee's philosophies. If the mentee wants to reject the advice, it is important to be honest about that with the mentor and see if an alternative path can be selected. Another potential pitfall for the mentee is to avoid making decisions.[7] Good mentors make themselves available, listen and ask questions, provide feedback and suggestions, and track the progress of the mentee.

After finding a mentor, it is critical that the mentee continue to monitor the relationship to determine if it is a healthy one. If the mentor demands that the mentee blindly follow advice, this may not be reasonable and the relationship may need to end. Mentees should avoid mentors who take credit for work done by the mentee or use the mentee for free labor without giving credit, as on a research project. It is, however, both permissible and necessary for the mentee to expect to work on a project if research is part of the relationship or they have accepted an invitation from the mentor to be part of a project. Then, the mentor should make the mentee one of the authors on any published manuscript(s) as an acknowledgment for the work performed by the mentee.[7]

If the relationship is not going well, a signal is the reluctance of either the mentee or mentor to schedule meetings or to let time go by without communicating. It means that the parties are letting the relationship die. A more graceful way to end the relationship is for the mentee to contact the mentor, thank the person for their help, and perhaps tell the mentor of future plans/activities. If the mentee has accepted the invitation to participate in a research project or other activity, it is imperative that the mentee either complete the assignment or contact the mentor and explain why this is impossible. This should not be an option for the mentee unless a true emergency or unforeseen event has occurred.

Letter of Recommendation

Finding someone to write a letter of recommendation for application to a residency program is different than finding a mentor. The person with the most direct knowledge of a medical student's performance is the individual best suited to write a letter of recommendation to programs to which the student is applying. Garmel[8] discussed in some depth the politics of finding the appropriate physician to write a letter of recommendation. That having been said, a student may wish a mentor to write a letter of recommendation when the mentor is aware of the student's work ethic, the mentee has a clear understanding of goals related to the medical specialty, and the mentor knows how the medical student arrived at the choice of specialty. This letter would then be in addition to other letters of recommendation furnished by the student to training programs.

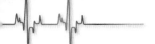

Summary

Finding a mentor has many values and may lead to a life-long relationship that is of worth to both individuals. Mentees may, and often do, have more than one mentor during the course of their careers and lives. The relationship is often helpful in clarifying goals, increasing productivity, and career advancement. A less tangible, but no less important, value is the intense satisfaction both individuals attain from the relationship. In the very best of situations, the mentor is indeed the "purveyor of dreams," and together they attain the goals and aspirations of the mentee.

References

1. Sambunjak D, Straus SE, Marusic A. Mentoring in academic medicine: a systematic review. *JAMA*. 2006;296:1103-1115.
2. Berk RA, Berg J, Mortimer R Walton-Moss B, Yeo TP. Measuring the effectiveness of faculty mentoring relationships. *Acad Med*. 2005;80(1):66-71.
3. Illes J, Glover GH, Wexler L, Leung AN, Glazer GM. A model for faculty mentoring in academic radiology. *Acad Radiol*. 2000;7(9):717-724; discussion 725-716.
4. Wise MR, Shapiro H, Bodley J, Pittini R, McKay D, Willan A, Hannah ME. Factors affecting academic promotion in obstetrics and gynaecology in Canada. *J Obstet Gynaecol Can*. 2004;26(2):127-136.
5. Palepu A, Friedman RH, Barnett RC, Carr PL, Ash AS, Szalacha L, Moskowitz MA. Junior faculty members' mentoring relationships and their professional development in U.S. medical schools. *Acad Med*. 1998;73(3):318-323.
6. Turban D, Dougherty T. Role of protege personality in receipt of mentoring and career success. *Acad Manage J*. 1994;37:688-702.
7. Rose GL, Rukstalis MR, Schuckit MA. Informal mentoring between faculty and medical students. *Acad Med*. 2005;80(4):344-348.
8. Garmel GM. Mentoring medical students in academic emergency medicine. *Acad Emerg Med*. 2004;11(12):1351-1357.

chapter 55

Women in Emergency Medicine

Wendy C. Coates, MD, FACEP

Professor of Medicine, David Geffen School of Medicine at UCLA, Director, Medical Education

Harbor-UCLA Medical Center, Department of Emergency Medicine

In the twenty-first century, the notion of gender differences in a professional career seems implausible. Despite the many advances that have taken place in recent decades, there remain issues that women face at a higher frequency than their male counterparts in emergency medicine training and practice. These are multifactorial and range from biological issues, to personal and professional choices, to societal concerns.

Biological and social considerations related to child bearing, and subsequently to parenting, impact women. The optimum age to become pregnant coincides with the most physically and intellectually demanding phase of professional training—residency. In addition to health concerns related to the postponement of child bearing, the female resident frequently must confront the impact her pregnancy has on her ability to perform her job effectively and the perception of her colleagues and residency director. Although it is inappropriate for the residency interview to probe female applicants about family planning, it may be wise for the applicant who is considering pregnancy to select a program that has an existing formal policy on maternity leave and work redistribution. With advance planning, the schedule can be manipulated to enable delayed graduation, elective time, and use of sick-time or the Family Medical Leave Act. Women who have an uncomplicated pregnancy may find it helpful to arrange shift trades with colleagues so their workload near the end of pregnancy is lighter.

Once the baby is born, the woman may choose to breastfeed the infant. One must consider in advance how time will be allotted during an emergency department shift at regular intervals for pumping of breast milk in a private location and where the milk will be stored. It is incumbent on colleagues and supervisors to be accommodating in this choice. In exchange, it is important that the new mother be aware that others support her needs and that she not exceed her fair share of time away from the department.

It has been described in the popular press that in today's society, women often bear a greater burden of child rearing than do men. This is an issue that persists throughout the lifetime of the child and is likely to impact the career path of many women. In an article in the *Harvard Business Review*,[1] the authors reveal an alarming statistic that women who are able to enter into a competitive professional environment at the same rate as their male counterparts frequently leave the "fast track" due to family concerns and find it difficult to return to their initial career trajectory. This has implications for immediate and future salary, including eventual retirement income. As women leave the workforce, even temporarily, their position in line to assume leadership roles is interrupted, and their final career level is lower than it could have been. These women have made a conscious choice to alter their careers to spend more time with their children, but fathers are not suffering the same economic and professional fates.

Many people enjoy flexibility in scheduling within the specialty of emergency medicine. It may be suited to women's lifestyles and may reduce some of the following institutional and personal difficulties that full-time workers with standard schedules face. Across all specialties, gender disparities prevail. Although this problem has not been studied formally within the specialty of emergency medicine, the female applicant should consider the implications of part-time work on partnership or academic tenure tracks. Institutional data spanning many disciplines reveal barriers such as lower comparable salary, lack of academic or organizational advancement, and fewer leadership positions than male counterparts. Personal factors such as equal talent and commitment on the part of women suggest that discriminatory patterns might still be in effect in career advancement. Women report less flexibility than men in job advancement offers. In addition, there seems to be a gender disparity in promotion, leadership opportunities, and salary within some institutions.[2] Women accounted for half of entering medical school classes in 2006; however, in 2005 they comprised only 15% of full professors and 11% of all department chairs in academic settings. It is important to participate in personal and professional mentoring relationships to garner support and learn effective strategies for advancement and recognition. The Association for American Medical Colleges (AAMC) has recognized the need to support women in their quest for leadership through active mentoring programs.[3]

Women in emergency medicine face other gender-based issues. Anecdotally, women in training have reported that they must first prove they are equal before they are able to prove to their colleagues and superiors that they excel. In some cases, women struggle with their authority with nurses and ancillary staff. Some patients are confused that the woman was actually their physician. Although these problems have improved significantly throughout recent years, they are still present in some locations. Hard work, pleasant demeanor, and a good sense of humor are often sufficient to circumvent lasting difficulties and will serve to reduce this problem for women of future generations. It is important not to blame every occurrence on gender. In some cases, an injustice that is perceived to be gender based may actually apply to all members of a group, such as an intern class rotating on another service. Good communication with the residency leadership or department chair is a necessary component for success.

A working professional woman should recognize that her freedom arises from her ability to make choices. In some instances, her choice may support her career, while at other times, it may favor her family. Acceptance of the fact that a woman can do "anything" but cannot be expected to do "everything" enables peace of mind and a realistic view of life.

References

1. Hewlitt SA, Luce CB. Off-ramps and on-ramps: keeping talented women on the road to success. *Harv Bus Rev.* 2005(3).
2. Wright AL, et al. Gender differences in academic advancement: patterns, causes, and potential solutions in one US college of medicine. *Acad Med.* 2003;78:500-508.
3. Bickel J, et al. Increasing women's leadership in academic medicine: report of the AAMC Project Implementation Committee. *Acad Med.* 2002;10:1043-1061.

chapter 56

Minorities in Emergency Medicine

Jocelyn Freeman Garrick, MD, MS

EMS Base Director, Alameda County Medical Center, University of California, San Francisco

Minority populations are the fastest growing segments of the U.S. population.[1] In 2004, according to the U.S. Census Bureau, persons who identified themselves as Asian, black, Hispanic, Pacific Islander, or American Indian comprised 35.0% of the population, and, by 2050 the bureau projects these groups will comprise 47.2%. Thus, physicians of the next century will provide care to a population whose characteristics will differ markedly from those of the population in the United States today, and who may have significantly different patterns of disease and health care needs. In 1998, the Council on Graduate Medical Education (COGME) charged that two things must be done to prepare for this population shift: increase the number of minority physicians and train physicians to be culturally competent.[2]

Data from 2000[3] regarding emergency medicine residency training programs reveal that a disparity exists for underrepresented minorities. Underrepresented minorities are classified by the Association of American Medical Colleges (AAMC) as black Americans, Native Americans, Puerto Ricans, and Mexican Americans. Blacks make up 13% of the U.S. population and compromise 5% of the total number of emergency medicine residents; Hispanics, 14% of the U.S. population and 4% of emergency medicine residencies; and Native Americans and Pacific Islanders in combination, 1.2% of U.S. population and less than 0.4% of emergency medicine residents. Data[5] also reveals that all underrepresented minorities in combination represent approximately 6% of emergency medicine faculty. This disparity is not unique to emergency medicine as a specialty and is found among all disciplines in medicine. Efforts to increase the number of underrepresented minorities in emergency medicine via mentorship, community involvement, and pipeline programs must continue. As the front line of care, emergency physicians are the gatekeepers who are charged to provide quality care for the United States' diverse patient population.

Resources

There are several organizations and resources available to the emergency physician who has an interest in working with underserved populations and/or minority health.

National Medical Association (NMA), Emergency Medicine Section. NMA (nmanet.org) is committed to improving the quality of health among minorities and disadvantaged people through its membership, professional development, community health education, advocacy, research, and partnerships with federal and private agencies. Throughout its history, NMA has focused primarily on health issues related to African Americans and medically underserved populations; however, its principles, goals, initiatives, and philosophy encompass all ethnic groups.

Society of Academic Emergency Medicine (SAEM), Diversity Committee. The goals of this committee are to assist with recruitment of underrepresented minority applicants to emergency medicine as a specialty, to provide cultural competency literature to emergency medicine residency programs, and to create avenues for research that addresses racial/ethnic concerns. Additionally, SAEM (www.saem.org) has created a Underrepresented Minorities Research/Mentorship Task Force to assist underrepresented minority medical students and residents who are pursuing academic careers.

National Hispanic Medical Association (NHMA). Established in 1994 in Washington, DC, the NHMA is a nonprofit association representing 36,000 licensed Hispanic physicians in the United States. The mission of the organization is to improve the health of Hispanics and other underserved populations. As a rapidly growing national resource based in the nation's capital, NHMA provides policymakers and health care providers with expert information and support in strengthening health service delivery to Hispanic communities across the nation. At its inception, NHMA held strategic planning meetings with physicians in five cities of the country, identifying the most critical issues they were facing, and took steps to define a blueprint of future activities in the following areas: delivery system, medical education, research, policy, and communications. In 1997, NHMA began convening its Annual Hispanic Health Conference in March each year in Washington, DC.

Association of American Indian Physicians (AAIP). The AAIP (www.aaip.org) was founded in 1971 as an educational, scientific, and charitable nonprofit corporation. At the time of its founding AAIP's primary goal was, and remains to improve the health of American Indian and Alaskan Natives. Today, AAIP fosters forums where modern medicine combines with traditional healing to provide care for American Indian and Alaskan Native communities.

Summary

To prepare for the culturally diverse population in the United States, teaching hospitals and national organizations must actively mentor and recruit underrepresented minorities. Additionally, community outreach and involvement in your local communities are pivotal. There are numerous resources available to students and physicians alike who serve an underserved population.

References

1. U.S. Census Bureau report 2004.
2. Council on Graduate Medical Education. *12th Report, minorities in medicine.* May 1998.
3. Association of American Medical Colleges. *Data book: statistical information related to medical schools and teaching hospitals.* Washington, DC: AAMC; 2000.
4. Scott CJ, Martin M, Hamilton G. Training of medical professionals and the delivery of health care as related to cultural identity groups. *Acad Emerg Med.* 2003;10:1149-1152.
5. James T. Women in academic emergency medicine. Diversity Interest Group position statement. *Acad Emerg Med.* 2000.

section six

VI

Emergency Medicine Wellness in Residency Life

chapter 57

How to Survive as an Emergency Physician: Take Care of Yourself!

Kristin E. Harkin, MD, FACEP
Past President, EMRA
Assistant Professor of Medicine, Division of Emergency Medicine
Weill Medical College of Cornell University; New York-Presbyterian Hospital

Be grateful for each new day. A new day you have never lived before. Twenty-four new, fresh, unexplored hours to use usefully and profitably. We can squander, neglect, or use it. Life will be richer or poorer by the way we use today. Finish every day and be done with it. You have done what you could; some blunders and absurdities crept in; forget them as soon as you can. Tomorrow is a new day. You shall begin it well and serenely and with too high a spirit to be encumbered with your old nonsense.

—Ralph Waldo Emerson

Physicians, by definition, are promoters of wellness. Yet, it requires a conscious, concerted effort for a physician to maintain one's own health and well-being. It is a necessity that seldom is taught in training. In short, *wellness* is the quality or state of being in good health, and all that good health incorporates (body, mind, and spirit).

Well-being is influenced by personal happiness and professional satisfaction. You know you are professionally satisfied when most of the time you look forward to going to work during your commute into the workplace.

A True Calling

May my love of the art of medicine inspire me to seek at all times to expand my knowledge and to see within each of those in need only the human being.
—The Physician's Prayer

You should sincerely love the job you choose and feel good about the work you do. Otherwise, it is not fun, and you will not last. Medicine is a vocation. It is not your identity. Do not get trapped into thinking that your paycheck defines your self-worth or the perceived status of your position determines your real value.

Your Values, Your Decisions

It took me a long time not to judge myself through someone else's eyes.
—Sally Field

Your personal happiness and self-fulfillment are what matter most. Decide on the values that are most important to you, and live by them always. Never compromise them or give them up—even when it seems as though that is the only way to get what you want. You may win in the short term, but never in the long run.

It may be difficult to take an objective look at our lives and reflect on the decisions that we have made thus far in life. Ruminating over the choices we have made in our professional decisions and, even more important, our personal ones that have shaped our lives today is not easy. Forgive yourself when you fall off track and realize that all you need to do is your best! Are you aligning your career goals with your personal ones? It is important to really plan a strategy for cultivating a successful, meaningful career in emergency medicine.

Time Management

Sometimes you're ahead, sometimes you're behind...the race is long, and in the end, it's only with yourself.

—Baz Luhrmann

Time management is the best gift you can give yourself. Emergency physicians are masters of multitasking. However, one of the hardest phrases everyone needs to learn is how to say "no." Do not fall into the trap of overcommitting yourself in every aspect of your life. Each opportunity is just that—an opportunity to succeed or fail. If the task or project is not in accord with your personal mission statement, then tactfully decline. Granted, some obligations must be honored and some sacrifices must be made. Still, it is wiser to not go overboard and pay the price of disappointing them and, more important, yourself in failing to do a good job or failing to balance your other, more significant projects in life. When appropriate, delegate tasks and, finally, avoid procrastination. Plan your career; do not let it plan you.

Lifestyle

You have to have emptiness before it can be filled. You have to exhale before you can inhale.

—Tom Yeomans

Physicians are experts in delayed gratification. Many long years have been sacrificed to train for the job you practice today. Nevertheless, delayed gratification should not last perpetually and become a way of life itself. It is easy to let a career in medicine consume you.

At the same time, it is tempting to overindulge because of this delay in attaining fulfillment in many aspects of life. There is no worse feeling than being locked into a lifestyle above your means where you are forced to work extra hours to maintain it, yet not have enough time to live and enjoy it. There is a never-ending sense of emptiness that is always looking to be filled, often by material goods, which simply results in working more and living less. Think twice before you sign on the dotted line and question whether you really need the most lavish home or the fastest sports car. Living above your means is a definite prescription for unhappiness.

Health

Be kind to your knees, you'll miss them when they're gone.
Enjoy your body...don't be afraid of it, or what other people think of it, it's the greatest instrument you'll ever own.

—Baz Luhrmann

You only have one you, and you are the only one who can take care of it. Simply put, your health is an absolute priority. There is no leeway or latitude here. You cannot function successfully, over a lifetime, at the high levels of physical and mental stress that the emergency department demands without taking care of yourself. Often, physicians care less for themselves than they do for their own patients. Time constraints may restrict and frank denial may cloud physicians into not taking care of themselves.

It is a conscious decision to choose life-enhancing options and requires emotional dedication to follow through with these pledges and promises. Changing one's old habits requires a firm commitment that is tested daily. The rewards of these conscious choices are

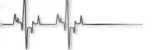

a sense of energy, well-being, and freedom. Through out it all, don't forget to breathe. Oxygen is the best nutrient you can give your cells.

Stress

The way I see it, if you want the rainbow, you gotta put up with the rain.

—Dolly Parton

Emergency medicine is not easy! It is stressful. In general, patients do not come to us when they are happy. They are sick and stressed. The knowledge base is extensive. The stakes are high. It is an overstimulated, pressured, overcrowded environment. Difficult consultants, staff members, patients, and patients' family members may make the practice of emergency medicine physically and emotionally draining. System failures with computers, labs, and radiology further complicate the shift. The hours may be very isolating. Then, one of the worst slaps in the face, is to fear being sued ... even when doing our very best. You may wonder at times why enter this specialty!

Thus, it is easy to understand how one could loose perspective. If you're going to loose it, make sure it is for a good reason. If not, move on. Put things in perspective—will it really matter in a month? A year? Five years? Respond, do not react—do not let your emotions get ahead of you. You choose your response, your attitude, and thus the way you allow life to impact you! You decide how something is going to affect you, not someone else. You can decide not to let certain things bother you, especially those over which you have no control. Know what you can and cannot change, and do not get frustrated by the latter.

Aging

People grow old only by deserting their ideals. Years may wrinkle the skin, but to give up interest wrinkles the soul...

—Douglas MacArthur

There is no secret to aging well. Aging is unavoidable. You can embrace it or fear it. The later makes it harder to accept the constraints that come with time. Continued growth is vital. Grow in every capacity. Stretch yourself- physically and intellectually. Read for work but also enjoyment. Cultivate your interests both inside and outside of medicine. Enjoy a sense of giving. Live with intention. Learn to prize what is of real value.

Welcome the satisfaction that comes with a life well lived. Smile at the wrinkles. Overlook the failures. Enjoy the power and beauty of true wisdom, inner peace, and the quiet that only comes with age. Be open to career transitions and alternative work opportunities in emergency medicine. Be willing to make modifications. Opportunity knocks every day—it's just a matter of recognizing it.

Longevity

To leave the world a bit better whether by a healthy child, a garden patch, or a redeemed social condition;
To know even one life has breathed easier because you have lived.
This is to have succeeded.

—Ralph Waldo Emerson

We are fortunate enough to truthfully do this every day and feel the incredible, unrivaled rewards of relieving someone's pain. It really does not get any better than that. It is a gift that we all have been given, worked to develop, and continue to practice every day.

It Really Is Your Life!

No one else can live a single moment of your life for you. That you must do for yourself.

—Shad Helmstetter

Never forget that you are the one in control of your life! The best way to predict your future is to make it. You have to fall a few times before you learn to walk. You have got what it takes—it has been in you all along, just waiting for you to find it. Your career should touch your heart and feed your soul in meaningful ways. It should delight your inner being. Very simply, you will never be what you were meant to be if you are not having fun.

In closing, I agree with Gary Kowalski that we can learn a lot from dogs. He summarized their virtues in *The Souls of Animals*

The Virtues of Dogs

Make friends easily
Don't hold a grudge
Enjoy simple pleasures
Take each day as it comes
Never petty
Remind us of the importance of frolicking, play, and exercise
Never anxious about their public image
Uncomplicated, genuine, and glad to be alive
Give unconditional love—never bark or growl at those they love

—Gary Kowalski[1]

Bibliography

Harkin KE. *It's your life! Live it well!* Section News: Section of Young Physicians. American College of Emergency Physicians, 2004;10:2:3-12.

Harkin KE. Physician wellness. In Aghababian R, et al, eds. *Essentials of emergency medicine.* 2nd ed. Boston: Jones and Bartlett Publishers; 2006:1019-1023.

Harkin KE. *Taking care of yourself.* Empire State EPIC. New York State Chapter American College of Emergency Physicians 2004;21:3:04:8-11.

Koltonow SH. Physician well-being. In Tintinalli JE, Kelen GD, Stapczynski JS, eds. *Emergency medicine: a comprehensive study guide.* 5th ed. New York: McGraw-Hill; 2000:1943-1948.

Margulies JL, Pollack ML. Developing a healthy lifestyle. In Andrew LB, Pollack ML, eds. *Wellness for emergency physicians.* Irving, TX: American College of Emergency Physicians; 1995:24-26.

Perina DG, Chisholm CD. Physician wellness in an academic career. In Hobgood C, Zink B, eds. *Emergency medicine: an academic career guide.* 2nd ed. Irving, TX: Society for Academic Emergency Medicine and Emergency Medicine Residents Association; 1999:53-58.

Pollack ML, Pollack FS. Health, diet, and exercise. In Andrew LB, Pollack ML, eds. *Wellness for emergency physicians.* Irving, TX: American College of Emergency Physicians; 1995:21-23.

Slapper DD, Mazur N. Career planning and longevity. In Andrew LB, Pollack ML, eds. *Wellness for emergency physicians.* Irving, TX: American College of Emergency Physicians; 1995:3-7.

Whitehead DC. Using circadian principles in emergency medicine scheduling. In Andrew LB, Pollack ML, eds. *Wellness for emergency physicians.* Irving, TX: American College of Emergency Physicians; 1995:8-13.

Reference

1. Kowalski G. The souls of animals, 2nd ed. Novato, CA: New World Library; 2006:18-19.

chapter 58

Professional Development:
A Lifelong Process

Glenn C. Hamilton, MD, FACEP
Professor and Chair, Department of Emergency Medicine
Wright State University, Boonshoft School of Medicine

Matthew C. Tews, DO
Assistant Professor of Emergency Medicine, Medical College of Wisconsin

It's All About the Plan!

Professional development is an active process of expansion and change in one's skill sets and understanding over a lifetime. It is not something you do once, and then check off your list and forget. It requires continued, deliberate efforts to learn new skills and develop new ideas, and then incorporate them into your day-to-day life and work. This is an ongoing process throughout your career, no matter where you start from or where you end up. All it requires to start is a plan. Sitting down and deliberately writing out your short and long-term goals with a plan for each one is a simple way to get started. This lays out a framework from which you can focus and prepare your professional direction. This list you develop is dynamic, not static, and can change as your interests and career paths change. As you set out to plan your career, there are a number of things you can do to prepare yourself for your career that are discussed in this chapter (see table page 203). The planning of your professional development is the key to a successful career and professional fulfillment.

Building the Foundation

Professional development starts in medical school. Regardless of the specialty you are considering, a foundation of basic medical knowledge must be established before clinical exposure and experience. The first 2 years of medical school lay this foundation with the last two years designed for application of this knowledge. This is a time-tested process designed and organized by others for your planned professional development. The importance of building this base of knowledge cannot be overemphasized, especially when considering a field as diverse as emergency medicine.

Armed with a foundation of medical knowledge on graduation from medical school, you are ready to enter into residency. At this time, there is a transition of responsibility away from someone else planning your entire professional development to an increased responsibility on you for your continuing education and growth. There are three areas that should serve as the focus of your educational development during residency:

Textbook Reading

Textbook reading is the basis for your knowledge of medicine. To never open a textbook is to cheat yourself out of knowledge, ideas, and trends that have been well established in your field. Recent textbooks are an excellent base of information whose principles hold true for most concepts and facts you learn from them.

Most residencies require you to read through at least one major emergency medicine textbook during residency. *Rosen's Emergency Medicine: Concepts and Clinical Practice*[1] is commonly used. Take the time to read each chapter and learn the basic concepts and principles of emergency medicine in each subject area. If your program does not require a weekly or monthly reading of a major textbook, choose one for yourself and devise a plan to read it during residency, one chapter at a time.

Contemporary reading is not limited to hardcover textbooks in print. Online resources such as MD Consult have many textbooks available, and internet sites, such as UpToDate, have extensive reviews of subjects relevant to emergency medicine.

Tailored Reading

As a student, the purpose of reading a textbook or going to a lecture was to pass a test, or even to pass a rotation. This is not the case during residency. One of the biggest changes from being a student to being a resident is the purpose of your reading. Your focus changes to patient-driven reading and learning. Develop the ability to take a question that arises during patient care, search the literature for relevant information, and then determine if you can apply the information to your patient. This ability to routinely search for and then integrate current medical literature into your patient care is essentially evidence-based medicine. Become familiar with the resources in your hospital library or online so that you can find the answer you need in a timely fashion, even when working in the emergency department.

Patient Interactions

Nothing teaches you like experience. In your undergraduate medical education, you had the opportunity to be the "fly on the wall"—to observe practicing physicians in their patient encounters. You saw the good and the not-so-good of patient care.

As a resident, this somewhat passive role suddenly becomes a very active one. You will be performing histories and physicals, talking with families and physicians, and performing this role day in and day out. This is the one opportunity in your career to be "the doctor" but to always have a more experienced attending as your backup. See as many patients as you possibly can during residency, even the ones no one else may want to see. This will develop you as a clinician and a professional, and you will gain the confidence you need to practice medicine when you are finished with your training.

Testing the Academic and Administrative Waters

The purpose of your training is to become a clinically competent emergency physician. Your time in residency is heavily geared towards meeting this goal. However, it comes as a surprise to young physicians that in their first job they may have certain administrative requirements in addition to their clinical duties. Depending on the type of job you take, there may be academic expectations, such as teaching medical students, giving lectures, or even some form of writing. Your life after residency consists of much more than just clinical work and your training is the ideal time to explore and learn some of these skills. You may find that you like them enough to pursue them as a career. There are four core areas that you should experience during your training.

Administrative

Involvement in administration can be one of the most important roles you can have in your hospital or emergency department in the real world. These positions will help develop and maintain relationships between your department and hospital or university administration. You are also in a position to change policies and procedures in your practice environment. For example, every hospital has a code committee, formed to determine what the response will be to a "code blue." Often an emergency department physician or resident will respond to codes on the floor. Being part of this committee will allow you to have input on how this process plays out in the hospital. Committees will also allow you to interact with other physicians and hospital administrators, who you otherwise may never talk with, or only speak with on the phone. It is important to build these relationships.

There are a number of ways to get experience with administrative skills during your training. Become involved in a specialty organization for emergency medicine, such as the Emergency Medicine Residents Association (EMRA). They offer opportunities to be involved in committees and interest groups, being a chapter representative from your program, or even running for their board of directors. This is an excellent way to become involved at the local, state, or national level.

Another way to gain administrative experience is as a chief resident in your residency. Being a chief resident will come with duties such as scheduling resident shifts, scheduling lectures for weekly didactic sessions, and dealing with resident complaints and problems that arise throughout the year. Chiefs also are the liaison between the residents and the faculty, and they may even attend faculty meetings during their chief year.

Teaching

Your training will naturally afford you many opportunities to teach, often informally. Whether you realize it, as a physician, you will be teaching frequently. You will be teaching your patients about their disease, teaching medical students or residents at the bedside or even teaching your colleagues new techniques or about a subject you are knowledgeable in. You will also inevitably be giving formal presentations to a variety of groups, from students to administrators. It is important to learn how to communicate your ideas and thoughts in a clear and concise manner.

When approaching any type of subject you are teaching during training, your goal should be to learn how to research a topic, prepare the lecture and to present to a specific audience using current technology, such as PowerPoint. Most residencies prepare you for this by requiring you to give lectures to your fellow residents. Examples include formal topic presentations at your weekly conferences or an M&M report. There is often opportunity to present other lectures on a voluntary basis.

When you give a lecture, keep track of when and where you gave the lecture and include it in your curriculum vitae. Be sure to collect some form of audience feedback, such as an evaluation, to prove your teaching effectiveness. This may be crucial to your promotion someday, especially if you work in the medical school environment, so get in the habit of doing this now. Constructive feedback will also help you develop your presentation skills.

Writing

Write something as a resident. It can be a high-quality lecture handout, a case report, a subject review, or an original research project. This skill of putting your thoughts onto paper is learned with repetition and practice. Invite your peers or faculty to review your work. The more critiquing, editing, and revisions you experience, the better your work will be and the closer you will be to publishable material. You may already have this as part of your training. For example, your program will likely require a written form of a research project before you graduate. You will have to perform a literature search, create an outline of your project, and then write and reference the paper. Publishing is usually not a requirement for your project or for residency, but having your name on a paper in a peer-reviewed journal can be beneficial in finding a job. If you cannot get your work into a peer-reviewed journal as a resident, such as *Annals of Emergency Medicine* or *Academic*

Emergency Medicine, search for non-peer-reviewed forums, such as specialty organization newsletters. Some journals also have sections reserved solely for residents such as "Residents' Perspective" in *Annals of Emergency Medicine* or the "Residents' Clinic" section in *Mayo Clinic Proceedings*. You can also write a case report, a visual diagnosis, or a subject review article. Be sure to work with a faculty member who has experience with writing and publishing. They may be able to guide you as to a publication to submit your work.

Research

The opportunity for research in emergency medicine is extensive. No other specialty gives you such a breadth of practice issues, clinical diseases, and pathology to draw from to study. However, a common misconception is that research has to be an original, double-blinded, placebo-controlled prospective study. Time is usually limited during training to complete this kind of project from scratch. Instead, find a faculty member or mentor who already has an established study or idea, and work on it with them. Most faculty are more that happy to have help with their project, and some may even let you run with it, staying close for guidance and overcoming the hurdles that are inevitable in research.

Typically, the goal of research during residency is to graduate from your program. Use it for more than just a requirement to finish your training. Use it as an opportunity to develop another skill set to grow as a physician. Research can change your perspective on emergency medicine and can teach you how to read the scientific literature with greater understanding. But do not do it alone—collaboration is crucial to learn while doing research.

Planning a Career Rather Than Consuming It

The progression of your career should be planned at intervals to allow you time to develop the skills and experience you need to mature as a professional. You will not become the director or chair of an emergency department during your first year after finishing residency. This type of position requires experience, knowledge, and understanding of the politics of the institution you are in to be effective. You do not need to climb the ladder and get to the top as quickly as you can. There are benefits to "paying your dues" such as developing some basic skills in education, administration, or any other job to prepare you for positions of leadership at the highest levels. Preparing a plan and taking the time to reach these positions will avoid burnout and will hopefully promote a sense of career satisfaction.

As you are planning your career, consider what your "specialty" or niche is going to be. At the culmination of your residency training, you will be considered a "generalist" in emergency medicine. You will learn to do a lot of things well. But defining a particular interest or focus within emergency medicine early on can help you plan a successful career. As you progress in your training, take note of the topics or rotations you enjoy and considering pursuing them for a career. For instance, if your interest lies in toxicology, learn about the opportunities available for training in a fellowship and the job market for a toxicologist in the region you would want to practice. Spend time developing these skills on rotations during residency. Or, your interest might be neurosurgical emergencies. Study these topics and become involved in national organizations that deal with these issues. Whatever interest you have in emergency medicine, consider turning it into the basis for your career work early on to see if you really like it.

Once you have determined what you may want out of your career, take the time to plan how you will do this. Carefully define short and long-term goals. It is helpful to sit down and imagine where you would like to be in 1, 3 and 5 years, and then plan a course of action of how to get there. Include activities such as extra training, key people you would like to meet, or committees or groups you want to be involved in. Once you have thought this through and have a written plan, sit down and discuss it with your mentor, residency director, or a respected colleague who has formed a successful career. They often have knowledge and wisdom from their prior experiences, and may know people in their institution or across the country to help you succeed. They can help you lay a roadmap to your ideal destination.

As you plan your career, it is important to keep in mind that everyone moves at a different speed. You will likely not be at the same place at a given time as your mentor was, as a colleague is, or even when you planned to be. So be patient and revisit your goals and plans at 1, 3, and 5 years to see what has changed or has been accomplished, and adjust them accordingly.

As a final phase of your planning and as you look into the future, plan to be different. When you reevaluate your career, you do not want to be the same person you were 1, 3, or 5 years earlier when you made your initial plans. The goal is to have grown and matured as a physician, building on what you have done, and not be stuck in the same rut. Keep your career fresh and moving in a forward direction. Try new activities and push yourself to meet your goals so that you can build on this ever-expanding foundation of knowledge and skills. Do not disregard opportunities to learn or try a new job ... you may actually like it. But do not overburden yourself with activities that will not help accomplish your goals. You will only be wasting your time. Additionally, remember that your answer should be "yes" when asked to do something that is in line with your goals and objectives. You never know where it may lead.

Summary

Professional development is a life-long pursuit that starts in medical school. It progresses as you develop and try new experiences, with the goal of finding a focus for your career. All it takes is a plan to get started. Stephen Covey, in his book *The Seven Habits of Highly Effective People*,[2] summed it up best when he said, "Begin with the end in mind." If you can do this and look into the future and determine where you want to be and how you can accomplish it, then you are on your way to developing a successful and satisfying professional career.

References

1. Marx, J, Hockberger R, Walls, R eds ,*Rosen's Emergency Medicine: Concepts and Clinical Practice, 6th Edition, New York, Mosby, 2006*
2. Covey SR. *Seven habits of highly effective people: powerful lessons in personal change.* New York: Simon and Schuster; 1989.

Bibiography

Lakein A. *How to get control of your time and your life.* New York: New American Library; 1973.

Stead LG, Sadosty AT, Decker WW. Academic career development for emergency medicine residents: a road map. *Acad Emerg Med.* 2005;12(5):112-116

Professional Development Opportunities in Training

Medical School
    First two years
        The basics of medical knowledge
        Exposure to clinical medicine
    Clinical years
        Application of basic medical knowledge
        Specialty exposure
        Reading medical literature

Residency
    Specialty focused learning
    Planning a career, not just rapidly consuming it
        Moving up the ladder with different levels of experience
        Know what you want
        Everyone moves at a different speed
    Networking
        Interacting with other physicians and determining their career path taken
        Job planning should occur early
    Becoming involved
        Local organizations
        National meetings and organizations
    Research
        Residency requirements
    Reading
        Textbook vs. Tailored reading
        Keeping up with the literature
    Scholarly Writing
        Goal of at least one peer-reviewed publication from research project
        Finding faculty to work with
    Speaking
        At least one prepared lecture per year to your peers, students and residents
    Finding a mentor
        A mutually beneficial relationship
    Leadership
        National organizations, chief resident, committees
        Administration
    Academic Medicine
        Fellowship Training, Educational and Research tracts
    Continuing Medical Education
        A lifelong process

chapter 59

Sleep Aids, Stimulants, and Drug and Alcohol Use in Residency

Joseph Chiang, MD
Department of Emergency Medicine, Mount Sinai School of Medicine

Andy Jagoda, MD, FACEP
Professor and Vice Chair, Medical Director, Department of Emergency Medicine
Mount Sinai School of Medicine

Lynn Ji, MD,
Department of Emergency Medicine, Mount Sinai School of Medicine

As graduating medical students embark on the next step of their training, many wonder if they are ready to deal with the stresses and challenges of professional practice. The combination of physical and emotional stress with high-acuity and high-volume emergency practice poses real threats to one's wellness. *Wellness* can be defined as "complete physical, mental and social well-being and not merely the absence of disease or infirmity." This also includes the ability to lead a "socially and economically productive life."[1] To be "well" allows medical residents to confront the challenges and stresses of their lives, whether they are personal or professional, without internalizing them. This allows for the resident to provide the best care possible for patients without bitterness, enmity, and the risk of burnout.

Studies on wellness suggest that there is a basis for concerns regarding the impact of residency training on well-being. One study reported a high incidence of hostility, indifference, inhibition, and nervousness, and depression with suicidal ideations in housestaff.[2] Housestaff's mood and stress clearly have implications on interaction with patients and colleagues, and on personal life.[3] Day/night shift changes, overcrowding, and ever-increasing illness acuity make emergency medicine training particularly stressful. Residents undergo 10 to 12 hours of intense information processing, with frequent changes from nocturnal to diurnal schedules. The effects of this schedule may best be illustrated in the increase of motor vehicle accidents after night shifts.[4]

Emergency medicine has led the way in advocating for resident work hour changes. The push for changes began in the mid-1980's with the Ad Hoc Advisory Committee on Emergency Services formed to study the famous Libby Zion case. The committee, better known as the Bell Commission, recommended the following:

Physicians should not work more than 12 consecutive hours in the emergency department (with a census of greater than 15,000)

Housestaff should not work more than 80 hours/week over a 4-week period

Housestaff should not be scheduled to work for more than 24 consecutive hours, to be separated by no less than 8 nonworking hours, and with at least one 24-hour period of nonworking time each week

As a direct consequence of the Bell Commission and other initiatives, the Accreditation Council for Graduate Medical Education (ACGME), which regulates the total number of resident work hours for both clinical and education activities, mandated regulations in resident work hours and supervision. Not surprisingly, preliminary studies demonstrate an improvement in resident mood.[5] However, even with work hour regulations, residents are still working at a pace per week double that of the federally imposed limits on other professions that affect the public (i.e., regulated transportation).

This chapter examines the body of literature describing dysfunctional behaviors associated with residency training and the risks associated with inappropriate coping mechanisms.

Stimulants

Sleep deprivation and the intensity required during emergency department shifts tempt many residents to use stimulants to remain vigilant and functional. Chronic stimulant use, with or without sleep deprivation, can result in tension and/or migraine headache, which leads to frequent analgesic use, and a vicious cycle of polydrug abuse can be established. Often, when the hazards are realized, sudden discontinuation of stimulant use can lead to withdraw headache, which increases the demand for more analgesics. The cycle continues.

Several central nervous system stimulants have been tested for their effectiveness in improving performance. High-dose caffeine, modafinil, and D-amphetamine have proved to be effective in reducing sleepiness when measured with polysomnography in individuals following reduced sleep for less than 2 days.[6-9]

Caffeine. The most commonly used stimulant is caffeine, which promotes alertness and can improve vigilance.[10] It is a substance that exists in many forms in daily life, such as coffee, tea, chocolate, and soft drinks. Purer, concentrated formulations have also been made available over the counter in products such as NoDoz, Tirend, QuickPed, Vivarin, Caffedrine, Durvitan, and Pro-Plus. As benign and ubiquitous as caffeine is, overdose is an acknowledged disease process reported in literature. The National Institutes of Health advises consumers that symptoms of caffeine overdose range from insomnia, dizziness, irritability, and urinary frequency, to fever, vomiting, diarrhea, gastric ulcer, muscle fasciculation, to altered mental status, convulsions, rhabdomyolysis, cardiac arrhythmia, and even death.[11,12] Withdrawal symptoms such as headache, anxiety, or muscle tension can present within 12 to 18 hours after abrupt discontinuation following several weeks of continuous intake.

Modafinil. A newer prescription medication, modafinil (Provigil) has been Food and Drug Administration approved to improve wakefulness in patients with pronounced daytime sleepiness, such as narcolepsy and shift-work sleep disorder. Its use in narcolepsy has been well tolerated, but its effectiveness for shift work sleep disorder requires further exploration.

The most common side effects include headache, upper respiratory tract infection, nausea, nervousness, anxiety, and insomnia.[13]

Ultimately, the most effective countermeasure for sleepiness is ... sleep! A 2- to 8-hour nap prior to 24 hours of wakefulness improves vigilance and minimizes lethargy for 24 hours.[14] Short naps, as concise as 15 minutes, at 2- to 3-hour intervals during 24 hours of sleep deprivation can significantly improve performance.[15] The American College of Emergency Physicians (ACEP) recommends that after a night shift, physicians consider wearing sunglasses to keep away morning light, eating lightly before going to sleep, and sleeping first prior to exercising to promote wakefulness.[16] During the night shift, working in a well-lit area has been reported to improve performance.[17] Similar suggestions have been given to internal medicine residents recovering from a 30-hour call; that is, maximize exposure to light during the day and sleeping at night to maintain circadian rhythm. This maximization of external environmental cues for speedy circadian phase adaptation has been practiced to great effect by air travelers dodging jet lag for the past century.

Sedatives/Hypnotics

Emergency residents have the distinctive experience of having to work consecutive nights. In order to facilitate adaptation to changing sleep patterns, many residents resort to pharmacological assistance, including benzodiazepines and benzodiazepine receptor agonists.

Zolpidem. Zolpidem (Ambien) may be the optimal choice for sleep periods of less than 8 hours. This imidazopyridine benzodiazepine receptor agonist has a short half-life of 2.5 hours and provides short-term sleep promotion while minimizing the possibility of post-nap hangovers as the emergency resident wakes to prepare for the next night shift. A further advantage of zolpidem is its proved efficacy and safety record used in normal, elderly, and psychiatric populations with insomnia. Withdrawal symptoms, issues of dependence/abuse, and drug interactions are minimal.[18][i]

Temazepam. Residents attempting to restore a sleep pattern may use temazepam (Restoril), which has a 9-hour half-life. Temazepam is best suited for sleep-maintenance, as users may be plagued by early awakening when short-acting hypnotics are used. Interestingly, absorbance, half-life, and distribution result in shorter efficacy for daytime administration compared with nighttime administration.[19]

Users of both zolpidem and temazepam need to be certain of the guarantee of uninterrupted sleep prior to resumption of clinical duties as both can produce drowsiness and psychomotor dissociation from sleep truncation; do not use it during off-service calls! Temazepam also demonstrates dose-correlation in drowsiness and along with higher rates of tolerance and withdrawal symptoms.[20]

Zaleplon. Another popular medication on the market is Zaleplon (Sonata), which is most suitable for the initiation of very short naps (half-life of 1 to 2 hours). While it may not prevent early afternoon awakenings, it can be a great tool in facilitating early sleep initiation of sleep for early predawn awakenings or a shift-schedule change.

Diphenhydramine. Anecdotal evidence has demonstrated pronounced residual drowsiness, ataxia, and dry mouth and throat associated with diphenhydramine use (Benadryl', Sominex) due to its anticholinergic effects: consequently, this is not a recommended sleep aid. More significantly, diphenhydramine seems to decrease cognition as seen in studies involving elderly adults suffering from insomnia.[21,22] While most housestaff known to the authors do not fall in the category of "elderly adults," arriving at work with the threat of being drowsy and decreased decision-making ability make this sleep aid option unappealing.

Triazolam. Use of triazolam (Halcion) has decreased due to reports of drug-related memory impairment, anxiety, and depression. Because of these concerns, the U.S. Air Force has discontinued triazolam as one of its recommended medications.[23]

Melatonin. Melatonin emerged in the 1990s as an attractive alternative to adjust to sleep-wake cycle disruption. Many mammalian biological functions are circadian and usually synchronized to the 24-hour solar cycle. The current hypothesis is that exogenous melatonin taken in the late afternoon produces a phase advance, moving the clock forward by an additive effect with endogenous melatonin. In the early morning, exogenous melatonin causes a phase delay, moving the circadian rhythm backwards by antagonizing the effect of bright light. A meta-analysis of travel-related sleep alternations concluded that melatonin increased total sleep time in subjects.[24] Unfortunately, studies looking at melatonin as a sleep aid for residents adjusting to different schedules have been disappointing at best.[25,26]* A MEDLINE search found no reports of significant adverse effects, other than abdominal cramping, when melatonin was taken in physiological doses of 3 to 6 grams. However, no long-term, large controlled studies exist regarding adverse effects.

---

*It is important to note these studies mainly looked specifically at residents' moods, sleep quality, nighttime/daytime sleepiness, attention, etc., not the hours of sleep.

Alcohol

With the stressful lifestyle of residents, an offer for "a drink, or two" often results in many takers. While the occasional drink is socially acceptable, the imperative exists to recognize the dangers of dependence and abuse. One study indicated that among emergency medicine residents, 12.5% had answered positively to one of the CAGE questions [a validated questionnaire named after its four questions used to screen patients for alcoholism], while program directors suspected alcoholism in only 1.0% of residents.[27] Furthermore, physicians as a whole appear to use alcohol at a rate greater than their gender and age counterparts.[28] While the data do not suggest there is rampant alcohol abuse and dependence among the housestaff, incoming residents must guard against the dangers posed by alcohol to themselves and their patients.

Other Substances

Housestaff use of illicit drugs has been reported to be as high as 8.8% for marijuana and 1.0% for cocaine. In one study, emergency medicine residents were identified as having one of the highest rates of substance abuse when compared to residents in other specialties.[29] The use of cocaine is troubling for many reasons, including the associated risk of vascular catastrophes, myocardial infarction, and renal failure (chronic use leads to a 7-fold increase in myocardial infarctions and in the hour immediately after its use, a 24-fold increased risk).[30] Cocaine and its variants also create chronic tolerance, leading to increased dosage on subsequent uses.

Marijuana, benzodiazapines, opioid, and other "downers" do not possess the nefarious reputation of cocaine but still possess their own side effects (e.g., respiratory depression and anoxic injury with opiods and withdrawal seizures from benzodiazepines).[31] A startling finding has been a high rate of self-treatment with benzodiazepines and opioids.[32] This leads not only to more opportunities for abuse and dependence but also to increased danger to physicians and their patients.

Emergency medicine has led the way to "assist the impaired emergency physician and to promote the well-being of all emergency physicians through education, information, and collaborative processes."[33] For example, ACEP has used evidence-based medicine to recommend programs that promote overall well-being through shift-work schedules based on the circadian rhythm, time-off for serious family issues such as sickness and even initiation of adoption, and so on. ACEP also has encouraged programs to provide medical treatment for the impaired physician and allow the resident to return when they are able.[34] The American Medical Association's Federation of State Physician Health Programs Web site (http://www.fsphp.org/6020.html) offers a state-by-state listing of medical society resources for impaired physicians and their colleagues who desire intervention. Many other emergency medicine professional Web sites also offer sections for residents' assistance in dealing with issues of dependence.

Summary

Graduating medical students are surely aware by now of the pressure and anxiety residency training may cause. They should be reassured that they are following the footsteps of thousands before them, the majority of whom have graduated from their training programs to lead a fulfilling career. With a careful eye on their own wellness, and on the pitfalls of inappropriate coping mechanisms, the same can be achieved for them.

References

1. World Health Organization Constitution. Available at http://www.searo.who.int/EN/Section898/Section1441.htm.
2. Asken MJ, Raham DC. Resident performance and sleep deprivation: a review. *J Med Educ.* 1983;58:392-388.

3. Daughterty SR, Baldwin DC. Sleep deprivation in senior medical students and first year residents. *Acad Med*. 2002;347:1259-1255.
4. Steele MT, et al. The occupational risk of motor vehicle collisions for emergency medicine residents. *Acad Emed Med*. 1999;6:1050-1053.
5. Kiernan M, et al. 24 Hours on-call and acute fatigue no longer worsen resident mood under the 80-hour work week regulations. *Curr Surg*. 2006;5/6:237-241.
6. Newhouse PA, Belenky G, Thomas M, Thorne D, Sing HC, Fertig J. The effects of D-amphetamine on arousal, cognition, and mood after prolonged total sleep deprivation. *Neuropsychopharmacology*. 1989;2:153-164.
7. Rosenthal L, Roehrs T, Zwyghuizen-Doorenbos A, Plath D, Roth T. Alerting effects of caffeine after normal and restricted sleep. *Neuropsychopharmacology*. 1991;4:103-108.
8. Reyner LA, Horne JA. Early morning driver sleepiness: effectiveness of 200 mg caffeine. *Psychophysiology*. 2000;37:251-256.
9. Wiegmann DA, Stanny RR, McKay DL, Neri DF, McCardie AH. Methamphetamine effects on cognitive processing during extended wakefulness. *Int J Aviat Psychol*. 1996;6:379-397.
10. De Valck E, Cluydts R. Slow-release caffeine as a countermeasure to driver sleepiness induced by partial sleep deprivation. *J Sleep Res*. 2001;10:203-209.
11. Wrenn KD, Oschner I: Rhabdomyolysis induced by a caffeine overdose. *Ann Emerg Med*. 1989;18(1):94-97.
12. Janeen R. Azare, PhD, MSPH, Department of Medicine, Memorial Sloan-Kettering Cancer Center, New York, NY. Review provided by VeriMed Healthcare Network. http://www.nlm.nih.gov/medlineplus/ency/article/002579.htm Updated 4/4/2006
13. Schwartz JR, Nelson MT, Schwartz ER, Hughes RJ: Effects of modafinil on wakefulness and executive function in patients with narcolepsy experiencing late-day sleepiness. *Clin Neuropharmacol*. 2004;27(2):74-79.
14. Horne JA, Reyner LA. Counteracting driver sleepiness: effects of napping, caffeine, and placebo. *Psychophysiology*. 1996;33:306-309.
15. Bonnet MH, Arand DL. Impact of naps and caffeine on extended nocturnal performance. *Physiol Behav*. 1994;56:103-109.
16. Home JA, Reyner LA. Counteracting driver sleepiness: effects of napping, caffeine, and placebo. *Psychophysiology*. 1996;33:306-309.
17. Carter CL. Innovative scheduling strategies can make a world of difference. In *American College of Emergency Physicians reference and resource guide*. Irving, TX: ACEP; 2006.
18. Lee C, et al. A compromise phase position for permanent night shift workers: circadian phase after two night shifts with scheduled sleep and light/dark exposure. *Chronobiol Int*. 2006;23(4):859-875.
19. Mitler MM, et al. Hypnotic efficacy of temazepm: a long-term sleep laboratory evaluation. *Br J Clin Pharmacol* 1979;8:63S-68S.
20. Roth T, Roehrs T. A review of the safety profiles of benzodiazepine hypnotics. *J Clin Psychitary*. 1991;52(9, suppl):38-47.
21. Basu R, et al. Sedative-hypnotic use of diphenhydramine in a rural, older adult, community-based cohort: effects on cognition. *Am J Geriatr Psychiatry*. 2003;11(2):205-213.
22. Glass JR. Acute pharmacological effects of temazepam, diphenhydramine, and valerian in healthy elderly subjects. *J Clin Psychopharmacol*. 2003;23(3):260-268.
23. Caldwell JA. Fatigue in military aviation: an overview of U.S. military-approved pharmacological countermeasures. *Aviat Space Environ Med*. 2005;76:C39-C51.
24. Herxheimer A. Melatonin for the prevention and treatment of jet lag. *Cochrane Database Syst Rev*. 2002;CD001520.

25. Jockovich M. Effect of exogenous melatonin on mood and sleep efficiency in emergency medicine residents working night shifts. *Acad Emerg Med.* 2000;7:955-958.

26. Cavallo A. Melatonin treatment of pediatric residents for adaptation to night shift work. *Amb Pediatr.* 2005;5:172-177.

27. McNamara RM, et al. Chemical dependency in emergency medicine residency programs: perspective of the program directors. *Ann Emerg Med.* 1994;23:1072-1076.

28. Hughes PH, Brandenburg N, Baldwin DC, et al. Prevalence of substance use among US physicians. *JAMA.* 1992;267:2333-2339.

29. Hughes PH, et al. Resident physician substance use, by specialty. *Am J Psychiatry.* 1992;149:1248-1254.

30. Pagliaro L, Pagliaro AM. *Pagliaros' Comprehensive guide to drugs and substances of abuse.* Washington, DC: American Pharmacists Association; 2004.

31. Shewan D, Dalgarno P. Evidence for controlled heroin use? Low levels of negative health and social outcomes among non-treatment heroin users in Glasgow. *Br J Health Psychol.* 2005.

32. Hughes PH, et al. Resident physician substance use, by specialty. *Am J Psychiatry.* 1992;149:1248-1254.33.

33. American College of Emergency Physicians Impaired physician Policy Statement: http://www.acep.org/webportal/PracticeResources/PolicyStatements/PhysicianWell Being/PhysicianImpairment.htm

chapter 60

Dealing With Peers

Parag Paranjpe, MD
University of Miami School of Medicine

Thomas Perera, MD
Program Director, Jacobi Montefiore Emergency Medicine Residency, Albert Einstein College of Medicine

After the stress of the preclinical years and Step 1, beginning the clinical years is viewed by most medical students as an eagerly anticipated and exciting time in their lives. As you put away the Krebs cycle and move into the clinical arena, there are some changes that you should make. Third year marks the beginning of a change in world view for most medical students. Standardized exams are now only part of what you will be graded on. You will be evaluated on your performance in whatever medical role you are placed.

Many of these roles require a level of teamwork for which many years of preclinical competition have not prepared you. It is time to put away your copy of Machiavelli's *The Prince* and buy a copy of Dale Carnegie's *How to Win Friends and Influence People.* A positive "can do" attitude and the ability to get along with anyone are what will make you a valuable part of the medical team. Maintaining good relationships with your peers will be an essential part of this formula. As they move through the clinical years, medical students are put through many stressful experiences in the clinical arena, as well as in their personal lives. If one of your peers has an emergency and needs a favor or a shift switch, you should try your best to help. If you get a reputation for being helpful, people will go out of their way to help you. You never know when you might need a favor.

Dealing With Peers: General Rules

- Keep your commitments and promises.
- Do not play the blame game.
- Share credit for your accomplishments.
- Never blindside a peer, supervisor, or nurse.
- Be mindful of your nonverbal communication.
- Help your peers succeed.

Dealing With Peers: On the Third Year Clerkships

You are not directly competing with your peers in third year. You are working with them to do well. What the student must realize is that the key to a successful medical team is good teamwork. Good teamwork can save the student time, increase the entire team's effectiveness, and make everybody look good. A successful medical outcome or patient interaction reflects well on everyone. Even the exams in third and fourth year are usually scored against a national average or against scores accumulated over the years. Therefore, your score will not affect your peer's score and you can work together to succeed.

In the clinical arena of third year you learn from what you see. Time limitations and random chance make it impossible to see the entire spectrum of pathology during your clinical time. There is a lot you can learn by discussing cases with your peers. Sharing knowledge and teaching from one case in exchange for what another student has seen in another case will allow you to learn a lot.

Last, avoid being seen as cutthroat. Attending physicians and housestaff can all spot "unsportsmanlike conduct" a mile away. Remember, they were once in medical school, and they had to deal with the same situations you are in now.

Dealing With Peers: On the Emergency Medicine Rotation

Dealing with peers on the emergency medicine rotation is much the same as dealing with peers on the third year core clerkships. Emergency medicine is a team sport, with attendings, residents, nurses, technicians, and medical students playing different but equally important roles. Having good teamwork on the emergency medicine rotation is of central importance to your success. Programs are looking for bright, motivated residents who are interested in learning and get along well with their peers. Nothing makes a student look better in the eyes of a program director than discovering that the student helped a classmate. Programs will have you for 3 or 4 years, and they are looking for personalities that can get along with the other residents. One of the questions on the standard letter of recommendation for emergency medicine asks how the medical student rates in their "personality; ability to interact with others." This clearly shows that the ability to deal with peers well is looked on as an important trait in our specialty.

Often, it may seem to the medical student as if he or she were in direct competition with their peers on the emergency medicine rotation. Nothing could be further from the truth. There are a lot of emergency medicine programs. The programs in which you are interested will not be the same as those your peers are interested in; there is plenty of room for everyone. In the 2005 match, there were 1332 categorical emergency medicine positions available, but there were only 1138 U.S. senior medical students applying for those positions. In addition, there were 403 "other" people (foreign medical graduates, etc.) applying, for a total of 1541 applicants for 1332 positions. However, of the 1138 U.S. seniors, only 78 (6.85%) did not match.

Most important, other medical students on the emergency medicine rotation are going to be your professional colleagues for the rest of your career. Emergency medicine is a relatively small field. You will run into all of your colleagues at some point in your career, and the friends you make in medical school may help you get the job of your dreams later in life. The emergency medicine rotation is a time to showcase yourself, and working well with your peers is a vital part of your success.

Dealing With Peers: Relationships

One survey in 2002 found that a quarter of long-term relationships start at work. We are often told not to mix our work life with our personal life, but this is not always possible. There are many successful relationships that occur between residents who work together, due to mutual attraction, compromise, understanding, and maturity on both sides. Keep in mind, however, that there are many aspects of residency that are not optimal for any relationship. These including scheduling, sleep deprivation, and stress.

Do not get involved with anyone at work without looking closely at the possible consequences of your actions. You will be spending many hours with your coworkers and tainting it with a poorly thought out romance can make your life more difficult for years. The key to success is to discuss the relationship and its ramifications with your potential partner and come to an understanding before moving forward.

Dealing With Peers: Problem Peers

What if there is someone with whom you do not work with well? First, do not let one event or interaction make for a bad relationship with anyone. Everyone has bad days. People often behave badly at work when faced with adversity or stress. Try to be understanding of your peers.

If interactions continue to be strained, ask yourself why there is tension. Is it because of something relatively minor, such as a personality clash or different styles of doing things? Is the reason more substantial, such as dishonesty or unreliability? If the the strain is due to a personality clash, or something equally minor, then a little self-reflection is in order. Will changing the way you act change your interactions with that person for the better? In these instances, a little compromise can go a long way.

Explore what you are experiencing with a trusted friend or colleague. Have the other person look objectively at the situation and offer support and advice. Do not start whining to everyone, however, as this will lead people to see you as a complainer.

If you feel the situation warrants it, speak to the problem peer about it in a private, nonthreatening, nonaccusatory way. Ninety-nine percent of the time, this will settle the difference, and the rest of your rotation can move along smoothly.

Consider a follow-up discussion after some time has passed to either discuss the improvement or lack thereof. Of course, you must decide whether a follow-up conversation will have any impact and if you want to continue to confront the difficult person by yourself. This discussion can be very effective at changing behavior.

If, this does not settle the problem, then you must consider if you feel the difference is problematic enough to go up the chain of command. This is something you must decide on a case-by-case manner. When all else fails, try to limit the difficult person's access to you. Whatever happens, always remember that losing your cool in your interactions with the problem peer will not make the problem better.

Summary

The clinical years of medical school can be a very exciting and rewarding time, and working effectively with your peers will greatly enhance your experience. Healthy peer interactions are always in your best interest. This is especially true for your interactions with your peers who are also choosing careers in emergency medicine. Armed with a little self-reflection and compromise, most difficulties you have with problem peers can be resolved. In regard to those of you who would like further training in dealing with peers, Dr. M. Ang at the University of Chicago has put together a course to prepare students for professionalism in the workplace.[2] Although the seminar deals mostly with conflicts with patients, it provides insights into the student's own communication style and how that may affect interpersonal interactions. Embrace teamwork and be accepting of the faults and foibles of your peers. It is important to remember that at the end of the day, you are now a medical professional.

References

1. Jolly P. Charting outcomes in the match. July 2006, AAMC and NRMP. Available at https://services.aamc.org/Publications/showfile.cfm?file=version68.pdf&prd_id=159&prv_id=189&pdf_id=68.
2. Ang M. Advanced communication skills: conflict management and persuasion. *Acad Med.* 2002;77(11):1166.

chapter 61

Optimizing Communication in the Emergency Department: Working with Consultants

Caesar Djavaherian, MD, MS
Instructor of Medicine, Division of Emergency Medicine, Weill Medical College of Cornell University
New York-Presbyterian Hospital

Stuart Kessler, MD, FACEP
Associate Professor of Emergency Medicine, Mount Sinai School of Medicine
Clinical Director, Elmhurst Hospital Center Emergency Department

Training in emergency medicine is comprehensive, yet the breadth of presenting diseases, the occasional need for specific expertise, the time limitations imposed on emergency physicians due to patient volume, and hospital policies necessitate frequent interactions with consultants. Unfortunately, communication with consultants can be one of the most challenging aspects of the practice of emergency medicine. Although the ability to communicate effectively with consultants may take years to perfect, using certain strategies to guide your interactions will dramatically optimize your conversations and ensure that the consult will meet your expectations in terms of providing necessary information and improving patient care.

When calling a consultant, the emergency physician must first clearly communicate the purpose of the consultant's involvement in the case. Generally, consultants are called to provide specialized knowledge, continuity of care, including admission and/or outpatient follow-up, or postprocedure management. This may include helping to determine a specific diagnosis or just optimizing a treatment plan. The emergency physician will also need to decide whether the consultant needs to evaluate the patient in person in the emergency department, in the hospital after admission, as an outpatient, or, in rare situations, based solely on a telephone conversation. This decision will depend on the acuity, natural history, and prognosis of the disease process. The emergency physician is often acting in a role of patient advocate as well as physician as the emergency physician attempts to efficiently determine the patient's diagnosis and best treatment options. Establishing the consultant's role in the patient's care helps set the framework for the remainder of the conversation.

The emergency physician must then pose a specific, well-defined question or limited series of issues for the consultant to address. The conversation should be limited to pertinent positive and pertinent negative information to the to help the consultant hone in on their expected role and responsibility for the patient's care. This form of communication is a dramatic shift from the typical patient presentations taught in medical schools where a history, including past medical and surgical history, social and family history, as well as physical exam are communicated in detail. In the interest of optimizing communication with consultants, the emergency physician must anticipate and present only the relevant pieces of information consultants will need. Presenting overly comprehensive histories, physical exam results, and patient's emergency department course will not only make your interactions inefficient and time consuming but may distract the consultant from the needed primary task. One pearl that may close the gap between the requested information and what the emergency physician has the time to convey is to say that you will be happy to fill in the details once the consultant arrives in the emergency department.

Hospitals generally have protocols in place for the involvement of consultants in the care of patients presenting with certain acute disease processes such as severe traumas, acute myocardial infarction, and stroke. These mandates must be thoroughly understood and implemented by the emergency practitioner. The emergency provider should also be aware that protocols that direct or encourage specific consults often come with recommendations of time frames within which consultants must respond and complete their consultations.

In addition to consultant response time, the emergency physician should try to be aware of the level of training of the consultant with whom they are speaking. Although there may be limited options as to who will respond to a request for consultation, emergency physicians should be cognizant of the fact that the consultant's level of training may impact his or her ability to make valuable recommendations. If the emergency physician believes that the level of expertise of the consultant is not appropriate for the question on hand, then the emergency physician needs to determine if other options are available.

Each consulting service has its own method of communication and likely will pay attention to specialty specific clinical features. When speaking with all services, gender, age, pertinent history, and pertinent findings from a thorough examination of the involved region(s) of the body including abnormal vital signs and available test results should be communicated. After providing this information, each consulting service may require specific, and somewhat different, information. Clearly conveying clinical instability in any presentation is critical, as it will attach a level of urgency to the consultation. This helps consultants prioritize their multiple tasks and patient responsibilities and allows for the setting of time frames within which the patient must be evaluated. Some examples of these situations are as follows.

Medicine subspecialists including intensivists are often more interested in a patient's detailed history and physical exam compared with some surgical specialties. In the interest of time, the emergency physician can expedite such conversations by specifically detailing the relevant information within the history, physical exam, and diagnostic work-up.

Often, surgical consultants may request relatively less information regarding patients. Because some less experienced surgeon's foremost question is, "Do I need to operate on this patient?" a concise and up-front delineation of the reason for the consult may be valuable. This can be followed by an abbreviated, but relevant, history and physical. The results of diagnostic tests, such as radiographs or computed tomograph demonstrating free air or bowel obstruction, or critical physical exam findings such as that of an acute abdomen, crystallize the issue and are generally the most important part of the presentation.

When speaking with a neurologist regarding a suspected stroke, a potentially high-acuity diagnosis associated with a time-sensitive treatment, communicating the exact time of onset of symptoms is essential. This would be followed by neurological deficits, neurological history, any relevant medications, and vital signs. If available, the result of the computed tomography scan, and the finger-stick glucose result should be discussed. Other important historical features in the setting of an acute cerebrovascular accident would include tPA contraindications.

When speaking with the neurosurgery service, the emergency physician needs to communicate history, physical exam features, and potential diagnoses that first pertain to any possible need for emergent operative intervention. In such circumstances, a history of trauma, other neurosurgical history, noted neurological deficits, mental status, and pupillary exam are significant. If the result of a computed tomography scan or magnetic resonance imaging study is available, then it should be communicated as well. In situations involving possible spinal cord syndromes, findings regarding rectal tone, motor and sensory exam findings, including sensory dermatome deficits, are exceedingly important to communicate.

Important clinical features for the obstetric/gynecology consultant when a diagnosis of a ruptured ectopic pregnancy is being considered include the results of the pregnancy test and hemodynamic stability, as well as LMP and related obstetric/gynecology history and physical exam. When consulting for possible ovarian torsion, a history of large cysts in conjunction with severe intermittent lower abdominal pain helps make the diagnosis. Serum beta-hCG and emergency department/hospital ultrasound exam findings are very helpful if available at the time of consultation.

When consulting an ophthalmologist, history and visual acuity are key components to communicate. This information combined with a physical exam, often encompassing a slit-lamp exam and in some situations an intraocular pressure reading, will help categorize a patient into those requiring immediate attention and those who can be evaluated less urgently.

For orthopedic emergencies, results of imaging studies that identify the extent of the injury (e.g., degree of angulation, extent of displacement) are often the most important part of the presentation. Suspicion or evidence of a compartment syndrome, acute dislocation, complex or unstable fracture, or neurovascular compromise will complete the crucial parts of the presentation.

The otolaryngology consultant will in some clinical settings be very concerned with airway issues. When the clinical scenario involves potential airway compromise, it is very important to evaluate and describe any signs of airway compromise or patency by relaying findings such as voice change, stridor, or the patient's inability to control secretions.

In speaking with urologists, the physical exam including loss of cremasteric reflex, blood at the urethral meatus, or an exam consistent with an acute scrotum are crucial findings that need to be reported.

The understanding of when and why to request a consultation combined with the knowledge of how to systematically organize your presentation will allow you to optimize your interaction with any consultant. The emergency physician must not only be knowledgeable about the diagnosis and treatment of a wide variety of disease processes but must also exhibit an understanding of the clinical issues that each consulting service is concerned with when they receive calls. The emergency provider must have reasonable expectations of what the consult will add to the patient's care. There is little formal teaching on this subject leaving emergency practitioners with the need to pick up most of the nuances over years of practice in the emergency department. By following some of the ideas outlined above, you can reduce the anxiety and potentially negative interactions experienced when speaking with consultants. Hopefully, this will lead to mutual respect and trust with each consulting service and the best possible patient outcomes.

chapter 62

Working With Nurses and Alternate Practitioners

Michael Cassara, DO, FACEP
Department of Emergency Medicine, North Shore University Hospital

Andrew E. Sama, MD, FACEP
Department of Emergency Medicine, North Shore University Hospital

It is common practice in the United States to use nonphysician practitioners to deliver patient care and to perform specialized and often highly technical procedures in the emergency department. Medical students on rotation in the emergency department will undoubtedly encounter nonphysician practitioners, working as part of the emergency medicine team, or as partners with consultants from other specialties within the institution. It is wise for the prospective medical student rotator to develop a comprehensive understanding of the similarities and differences in education, training, clinical capabilities, and responsibilities of the various nonphysician providers most likely to be encountered. Knowledge of the competency, roles and responsibilities of this group of patient care providers will assist the medical student rotator in assimilating as a member of the patient care team and serve to enhance his or her clinical experiences and interactions during the duration of the emergency department rotation.

Nonphysician Practitioners

Nonphysician practitioners credentialed to practice in the United States include licensed practical nurses (LPN), registered nurses (RN), clinical nurse specialists (CNS), nurse practitioners (NP), certified nurse midwives (CNM), certified registered nurse anesthetists (CRNA), and physician assistants (PA). The most frequently encountered nonphysician practitioners in the emergency department are registered nurses, clinical nurse specialists, nurse practitioners, and physician assistants, as detailed.

Registered nurses are recognized as vital components of the emergency department workforce. They triage patients, perform direct patient care activities (e.g., patient assessments, periodic reassessments, medication administration, phlebotomy, specialized nursing care/interventions), ensure effective information transfer when the patient is admitted/discharged, and foster open communication between patients, their families, and the emergency physician. Select nurses, generally with advanced education, also serve as department administrators, assisting with managing and overseeing staffing, patient throughput, and resolving patient complaints and staff concerns. Some nurses have specialized roles in academic institutions, serving as investigators in clinical, basic science, or translational research, as staff educators, or as sexual assault nurse examiners (SANE). Most RN training programs confer a bachelor of science in nursing (BSN), although many associate degree programs still exist. Nurses with expertise with regard to the practice of emergency nursing may be credentialed as certified emergency nurses (CEN) by meeting the prerequisites of the American Board of Nursing Specialties and the Emergency Nurses Association.

Clinical nurse specialists came into being in response to changes in health care technology that required nurses with highly specialized knowledge and skills. Clinical nurse specialists provide patients with advanced clinical nursing care and are often engaged in educational activities instructing and educating hospital staff and patients on clinical issues. They provide direct patient care, educate staff and patients, consult with other professionals, and provide leadership and supervision. Clinical nurse specialists work in various environments according to their specialty, but most work in a hospital setting. To become a certified clinical nurse specialist, one must have completed a master's degree and on graduation be eligible to take the state certification exam for a CNS certificate as well as the professional certification exams for their specific area of study.

Nurse practitioners and physician assistants are recognized as "physician extenders and mid level providers." Their roles and capabilities vary based on location, institution, and individual education, training, and experience. Physician assistants and nurse practitioners in the emergency department most commonly provide patient triage and direct patient care under the supervision of emergency physicians. The medical director of the emergency department or a designee has the responsibility of providing overall direction of activities of nurse practitioners and physician assistants in the emergency department through formalized agreements. Select physician assistants and nurse practitioners may serve as department representatives responsible for quality management, performance improvement, service excellence, and/or benchmarking. They may also serve as investigators in clinical, basic science, and translational research, and as faculty for continuing medical education coursework. The requirements with regard to the education, certification, and licensure of nonphysician providers vary, depending on the training program and its curricular design, affiliation with a degree-granting institution, and state regulations. Most nurse practitioner and physician assistant training programs now confer bachelor and/or master's level degrees on successful completion. There is yet to be a standard universally recognized certification indicating that a nurse practitioner or physician assistant has acquired specialty expertise in emergency medicine.

Advanced-Level Nonphysician Practitioners

The distinguishing features differentiating nurse practitioners and physician assistants from other nonphysician practitioners (in addition to education and training) is the increased autonomy they are given with regard to patient care activities and their ability to bill patients (or insurance carriers) for their services.

Hospital and medical staff policies and procedures, bylaws, and other institutional, state, and federal rules and regulations very specifically define the nature and governance of nonphysician practitioner patient care activities and clinical privileges within a specific institution and region. In general, nonphysician practitioners are capable of providing a wide range of services to patients in the United States. The services must be medically necessary and within the predefined scope of practice for the individual nonphysician practitioner. As previously mentioned, most institutions and organizations require a specific delineation of privileges for nonphysician practitioners. These privileges may be exercised only within the department/division in which the nonphysician practitioner performs the majority of his or her patient care activities. Well-managed and comprehensive credentialing programs for nonphysician practitioners demand that all patient care providers demonstrate current competency, continued procedural proficiency, and proof of maintenance of certification/expertise (generally by meeting continuing medical education requirements and by participating in quality assurance/performance improvement reviews).

In many circumstances, health care services provided by nonphysician practitioners are recognized and reimbursed by insurance carriers, including Medicare, Medicaid, and nongovernment insurance programs. The detailed guidelines for practice are different for each state; emergency physicians, therefore, need to be cognizant of the state and federal licensing regulations and registration requirements for nonphysician personnel with whom they work, so that an appropriate structure for documentation, coding and billing exists.

Practice Models Supporting Advanced-Level Nonphysician Practitioners

The American College of Emergency Physicians (ACEP) endorses guidelines for emergency department's that employ nurse practitioners and physician assistants to care for its patients. The best practice models incorporating nonphysician practitioners are based on the "team" concept; nonphysician practitioners are integrated with and work alongside emergency physicians to ensure the most efficient, effective provision of emergent health care. The implementation of a successful practice model including nonphysician practitioners requires that the relationship between emergency physicians and nonphysician practitioners be formally defined; in particular, the scope of practice and the clinical privileges for each individual nonphysician practitioner must be clearly delineated and agreed on. Several different practice relationships and structures are possible. The structure of the relationship and the role of nonphysician practitioners in the emergency department are influenced by local and regional practice standards, state law, federal Medicare guidelines, needs of the patient population the emergency department serves, and the current competency, experience, and expertise of the individual nonphysician practitioner. Some nonphysician practitioner models of practice bestow more independence and clinical autonomy than do others. Most, however, expect the nonphysician practitioner to collaborate with the supervising emergency physician during the course of each patient encounter; specifically, the attending emergency physician is expected to evaluate the entirety of care provided and supervise the key portions of any procedures performed as each is occurring. This requirement for performing supervision is similar to that required of attending emergency physicians who work with medical students and residents. If a nonphysician practitioner is expected to perform direct patient care that is not contemporaneously supervised by a qualified emergency physician, then he or she should demonstrate specific experience and training in emergency care. Nonphysician practitioners should also be educated with regard to institutional and emergency department policies and procedures, their scopes of practice, and their delineations of privileges. Emergency department medical directors are expected to provide oversight of all nonphysician practitioner patient care activities; this responsibility includes implementing assessments and measures focused on quality assurance and performance improvement. Practice models that ultimately require emergency physicians to accept final responsibility for patient outcome and satisfaction usually represent the best means for ensuring high-quality patient care in the emergency department.

Working With Nurses and Alternate Practitioners

It is helpful for the medical student presenting to any patient care unit at the beginning of a clinical rotation to develop a productive, collegial relationship with the professionals working on that unit. Establishing excellent rapport with the professional staff working in the emergency department is essential for the successful assimilation of the medical student as part of the patient care team. This is much more challenging in the emergency department. Given the demanding and time-sensitive nature of emergent patient care and the wide variety of patient presentations one will encounter, medical students rotating in the emergency department who do not interact well with the professional staff may easily become overwhelmed, overworked, overlooked, or, worst of all, ignored losing an important opportunity to learn. Medical students whose professionalism, altruism, and interpersonal and communication skills enable them to integrate into the patient care team more quickly will undoubtedly be encouraged to participate fully within the entire spectrum of clinical opportunities available to emergency department rotators, and, as a result, will observe, experience, practice, and learn more emergency medicine.

Entering the emergency department as a medical student rotator is an exciting yet challenging learning experience. For many it will be the first time they encounter patients with high-risk, high-acuity medical problems since beginning their medical school training. The most important thing the medical student rotator must do when first presenting to the emergency department for a clinical shift is to introduce himself or herself to all staff members working on that shift. Medical student rotators should clearly state their names, their programs, and their year of training. Most academic institutions accept student rotators from prehospital provider training programs, nursing and other allied-health care professional training programs, and resident physician rotators from within and outside the department. Do not assume that the emergency department staff can distinguish the medical student rotators from these other student rotators.

It is important for medical student rotators to communicate professionally with everyone they meet (including the clerks, receptionists, transporters, and other ancillary staff working in the emergency department). Inappropriate, unprofessional medical student rotator interactions with emergency department staff usually have significant, long-standing consequences. More important, improved patient outcomes emerge when all members of the emergency department staff collaborate to provide care in accordance with a common set of core values that is patient-focused.

It is essential for medical students to familiarize themselves with the dynamics of relationships in the emergency department. Interactions with nurses are regular events during medical rotations as well as throughout one's career. Understanding the educational importance of those collaborative relationships and the true shared responsibility for patient care may be one of the greatest points a medical student can learn on rotation in the emergency department. Open communication, trust, and respect are the hallmarks of successful and productive relationships with all professionals and personnel in the emergency department.

Teaching intuitions where medical students, residents, attending physicians, and nurses collaborate is a great place for students to learn from nurses as well as their physician mentors. Most students learn quickly that nurses can help students integrate into the unit and serve as a functional team member without difficulty. Multidisciplinary case management and excellent physician-nurse relationships are practices in health care that medical students will learn to master as they progress in their careers.

One area of anxiety and stress for medical student rotators new to the emergency department is dealing with the "seasoned" registered nurses working in the unit. The value of positive nurse-physician interactions is well recognized. Medical student rotators working and learning within the complex clinical environment of the emergency department will observe and appreciate just how much nursing care is required for the prompt, timely, accurate, and safe execution of emergent health care decisions and interventions. A critical issue is to learn the importance of excellent interpersonal and communication skills (especially with nurses), and how those skills contribute to fostering the cohesion necessary for the smooth functioning of the patient care team. Medical student rotators should learn how to write orders on their patients (legibly and correctly), and how to inform nurses that they require execution. Medical student rotators should understand that many nurses have excellent clinical skills and an uncanny ability to promptly distinguish between patients who are acutely sick and those who are not; their recommendations and suggestions should not be discarded without due consideration. A truly shared responsibility for patient care between medical student rotators and nurses should exist.

Medical student rotators in the emergency department may also work alongside the aforementioned advanced-level nonphysician practitioners. Medical student rotator interactions with these providers will be similar to those with resident and attending-level physicians working in the emergency department. Medical student rotators may be expected to review their patients with these staff members, including the pertinent findings acquired in the patient history and on the physical examination prior to the emergency medicine attending formalizing the patient care plan.

Summary

Nonphysician practitioners continue to partner with emergency physicians across the United States to provide high-quality emergent patient care services. ACEP and other professional organizations encourage the continued collaboration of emergency physicians with nonphysician colleagues in the provision of comprehensive and prompt health care to emergency department patients. A positive working relationship and continued growth in mutual educational efforts will only strengthen a currently sound professional partnership between emergency physicians and nonphysician practitioners.

Emergency departments with teaching programs where medical students, resident and attending level physicians, and nursing staff are continuously working together as part of an integrated team are unique environments for medical students. The breadth of practitioners providing patient care, the depth of each practitioner's experience, and the wide spectrum of patient presentations make the emergency department a great place for a rotating medical student to receive a broad clinical education that transcends the experiences available on other inpatient units. Medical student rotators can learn from nurses and other advanced-level nonphysician practitioners as well as from their resident and attending-level physician mentors. Nurses, physician assistants, and nurse practitioners can help medical student rotators assimilate more easily into the patient care team and enable them to more readily serve as a functional team member with less difficulty. Embracing a multidisciplinary perspective and learning how to encourage the most productive physician-nurse interactions are essential skills medical students will need to master as they progress throughout their years of training if they are earnestly seeking a rewarding and successful career practicing emergency medicine.

More than ever, practicing emergency medicine in the twenty-first century requires emergency physicians to work well alongside a cohesive team of personnel dedicated to providing only the highest quality patient-oriented emergency care. The challenge of current and future health care providers is to continue to recognize and appreciate the importance of creating an environment where all members of the health care team can contribute toward excellent patient care; when this is achieved, positive patient outcomes are the result.

chapter 63

Handling the Toll of Emergency Medicine Practice

Joel Gernsheimer, MD
Department of Emergency Medicine
State University of New York Downstate Medical Center, Kings County Hospital Center

Rewadee Soontharothai, MD
Resident, Department of Emergency Medicine, Lincoln Medical and Mental Health Center

As a medical student considering the exciting field of emergency medicine, one might hesitate because of the stresses and subsequent burnout that are often associated with the practice of emergency medicine. The good news is that the burnout is much less than was previously thought and the stresses can be handled by understanding and practicing the concept of wellness.

Stresses of Emergency Medicine and Why Wellness is Needed

Emergency medicine is exciting, but also can be a stressful field. While working in the emergency department, there are constant challenges for the emergency physician. The environment is fast-paced and unpredictable. Quick, hard decisions have to be made, sometimes without all of the needed information. The emergency physician must be able to manage everything that comes through the door, from the highest-acuity patient in cardiac arrest to the lowest-acuity patient with an upper respiratory tract infection. The emergency physician must be able to multitask managing multiple patients at the same time. The emergency physician must interact with all patients who come to the emergency department, including difficult patients who may have multiple social and/or psychological problems and may be angry or even violent. In addition to interacting with uncooperative patients, the emergency physician sometimes interacts with uncooperative consultants who may resent demands on their time, especially during off hours. In addition, the emergency physician must practice in a "fishbowl" environment, where others get to second-guess initial decisions made in the emergency department. Furthermore, emergency medicine is a relatively young specialty, and in some institutions, it is not given the respect it deserves, leading to rules and regulations that may make it more difficult to work in the emergency department. Add all the above to the constant threat of litigation (emergency medicine has one of the highest rates of malpractice suits), and it is not hard to understand why emergency medicine practice can be so stressful.

In addition, the shift work (and lack of calls) that is envied by others can be a source of stress. Shift work, especially working night shifts, has been compared with smoking one pack per day of cigarettes in taking 10 years off one's life. It has been touted to contribute to higher rates of motor vehicle accidents, myocardial infarctions, divorces, suicides, substance abuse, depression, and mood swings among emergency physicians. It has even been said to contribute to a seven-fold increase in gastric and duodenal ulcer rates. This is probably because it disrupts the circadian rhythm of our internal biological clock. It also puts the emergency physician at a disadvantage when trying to relate to others, who commonly work Monday through Friday, 9 AM to 5 PM. The emergency physician must work long shifts, often at nights, on weekends, and on holidays leading to conflicts with family activities and social events, and to possible social isolation. Also, busy shifts may leave little energy to do more than go home and sleep, causing the emergency physician to miss personal, family, and social activities. Last, camaraderie among colleagues may be difficult to develop due to separation caused by shift work.

Emergency medicine residency training can be an especially stressful time in the development of the emergency physician. Trainees must acquire new knowledge and skills, take on new responsibilities, and learn to cope with changes in their environment and living patterns. Sources of stress include sleep deprivation, long hours, high patient loads, patient deaths, need to pass examinations, adjustment to attending physicians, and competition with peers, including competition for procedures. Thus, training in emergency medicine has its own challenges that must be handled. All of the above mentioned stresses can take their tolls and contribute to dissatisfaction, illness, and burnout among emergency physicians.

Recognizing and Avoiding Burnout

Figures vary on the rate of emergency physician burnout. It appears that burnout is more prevalent in non-emergency medicine-trained physicians and in those physicians who chose a career in emergency medicine by "default" than in those who really wanted to enter the exciting and rewarding field of emergency medicine and avidly pursued the proper training to confidently and competently practice emergency medicine. Therefore, to avoid burnout, it is important to decide that emergency medicine is a good fit for you and to obtain the best possible training you can to prepare you for the practice of emergency medicine. For students and residents who want to enter the field with the intention of making this their lifelong career, the statistics on burnout are not important. What may be of more pertinence is how to avoid becoming a statistic. In order to avoid burning out from the stresses of emergency medicine practice, the emergency physician must recognize early the signs of burnout:

Involvement in work turns into exhaustion, cynicism, indifference, and a burden.

Patience and compassion turn into anger, bitterness, and frustration.

The sense of teamwork both at work and in one's personal life turns to alienation and isolation.

The emergency physician must identify and accept what stresses are leading to burnout. This involves some honest self-inspection. The individual can then decide how best to deal with these issues and whether outside help is needed. With an understanding of the factors that are causing stress and leading to burnout, it is possible to take steps to promote wellness and repair the situation before it is too late.

Promoting Your Own Wellness

Working in the emergency department can be a thrilling and fruitful learning and working experience, but at the same time it has its challenges and stresses. To best profit from the experience, it is important to keep a balance in your personal and medical life. Here are some useful strategies for promoting your own wellness:

Get Enough Sleep and Rest

Shifts in the emergency department can offer constant excitement and may require some stamina. Thus, it is important to be well rested and ready for the challenge of working and learning in the emergency department. Shift work can disrupt circadian rhythms and the sleep cycle, so plan ahead and schedule time to sleep before a shift. Try to get a similar number of hours of sleep before a night shift as you would for a day shift. If you needed 8 hours of sleep to function well during the day, the same probably would be true for the night shift.

There are many strategies to get quality daytime sleep that you can try. First, good sleep hygiene helps. Try to find a dark, cool, and quiet setting (if possible). Consider investing in blackout shades, earplugs, and eye covers. Minimize interruptions during scheduled sleep hours by turning off telephones, pagers, and other noisy devices when possible. Get help from friends and family to decrease disruptions during sleep hours. In addition, because circadian rhythms can work against sleep, consider the following strategies. Get some sleep in the afternoon or evening prior to any night shifts. If doing a string of night shifts, try sleeping after the shift, then getting another nap before the shift. If you are planning to sleep before a night shift, try following your regular "before sleep routine" before going to sleep. This means that if you usually drink milk, take a shower, and then go to sleep—you would do exactly that before going to sleep prior to the night shift. Also, this may be a good time to try reading that sleep inducing medical textbook you have been trying to get through. Also, make sure to set an alarm before going to sleep. Then, when it is time to get up for the shift, turn on bright lights, eat, and follow your usual morning routine. Individualize the strategy that works best for you.

Eat Well

Remember the common saying "you are what you eat"? Well, in the emergency department it is important to remember to take a break and eat. During a busy shift, because meal times are not put into the schedule, it is easy to forget to eat; if you do not eat, it should not be a surprise that you will feel drained. In addition, it is often easy to forget about proper nutrition and grab the fast foods. However, be careful not to make it a routine. We should practice what we preach to our patients, including not smoking. Getting good nutrition will keep you in good shape for many more shifts to come, so plan on eating balanced meals.

Get Enough Exercise

Exercise is good for the body, mind, and soul. It will give you the stamina needed for the demands of the emergency department. So, schedule time to get regular exercise. All physical activities count, and it does not need to be in a gym. Consider taking a walk to the train instead of the bus, walking up the stairs instead of the elevator, walk your dog, or make your own list. Keeping in good shape will also come in handy when you are asked to do CPR on that long resuscitation case.

Make Time to Relax

Make time to clear your mind and relax, a time when you do not have to do something. Think of it as time to reboot your system. Consider a short version of this during a long and hectic shift, especially if you are feeling overwhelmed. This can even be done as part of your lunch break. It will leave you more refreshed to return to what you need to do.

Spend Time With Your Family and Friends

Due to the demands of medicine, it is easy to forget that we are more than just physicians. This is an unhealthy tendency. Life and relationships outside of medicine have a considerable impact on our wellness and is much needed for balance. Make time to be with those you care about. In times of stress, your relationships outside of medicine can become a priceless resource.

Make Time for Fun (Outside of Medicine)

Give yourself time to do what you enjoy, whether that is a hobby, shopping, or any other activity that makes you happy. It will make you a more balanced individual and leave you more refreshed for learning and working.

Use of Caffeine and Other Substances

The moderate use of caffeine in the form of one or two cups of coffee or tea can help with alertness during a shift. However, overuse of caffeine can cause nervousness, palpitations, and withdrawal headaches. Also, caffeine too close to planned sleep-time can disrupt needed sleep. Beware of the regular use or dependence on sleep inducing medications such as sedatives-hypnotics. It is usually best to avoid their use. Melatonin has been touted as being able to modulate the sleep-wake cycle, but this is still unproved, although it is thought to have few side effects. The key word here is *moderation*.

If you are using recreational substances, know that emergency physicians are not exempt from the issues of abuse and substance dependence. In fact, emergency physicians have a high rate of addiction. Get help! There are physician wellness programs available in most hospitals, which can help with substance dependence issues. The successful rehabilitation rates through these programs are high. Getting help may save your life and your license.

Study

This subject hardly needs to be mentioned because it is on the mind of all trainees, but it is mentioned here for encouragement. Reading will help improve understanding of the pathology that is seen in the emergency department, improve your emergency department experience, and increase your fund of knowledge. In addition, it will improve self-confidence and thus decrease stress levels. Reading about a disease you encountered during a shift is a good way to remember that disease process. It will help improve your test score, and further lower your stress levels. In addition, it will make your program director happy and lower his or her stress levels. is that enough encouragement?

Keep Your Eye on the Prize

When things get rough, try to remember why you chose the field of emergency medicine. Remember your goals and the good things you do, like saving lives and making a difference in the lives of your patients.

Summary

A career in emergency medicine is a constantly stimulating, challenging, and sometimes stressful endeavor. In order to keep a sense of fulfillment, emergency physicians need to learn and apply wellness skills early in their careers. Learning how to plan and balance life and career will improve a physician's sense of well-being. A happy and well physician is a better and more caring physician. In addition, keeping well physically, mentally, and emotionally will better ensure longevity in emergency medicine. Thus, the promotion of wellness is to everyone's benefit, including the emergency physician, their patients, family, friends, colleagues, and society as a whole.

Bibliography

Bintliff SS, Kaplan JA, Meredith JM III, et al. *Wellness book for emergency physicians.* Irving, TX: American College of Emergency Physicians; 2004.

chapter 64

Coping with the Unanticipated Personal Emergency

Jay Kaplan, MD, FACEP
California Emergency Physicians

The philosopher Albert Camus once wrote, "In the depths of winter, I finally learned there was an invincible summer." As human beings we will face crises in our lives that we do not foresee and cannot anticipate. Life throws curveballs at us when we least expect it, and so we need to learn how to prepare for and respond to those personal emergencies. Part of that preparation is developing support systems that we can rely on in times of crisis, and part is developing skills and flexibility to help us adjust to what falls in our path.

What are the kinds of unanticipated events that can cause personal crises? Sudden medical illness, acute trauma which leads to temporary or permanent disability, family tragedy such as the illness or loss of a loved one—all of these experiences can cause profound alterations in the way we perceive our lives and ourselves. Those are all acute sudden events that affect us. But personal crisis is not always caused by an acute event. Burnout is a loss condition created over a longer time, and because of this fact, it may be quite insidious. Once the "tipping point" is reached, a person may precipitate change or hurt as damaging as acute loss. Our reaction to a sudden change in circumstances mirrors the more chronic responses found in burnout: Our energy, involvement, and engagement in our lives are replaced by exhaustion and cynicism; the enthusiasm, patience, and compassion we had at the outset by anger, bitterness, and frustration; our feeling of fit and the excitement in being a part of a greater group are replaced by a feeling of lack of fit, by alienation, and by isolation.

We also need to understand that somatic symptoms of illness may also appear in response to sudden loss or change in circumstances. Headaches, chest pain, abdominal pain, and virtually any chronic illness/symptom may be exacerbated by the stress of personal emergency. In 1967, Thomas Holmes and Richard Rahe[1] created the concept of the Social Readjustment Scale, wherein different life events were given life change units depending on their potential impact on a person's life. For example, loss of a spouse was 100 points; divorce, 73; personal injury or illness, 53; being fired at work, 47. If a person accumulated more than 150 points in 6 months, he or she would have a 50% chance of major life-threatening illness or injury within the next 2 years; if greater than 300 points, the percentage would increase to 80%. Coping with personal disaster often involves not only emotional skills but also the need to take action with regard to physical symptoms.

People in the field of health care field, especially those who are physicians or becoming physicians, are accustomed to being in positions of control. We are health care givers who make choices ourselves about what is to be done and when; we are not familiar with or comfortable with being on the receiving end where others are making those decisions. Change is not easy, especially when it is change that is forced on us rather than change that we determine and manage. And sudden illness, acute disability, injury or illness of those we love—leave us feeling at least temporarily helpless.

Change = Loss = Grief. Grief has been variously defined. In 1974 in *The Handbook of Psychiatry, grief* was defined as "the normal response to the loss of a loved one by death."[2]

In 1984, Dr. Terese Rando, a noted grief specialist, researcher, and author, defined *grief* as the "process of psychological, social and somatic reactions to the perception of loss."[3]

In 1991, the Grief Resource Foundation of Dallas, TX, described a good working and practical definition of *grief* as "the total response of the organism to the process of change."[4]

Elizabeth Kübler-Ross in her landmark book *On Death and Dying* (1969)[5] and, more recently in another book co-written with David Kessler, *On Grief and Grieving: Finding the Meaning of Grief Through the Five Stages of Loss* (2005),[6] discussed the five stages that people go through in responding to catastrophic news/loss:

1. **Denial—The initial stage**: "It can't be happening."
2. **Anger**: "How dare you do this to me?!" (referring to either God, the deceased, or oneself)
3. **Bargaining**: "Just let me live to see my grandchild born."
4. **Depression**: "I'm so sad, why bother with anything?"
5. **Acceptance**: "I know that all happens for the best."

Kübler-Ross originally applied these stages to any form of catastrophic personal loss, such as the death of a loved one or even divorce. She also claimed these steps do not necessarily come in order, nor are they all experienced by all patients, although she stated a person will always experience at least two. The truth is that any change of circumstance can cause us to go through this process, and we do not have to go through the stages in sequence. We can skip a stage or go through two or three simultaneously, and we can go through them in different time phases. The intensity and duration of the reaction depend on how significant and permanent the change-produced loss is perceived.

The above five stages in fact define steps that we all go through in reacting and responding to sudden personal emergency. However, the real work in terms of moving forward begins in the fifth step. Some have suggested that grief work is best defined by the acronym TEAR:

T = To accept the reality of the loss
E = Experience the pain of the loss
A = Adjust to the new environment without the lost object
R = Reinvest in the new reality

This work begins when the honeymoon period is over, the friends have stopped calling, everyone thinks you should be over it, the divorce is finalized, "closure" has been effected, and everything is supposed to be back to normal. It is at this point that real labor begins.

So, what can we do to prepare ourselves for coping with sudden personal emergencies? We can develop those same skills that allow us to remain healthy and well and avoid burnout. One suggestion is to create a formalized "renewal investment plan" for ourselves, to help us remain healthy and enhance our well-being. RIP does not have to stand for "Rest in Peace." Some areas to include in your RIP are the following:

1. *Rest.* How much sleep do you need on a nightly basis? Plan to get it, even if that means setting an alarm clock or watch to tell you not when it is time to wake up but rather when it is time to go to sleep. Make certain that when you as a student or physician are working through the night you get enough rest and have the support of your family and environment to support your sleep time.
2. *Exercise.* What and how often—you should put this into your calendar. Most studies suggest that people who exercise early in the morning are more successful

in maintaining an ongoing and regular exercise program. Give yourself enough time to warm up, cool down and stretch in general in order to remain flexible in both mind and body.

3. *Family/significant other time.* Amid our harrowing and busy work lives we must ensure that we take the time to connect with those we love and who love us. As Gandhi once said, "There is more to life than merely increasing its speed" (and he said that more than 50 years ago).

4. *Build down-time into your schedule.* Time to "just be" rather than "do." We are human beings, not human doings. Let us not experience "pure terror at the thought of nothing to do and nowhere to go."

5. *Spirit.* Time and energy to relate to our humanity and to a power greater than ourselves. How do you connect to spirit and from what do you derive your sense of meaning in your life? Write out a mission statement for yourself, in a similar manner to the way that the organizations for which we work do.

6. Nutrition. How do you physically nourish your body? What kind of diet makes you feel great? Your body is your temple, not just a vehicle to carry you from place to place.

7. *Joy.* How do you emotionally nourish your self? Create a joy list—a list of things that you can do or how you can be that really brings you happiness and joyfulness. After you create the list, write down next to each entry the last time you did or experienced that particular event. It can be sobering to realize that it has been a very long time since you gave yourself a particular experience of joy or pleasure.

If you can consistently practice wellness in your life when things are going well, you will have developed skills and capabilities to respond to sudden changes in you or your family's wellness. In times of crisis, the above seven areas remain critically important in helping you move through your feelings and toward a grounded and healthy existence.

So the admonitions with regard to coping with personal emergency are as follows:

1. Do not isolate. reach out to those in your social network and share your feelings, no matter how difficult.

2. If you do not have people to whom you can turn, reach out to counselors or therapists who can help you deal with your crises. There are many skilled expert health care providers with great experience in helping us TEAR. If you are a religious person, turn to your faith-based leader for assistance and prayer.

3. If you are having somatic illness, make certain that you see your personal physician. If you do not have one, ask a friend for advice and who to see. Sometimes transient use of medication can be very helpful, as can reassurance that physician symptoms are not indicative of a serious ongoing illness.

4. Get enough rest and ensure that you eat nutritional food. Avoid alcohol or sedatives whenever possible.

5. Ongoing physical exercise is a great way to channel your anxiety and physical stressors.

6. While work can be helpful in terms of taking your mind off of your loss, do not over-work. Take the time you need to grieve.

Rocky Balboa in the memorable film of 2006 about the aging prizefighter of the same name said the following to his son: "It will beat you to your knees and keep you there permanently if you let it. You, me or nobody is going to hit as hard as life. But it ain't about how hard you hit, it is about how hard you can get hit and keep moving forward, how much can you take and keep moving forward. That's how winning is done!"

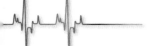

Bibliography

Albom M. *Tuesdays with Morrie.* New York: Doubleday; 1997.

Bach R. *Illusions: adventures of a reluctant messiah.* New York: Bantam Doubleday; 1977.

Grateful Members. *The twelve steps for everyone . . . who really wants them.* Center City, MN: Hazelden: 1994.

Kushner H. *When bad things happen to good people.* New York: Avon Books; 1981.

Moore T. *Soulmates: a guide for cultivating depth and sacredness in everyday life.* New York: Harper Collins; 1992.

Muller W. *Sabbath: restoring the sacred rhythm of rest.* New York: Bantam Books; 1999.

Rohn J. *Leading an inspired life.* Niles, IL: Nightingale-Conant; 1997.

Seligman M. *Learned optimism: how to change your mind and your life.* New York: Pocket Books; 1990.

References

1. Holmes T, Rahe R. The social readjustment scale. J Psychom Res. 1967;11(2):213-8.
2. Solomon P, Vernon D (Eds). *The handbook of psychiatry. Los Altos, CA: Lange Medical Publications*1974.
3. Rando T. Grief, Dying, and Death: Clinical Interventions for Caregivers. Champaign, IL:Research Press. 1984.
4. Dallas, TX: Grief Resource Foundation; 1991.
5. Kübler-Ross E. *On death and dying.* New York: Touchstone; 1969.
6. Kübler-Ross E, Kessler D. *On grief and grieving: finding the meaning of grief through the five stages of loss.* New York: Scribner; 2005.

chapter 65

Pregnancy and Breastfeeding During Residency

Heather Long, MD
St. Peter's Hospital Emergency Department

Karen Onufer, MD, FACEP
University of Medicine and Dentistry of New Jersey

You're pregnant! How wonderful, and exciting but you are probably thinking "Wait, I'm a resident. How am I going to do this?" Do not worry, you absolutely will, and you will do it with all the grace and confidence that made you the successful physician that you are today.

As I write this, I am looking at the smiley face of my 3-month-old son. I survived pregnancy and the emergency department, and you will, too. This is an amazing and exciting time, and I hope to share a few helpful hints that may make the transition from ER Doc to new Mommy a little bit easier.

Surviving the Symptoms

Once you have had that positive b-hCG test, your world will never be the same. This includes your life as an emergency physician. That first trimester is filled with such joy and anticipation, but also fatigue and nausea. Twelve hours in the emergency department can be tiring, but it only gets compounded when you are pregnant. No one really prepares you for how tiring pregnancy can be. I have never been a nap person, and I always thought naps were reserved for little kids. When you are pregnant, your view on naps will certainly change; all of a sudden you are more tired than you have ever been before. Twelve-hour shifts seem even longer than before. You may spend your days off catching up on your lost sleep, but that's just fine. Remember extra sleep is your body's way of telling you what it needs. You have a very challenging career, and with all the physiologic changes of pregnancy, it is very understandable to lay down for that nap.

My best advice is to sleep when you can, and nap if you need to. Running around the emergency department is hard enough, and now you have a little one taking some of that boundless energy away from you. Be sure to stay healthy and take care of yourself. Sleep, eat well, try to stay away from the waiting room vending machines, and do not be afraid to say no to something you cannot do because you are not feeling well.

This leads us to morning sickness. There are times when you may need to run to the bathroom between patients to vomit yourself! There may be times when you wonder why your nauseous patient is complaining—you are sure you feel ten times worse than she does. This, too, shall pass, so hang in there. It is time that you take all the advice you give your hyperemesis patients and start listening to some of it yourself. Be sure to eat and have those saltine crackers ready at all times. Drink plenty of fluids, stay hydrated, eat small meals, and rest assured that the nausea will end.

Be sure to wear your most comfortable shoes at all times. Your feet have may have hurt before, but your legs may now have pitting edema that you have never personally experienced. You may feel like a congestive heart failure patient and will have a new sympathy for those with dyspnea on exertion. I quickly learned to avoid lots of steps and the art of consolidating those walks to the radiography and computed tomography suites. You will learn the meaning of "cankles," in which your calf and ankles become one (I know it is not a real medical term, but it is amusing nonetheless). The good news is that most of your colleagues are very sympathetic to pregnant women, so take advantage of them giving you the one available chair—that will end the minute you get back from maternity leave! Remember to try to not stand when you can sit. I know it is hard in the emergency department, but you need to minimize the time on your feet.

Beware of the bad emergency department smells! We all know how bad some of the many scents of the emergency department can get, but pregnancy can bring these to a new level. Do not be afraid to tell your colleagues that you need to step away for a moment to cleanse the air; this, too, shall pass!

And finally, what is a discussion about the first trimester without mentioning those countless trips to the bathroom? I would run to the bathroom between trauma patients, as nothing is worse than trying to do an intubation, and worrying that you cannot hold it in any longer. Go to the bathroom when you have the chance; you have a very valid excuse and everyone will understand.

As the Big Day Approaches...

One big advantage of being an emergency physician, which I am definitely guilty of, is using the department ultrasound to peek at what my little one was up to during the day! As your baby gets bigger, and you do, too, you will be begin to wonder about what life will be like and how will I handle all of this?

Be sure to discuss maternity leave options with your superiors early on in your pregnancy. Knowing that you have your leave arranged will take a weight off your shoulders. Your colleagues will also appreciate being able to fill in the gaps while your gone by having plenty of notice of your time off.

Once your little one arrives, you will experience a love you have never had before. All of those tired days running around the emergency department are suddenly worth it, and you cannot imagine what you ever did before you had a baby. Well, you do remember one thing from your former life, which was sleeping more than 2- to 3-hour stretches at a time.

Sure, we've all pulled all nighters, and we've survived medical school, so how hard can this baby thing be? Well, the good news is that your night shifts are good preparation for baby sleep depravation. The bad news is that no one really tells you how tiring new motherhood can be. There are definitely days when I think that a 12-hour shift is easier than all this laundry, bottles, and diapers. But rest assured; your emergency department training of juggling ten things at once will definitely come in handy with your newborn. Your friends and family, and even you, will be amazed at how quickly you figure this baby thing out. Before you know it, you will be juggling all the things you need to do, and you'll have your own little schedule down pat.

Remember the advice to not stand when you can sit in the emergency department? Now, it is important to not be awake when you can sleep! Countless friends told me to sleep when the baby sleeps, and initially I did not listen. I thought I was stronger than that. I would take that time to catch up on bills, laundry, e-mails, etc... Well, after REALLY getting tired and worn down, I learned that the advice of all those mothers before us is really useful. Take the opportunity to sleep when you have it. Soon enough, those long baby stretches of sleep during the day will be over, and you will be chasing a crawling baby around the house (but that's a topic for another time).

It is also crucial to remember to take time for yourself. Try to take a shower everyday, put on your makeup, or whatever it takes to make yourself feel like yourself and not just a new mom. Ask your husband to watch the baby and run for a haircut, facial, to the mall, or whatever makes you feel like you have had a moment to yourself. Before long, you will be back at work and juggling a family, so take time for yourself to regroup when you need it.

Child care may be an issue for many returning to work. Most of us are not lucky enough to have family nearby who can care for our newborn when we return to our shifts. Be sure to look into your child care options early in your pregnancy. Your leave will go way too fast and you will be very busy juggling your newborn and getting used to your new way of life. Start planning your child care options early on in your pregnancy. Start interviewing day care centers, potential babysitters, nannies, or whatever child care options are available to you. Your newborn is now the center of your existence, and you cannot imagine going back to work and leaving him or her. The prospect of leaving your baby with anyone is terrifying; however, if you start early, you will feel much better if you have your child care lined up. Finding loving, responsible, and affordable daycare can be challenging, but you can do it; just start early.

One other bit of advice is to remember that you are a physician, but now you're a Mommy and do not try to both to your little one. Once my son was born, I think I forgot every bit of pediatric medicine I have ever learned. But when it comes to him, I am Mom and not Doctor Mom. Do not be afraid to call the pediatrician with questions, even if you think they are stupid and you should know the answer yourself. I remember cutting my little guy's finger with the nail clipper, and I do not know who cried harder, me or him! A few days later I thought it was getting infected (his finger was so tiny it was really hard to tell). I took him to the pediatrician , and not only was it fine, but it was such a simple visit that the physician did not even fill out the chart. I felt pretty silly, but the pediatrician had some good advice: "be his Mommy first, and not his doctor." You may be a physician but you do not have to know it all. You are a new mother, with a new baby, and sleep deprived to boot! Do not be afraid to ask questions or seek advice no matter how simple the problem may seem.

These are only a few words of advice from someone who has made it through pregnancy in the emergency department and is now surviving (and loving) being a new Mom and an emergency physician. You will quickly learn your own helpful hints and get plenty of advice from loving family and friends. Just remember that you are a successful, intelligent physician who can succeed at motherhood and your career. Best of luck and enjoy every minute!

Breastfeeding Survival Guide

Breast is best. This is what we heard throughout medical school and what we have been telling our pregnant patients. It is also best for physicians' babies, but what they do not teach us in medical school is how to juggle the demands of residency with those of breastfeeding. First of all, cut yourself some slack residency and new motherhood both place enormous constraints on your time and well-being, and inflicting guilt on yourself will not help the situation. Breastfeeding does not have to be an all-or-none proposition. You may continue to make enough milk to nurse your baby once or twice a day for months after you return to work just by continuing to breastfeed when you are able and by pumping once or twice a day. You may be able to freeze and store enough milk during your maternity leave to extend your breast milk supply for months. Having your partner give your baby a bottle while you get some much-needed sleep ultimately may allow you to continue to breastfeed for longer.

Most new mothers do not begin pumping and storing breast milk until at least 2 weeks after the baby is born—your nipples may still be too sore and you may be overwhelmed with the adjustments of new parenthood. Most lactation consultants recommend you introduce a bottle to your baby somewhere between 2 and 4 weeks of age. Introduce it earlier and you may confuse your baby; wait until later and your baby may refuse it. Getting your baby to take a bottle may require multiple attempts and you may need to try multiple different types of nipples before finding one your baby will accept.

If you are thinking of pumping once you return to work, research where to pump ahead of time as you may have just enough time in your day to squeeze it in without trying to find a private area in the hospital. Ask other residents and nurses for suggestions. A call room may be ideal, but if you have to travel the equivalent of two city blocks to get to it, it may not be practical. Some hospitals' postpartum wards have a room with a hospital grade pump where you can pump in privacy. You may want to buy a "hands free" bra to use while pumping so you can eat lunch, etc. while you pump instead of holding the cups to your breasts. Additionally, you can purchase a converter for your car's cigarette lighter so you can pump on the way to or from the hospital.

Below is a list of items and suggestions road tested by working moms. Items you should pack in your bag to bring with you to the hospital when you go into labor (or have with you for your home delivery) are italicized.

Lanolin ointment/cream. Apply to nipples before and after breastfeeding and in between sessions. You don't have to wipe off before feeding. (It gets all over their mouths and is really adorable). BRING to hospital.

Breast gel pads. Keep in refrigerator and apply in between sessions for temporary soothing. BRING to hospital.

Breast pumps. (1) Hand pump (» $35). Even if you do not plan to pump and store your milk, you should get one of these, and even if you buy the expensive electric pump, you should get one of these for when you are out and do not have time and/or access to the other pump, such as in a restaurant, on an airplane, or at work when you just have time to run to the bathroom. BRING to hospital in case your milk comes in while you are there—some babies initially have difficulty latching on when you are really engorged. You can pump a little off and it makes it more comfortable for both of you.

(2) Near-hospital grade electric pump (» $250) (or you can rent a hospital-grade pump or use your hospital's if permitted). These are fully automatic and a must if you plan to pump and store your milk. You will not be able to rapidly and effortlessly hand pump enough milk to store. You may prefer to wait to buy this (or send someone out) until after you have the baby and you are sure you and your baby are able to breastfeed as breast pumps are not returnable.

Freezer bags for breast milk storage are sold separately. Also sold separately and recommended are bags for microwave sterilization of breast pump parts; this is more convenient than running the parts through the dishwasher or boiling them every time you use the pump.

Nursing bras. You will need at least two in the beginning; once your milk comes in and you see how those fit, you can order more or switch styles. Buy bras as close to your due date as possible so the fit is a reasonable approximation. (Your cup size increases up to two sizes with engorgement and then decreases again after feedings. Nursing bras have expandable cups.) WEAR to hospital.

Nursing pads. Buy the most absorbable nursing pads you can find initially. Later, once your milk production slows down, you may be able to use thinner ones. Once you return to work, be sure to bring multiple extra pads with you as well as extra tops. BRING to hospital.

My Brest Friend nursing pillow (» $34). A wrap-around pillow for supporting baby and your back while you breastfeed.

Nursing stool (» $200). The stool eases pressure on your legs and on your lower back while breastfeeding. It is not a necessity but IT really makes you more comfortable.

Best piece of advice I got: In the beginning, it may be difficult to determine if your baby is correctly latched on. Lactation consultants will tell you if it hurts, it's not right. Well, when you first start breastfeeding, it does hurt when baby first chomps down (and "chomp" is what it will feel like), but then if your baby is latched on correctly, the pain quickly subsides. My medical school roommate used to count to 10, and if the pain had stopped by then, she figured the baby was latched on correctly. The good news is that after a few weeks, it stops hurting altogether. Nursing your baby, sharing that special closeness before heading off to the hospital or on returning from call, may be the highlight of your day!

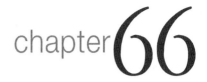

chapter 66

Gay, Lesbian, and Bisexual Issues in Emergency Medicine

Nicole Bouchard, MD
Faculty Advisor, Department of Emergency Medicine, New York-Presbyterian Hospital

Tejash Shah, MD
Resident, Department of Emergency Medicine, New York-Presbyterian Hospital

The topic of homosexuality in emergency medicine, and broadly in all of medicine, may be addressed from two perspectives: that of patient and that of provider. Although it is important for all physicians to be aware of this topic from each of these vantage points, it is the intention of this chapter to discuss only briefly the patient issues and to focus instead on the relevant issues facing lesbian, gay, and bisexual (LGB) medical students and residents.

The Gay, Lesbian, or Bisexual Patient

Although society has begun the evolution toward accepting homosexuality as a prevalent, normal form of sexual expression, this view is not yet universal. Surprisingly, this is as much a problem for providers as it can be for their patients.

It is imperative for every provider to consider the possibility of homosexual behavior in our patients. Because each patient may define this differently, we must ask inclusive questions to be most sensitive in recognizing this activity. Just as the questions one might ask a patient complaining of chest pain are similar between men and women, it is recommended that questions regarding sexual practice be similar between sexes. As an example, many effective physicians ask their patients whether they engage in sexual activity with men, women, or both. With practice, the tone of the question becomes unassuming and nonthreatening. It allows the patient to answer honestly, knowing the provider attaches no judgment to the answer and will use it only to ensure the best possible care. Additionally, many physicians choose to use the word "partner" whenever they ask about relationships, regardless of sexual orientation. This implies inclusiveness and is nonjudgmental, which will be appreciated by the LGB patient. Finally, if the situation requires a discussion regarding health care proxy, be up-front about asking whether the patient might have chosen the partner to fill this privileged role.

For patients, the problem is greater and more difficult to address. The Gay and Lesbian Medical Association estimates in their 2004-2007 Strategic Plan that there are at least "27 areas in which there is evidence that LGB people experience health disparities—outcomes that are worse than the general population." Their data indicate higher rates of smoking, depression, and certain cancers in the LGB population, with little new research being done to address these disparities.[1] This lack of research is perhaps one reason why many LGB patients distrust the medical profession. In turn, these patients may feel uncomfortable sharing their sexual practices with health care providers.

Gay, Lesbian, and Bisexual Physicians

Thankfully, because of efforts undertaken by physicians and activists before us, the path of the LGB physician, although still difficult, seems more maneuverable today. That said, there exist very unique issues the LGB student/resident faces on the road toward becoming a physician.

Medical School

If you are reading this chapter, you have already made it into medical school, passed your basic science courses, and, likely, have a good deal of clinical experience under your belt. You have realized great successes and have balanced your minority sexual preference with the challenges of working in a largely conservative profession.

If you chose to come out before medical school and were open during your application process, you might be interested to know that you are among only 5% of LGB applicants found to have done so in a study published in 2005. The same study found that of the medical students who planned to continue on to residency, only 33% planned on disclosing their sexual orientation during this selection process while 15% definitely would not. Of that 33%, about 25% were doing so to determine whether the program would accept their lifestyle, while another 25% wanted to find out if the environment within the program was acceptable for them. The majority of those that definitely would not reveal their sexual orientation during residency application were afraid that doing so would jeopardize their chances of matriculation into a chosen program.[2] Although this study is small, it highlights the difficult decisions that LGB students make throughout the residency application process.

The decision to be open regarding your sexuality while applying for residency is strictly personal. Those that argue in favor of being out have cited many reasons why they chose to do so. Most obviously, out residents want to be at a program where their sexuality will be honored and accepted. By being up-front about this important aspect of their lives, these LGB students feel they will be more likely to match at a program that is forward-thinking and one that has fewer issues regarding their lifestyle. If this strategy is effective, openness should also allay at least one of the many stresses of residency, one that is not faced by the majority of their colleagues. Finally, some residents report that being open upholds the principle of honesty and integrity so strongly valued by the medical profession. By doing so, they hope they will gain respect and trust.[2]

Obviously, as was seen in the study just cited, many medical students choose not to disclose their sexual orientation during the residency application process. Going even further, a 1994 study revealed that 30% of LGB medical students intentionally failed to report affiliations with organizations or activities that may identify them as gay or lesbian out of fear of homophobia.[3] Although this concern has lost much of its validity over the past 20 years, it unfortunately maintains some truth. A paper from the mid-1990s reports that "40% of general internists and 50% of internal medicine residents reported witnessing homophobic remarks in the workplace towards lesbians and gay men…," while still another reports that "one-third of family practice residents and psychiatry faculty were found to be homophobic."[4] There is no comparative literature available for the specialty of emergency medicine.

How you decide to manage your sexual identity through the residency application process remains strictly your decision. As you consider these ideas, though, remember that this aspect of you is only part of the larger picture you present. Having read through many emergency medicine residency guides, it was apparent to me that directors and their programs thought other aspects of a resident's application to be much more important. In residency, it is clear that qualities such as integrity, intelligence, an eagerness to learn, the ability to work well in teams, and motivation are appreciated and evaluated daily, regardless of your life outside work. Although this sentiment is based largely on personal experience, the same thoughts have been echoed by friends who are residents at many other emergency medicine programs.

Residency

Whether or not you decided to come out during the residency interview process, you have now matched and are practicing emergency medicine, one of the youngest and most progressive specialties in medicine. You are finally doing what you have waited so long to do but are starting to realize that you still face the challenge of being gay and choosing how out to be to your colleagues, coworkers, and patients. If you are in a relationship, you also face the challenge of managing that aspect of your life during this extremely stressful and demanding time. Hopefully, this chapter will help you start to formulate how you will go about making these decisions.

During training, you will obviously spend a tremendous amount of time with other emergency physicians and will naturally share some aspects of your life with these people. What you will have to decide is exactly how much you will reveal. Regardless of whether you were out during the residency selection process, now that you're here, working, it is wisest to assess each individual's responsiveness to and ability to accept your sexual preference. You may find it easiest to first come out to other LGB physicians, but do not be limited by this bias. Although these may be the most accessible people for you initially, you may also find the most important resources or mentors in those who are not.

It may be worthwhile to find out if your hospital has an LGB group with which you can become involved. It is difficult to find time in residency for things outside work, but such a group may help you throughout your training. This group can help you find resources within your community; find support among these people for those times when you need someone outside of your program with whom to speak; help with problems you might have in your relationship; and, if you are single, they may serve as a terrific dating pool. If such a group does not exist, find out how your institution might feel about your starting one—most academic programs are relatively open to resident groups that might make life more tolerable.

You did your research regarding the program's attitude concerning homosexuality during the interview process, but you may find that there are still some faculty/staff who do not respond positively toward your sexual preference. If at any time during your training you feel that your advancement or education is impaired due to a supervisor or colleague's attitude, you should seek out an intrainstitutional organization or individual, including the program director, who may be able to provide support. You should additionally research the organization's nondiscrimination policy and approach whichever people you feel comfortable with to aid you. Although this issue may consume you, remember the principles that helped you decide to become a physician—let these continue to guide you on a daily basis. Remember that it is the program's responsibility to train residents to the best of their ability and that residents are entitled to work in a nonhostile environment.

As a physician, you have the tremendous obligation to help people, regardless of their sexual preference. As an LGB physician, although these situations are few, you face the added challenge of dealing with people who may be LGB or who may have tremendous bias toward LGB people. Through observation of my more experienced seniors and attendings, I have learned that the best way to handle either of these situations is to remain professional and to have the goal of excellent health care in mind at all times. You have already demonstrated the capacity to empathize with your patients—usually without having to reveal anything about yourself—and should utilize this ability equally effectively with your LGB patients.

Conclusion

There is, unfortunately, no compelling evidence to help an individual decide whether to be open regarding his or her sexuality during medical training. One paper that studied a small sample of medical residents states quite eloquently: "we suggest that—whenever and wherever it feels safe—lesbian, gay and bisexual physicians join others in the workplace in the casual, honest conversations that pertain to career, family and personal choices... .

[These] informal conversations are a great aid to physician well-being. We also suggest that the colleagues of [LGB] physicians listen respectfully to this shared information, realizing the cost at which it has been spoken... . For those who are not ready to come out, because of either a real or perceived threat to their livelihood, family or personal safety, we advise tolerance and patience within the [LGB] physician community."[4]

References

1. Haller K, et al. GLMA Strategic Plan 2004-2007.
2. Merchant R, et al. Disclosure of sexual orientation by medical students and residency applicants. *Acad Med.* 2005;80:786.
3. Burke B. The well-being of gay, lesbian and bisexual physicians. *West J Med.* 2001;174:59-62.
4. Risdon C, et al. Gay and lesbian students in training: a qualitative study. *Can Med Assoc J.* 2000;162:331-334.

chapter 67

Financial Planning

Rahul Sharma, MD, MBA
Department of Emergency Medicine, Weill Medical College of Cornell University
New York-Presbyterian Hospital

As you finish medical school, you are ready to move on to residency training and to the next major step in your career. You now become a real "grown up" and will be faced with key financial decisions regarding the future well-being of yourself and your family. It is never too early to start thinking of the issues one could face in the future. The following is a brief overview of various investment vehicles available to individuals in order to prepare for a sound financial future.

To start on the road to financial health, one needs to be efficient at cash management while keeping goals and priorities in check to avoid frivolous spending. You will be faced with several expenses such as the cost of living, loan repayment, insurance payments (automobile, home, disability, and life), and retirement planning. If you do not set your priorities straight and plan accordingly, you will be faced with additional burdens (in addition to the stress of residency). You should determine your goals and figure out where you see yourself financially over the course of the next few years. The key to successful financial planning is reducing debt and bad spending habits. One should try to use credit cards only when you are compelled to for emergencies and minimize the tendency to spend frivolously.

Financial Advisors

Before making any serious financial planning decisions, you should consider "investing" in a knowledgeable financial advisor. Physicians have been known to provide excellent medical care, but when it comes to financial planning and management, we have been known to not be the top in this category. Just as we spend several years reading medical literature, taking call in hospitals, and saving lives, financial advisors have also spent a significant time in the field of financial planning.

You should choose a financial planner based on recommendations of friends, family, and colleagues. You can also contact your state medical society to see if they have any contacts that specifically focus on financial planning for medical professionals. You should choose a financial advisor who is reliable and easily accessible and really understands your goals. You should take some time in choosing a financial advisor rather than jumping into a relationship that might not work. This will be a "marriage" between you and your financial advisor so make sure you take your time. Another consideration to look for is whether your financial advisor is a CFP. The certified financial planner (CFP) is a certification demonstrating the individual has completed a comprehensive education and training program.

Student Loans

Once you have completed medical school and have started your residency, the reality of paying off your loans is a scary thought. You can choose to have a "grace period" but this does not mean interest on your loans is not accumulating. If you went to a private medical school, your debt from student loans can approach $200,000. This loan repayment can drain your income and you must think about the best way to approach this. Consider consolidating your loans as it can reduce your interest rate and total repayment schedule. You should compare the various plans and rates and speak to your friends and colleagues to see what deals they obtained. You should try to pay off the higher interest rate loans as soon as possible and always try to make the full payment every period.

Disability Insurance

Residents and medical students often overlook this but it is never too early to start thinking of obtaining a disability insurance policy. Ask yourself: "What would happen if I were disabled and not able to perform my duties?" "Who would pay my bills?" "Do I have the outside support (i.e., family, friends, spouse) to help me in the long term?" Your ability to work and earn income is your most valuable asset, and you must protect yourself! Policies can be purchased on a group or individual basis. A group policy is typically offered through your employer as part of their employment package. However, these plans often have several limitations, and if you change your job, you cannot necessarily transfer the policy to your new position. Although group policies are cheaper, they usually contain restrictive definitions of disability. If you purchase an individual disability policy, it will be more expensive but will stay with you even if you change your job from one hospital to another. If you purchase a policy through your group or hospital, the policy is no longer valid if you leave. Moreover, you may then be subject to another health assessment and higher premiums on the new policy. Make sure to find out if the policy you are purchasing is an "own occupation" policy. Under an "own occupation" policy, if you become disabled, you will receive benefits as long as you cannot practice your own specific specialty. Be careful as some policies do not specify "own occupation" coverage. For example, if you are a practicing emergency physician and you become disabled, some policies may expect you to teach or do research because they did not specify own occupation. Some policies have specific definitions on disability, so be sure to look at this carefully.

The ideal policy should be noncancellable and guaranteed renewable and should not be allowed to have any restrictions or provisions added once purchased. This means that the company cannot cancel the policy, increase premiums, or add any clauses or restrictions to the policy as long as you continue to make your payments. Many policies also have a cost of living adjustment rider (COLA). This is extremely helpful if you become disabled for a significant amount of time (longer than 1 year) and you want the payments you are receiving to keep up with inflation. You should also try to buy a policy as early as possible because buying a policy when you are young and healthy has advantages. As you get older, the premiums become more expensive and your chances of being rejected increase, especially if you acquire a medical condition. Just as you shop around for any other type of insurance policy, you should speak to several companies that offer disability policies. Make sure you read the fine print, as there are significant differences between the various policies. Most disability policies provide income coverage up to 60% that of a practicing physician. It is important to note is that medical students and residents are allowed to obtain policies that are based on income potential rather than on their current earnings and thus would benefit if they were to become disabled. Also, you should ask about a future purchase option rider. This will allow you to increase your disability coverage regardless if your income increases or if your health fails.

Life Insurance

Life insurance is something one should consider obtaining regardless of where you are in training. If you have dependents such as a nonworking spouse and children, then obtaining a life insurance policy is crucial. If you are single with no dependents, then obtaining life insurance is less crucial. Many employers offer a basic life insurance policy with minimum coverage. However, if you have dependents, you should consider obtaining an separate policy. A financial advisor would be beneficial in helping you determine how much coverage you should purchase.

Retirement Planning

The key to retirement planning and investing is to start investing and planning as early as possible. The concept of compound growth is something that confirms early investing is the best investing. With early investing, you will get the most "bang for your buck." Remember that retirement plans are long term investments.

You should consider meeting with a financial advisor to discuss exactly what type of investments would be suitable and in line with your financial goals. Usually, investing in stocks carries the greatest risk, and this is why many retirement plans do not allow for individual stock purchases. Mutual funds are common as they are less risky due to the diversification they offer. *Diversification* is a term used in investing that can be easily summed up as "don't put all your eggs in one basket." A mutual fund usually has investments in stocks, bonds, and other investments. However, remember that mutual funds can also sometimes be risky, and it is important to study their individual long-term (5 to 10 years) performance.

Once you start your new job as a resident, you will probably be given the option to enroll in the institution's retirement plan. Depending on the type of institution (for-profit versus not-for-profit), you will be offered to participate in a 401(K) versus a 403(B) retirement plan. This will be an ideal opportunity to meet with a financial advisor to strategize over your long-term investment goals and decide how your disposable income can be invested.

Roth IRA

The Roth IRA is probably one of the best investing opportunities available for anyone who is eligible to participate. Unlike other traditional IRAs, the Roth IRA is a "tax-free" investment. Other IRAs are usually tax-deferred investments, and you pay taxes on them once you withdraw the contributions. With a Roth IRA, you pay no taxes on your investment as long as you wait (to withdraw) after you are 59½ years old. However, there are specific eligibility and contributions limitations for a Roth IRA, and that is why you need to act now. Your income must be less than $100,000 and your maximum contribution is around $4500 per year (these numbers usually fluctuate slightly from year to year). This is ideal for you to invest in during your residency because once you complete training and are earning an attending physician salary, you will no longer be eligible for the Roth IRA. Do not underestimate the investing potential of a Roth IRA, and definitely try to take part in this opportunity.

Summary

As you progress in your training, you will be faced with key financial decisions. Remember to invest smart, start early, and try to cut down on any frivolous spending habits. Having a knowledgeable financial advisor will also make your life easier, and this is probably one of the best investments you can make.

Emergency Medicine Medical Student Involvement

chapter 68

Emergency Medicine Interest Groups

Erica Douglass, MD
Denver Health Medical Center

Laura Oh, MD
University of Virginia Health System

Jennifer Provataris, MD
Jacobi Medical Center; Department of Emergency Medicine, Albert Einstein College of Medicine

Emergency medicine is a relatively young specialty, with tremendous opportunity for individual leaders to make a significant contribution to the development of clinical practice, research, education, and administration.

As a student interested in emergency medicine, it is important to not only develop your clinical skills and knowledge base but alsoto develop your leadership skills in parallel. One way to do this, and to gain exposure to the field prior to residency, is through participation in your school's emergency medicine interest group (EMIG). An EMIG is a student-run group that both promotes interest in emergency medicine and helps students determine "fit" of specialty. An EMIG facilitates educational experiences in emergency medicine, informs students about a career as an emergency physician, puts students in contact with the resources and people needed to successfully apply for a residency, and provides a network of support. Every student considering a career in emergency medicine should get involved in his or her school's EMIG in some capacity.

How Can You Get Involved?

If an EMIG exists at your school, becoming involved may be as simple as demonstrating interest by attending meetings, lectures, and clinics. Most EMIGs welcome members who wish to take on additional responsibilities and do not limit leadership positions to fourth-year medical students. Some of the more common board positions may include president, treasurer, skills clinic coordinator, and national organization liaison. Before you apply for a position, speak to the current officer of the position you are interested in, so that you best understand the job description, time commitment, responsibilities, and application process.

What If Your Medical School Does Not Have an EMIG?

If your medical school does not already have an EMIG, starting one is an excellent demonstration of your commitment to the field of emergency medicine. It may also provide you the valuable opportunity to interact with emergency medicine faculty and school administrators. Medical schools differ in their requirements for starting a new organization, so check with your Office of Student Affairs for guidance before beginning the process.

Once you have determined what needs to be done to create an EMIG at your school, you will need to find a faculty advisor. A good place to start the search is through the emergency department chair, who will be able to identify the faculty members most interested in student mentorship. Alternatively, most academic emergency departments have a faculty member in charge of undergraduate medical education. This person is an excellent resource and may be more accessible than the department chair. In addition to offering advice regarding EMIG activities, a faculty advisor can facilitate shadowing, mentoring, and research opportunities, as well as provide educational materials.

Communication Is Key

At the beginning of the year, it is important that the EMIG leadership meet with the faculty advisor to discuss goals for the year and how those goals will be met. Writing an organizational mission statement or reviewing it at this time ensures that everyone understands your EMIG's identity and purpose. Now is the time to have an honest discussion with your faculty advisor about what you perceive each other's roles, responsibilities, and level of involvement to be. One of the trickiest parts of running an EMIG is that it requires an understanding of where your organization stands in relation to your department and school. Your EMIG always acts as a representative of both, whether or not this relationship is formally recognized; therefore, keep them informed of your planned activities.

In addition to communicating well with your faculty advisor and administration, it is also important to communicate well with your peers. Writing a formal constitution detailing organizational structure, election procedures, etc., will increase your EMIG's life span—not only is it often a prerequisite for grant applications and recognition by your school as an "official" body, but it also provides guidelines that help ensure harmony among future board members and continuity of mission.

Ideas for Your EMIG New or Old

Whether your EMIG has been around for years or is just beginning, a critical component of success is frequent, well-timed, well-advertised events. Aim to sponsor at least one event a month in order to maintain a high profile. Because third- and fourth-year students are often busy with clinical rotations, most EMIG events will be attended by first- and second-year students beginning to explore career opportunities. With this in mind, popular events are generally those that satisfy this curiosity without conflicting with demanding academic schedules.

Lunch or dinner lectures can be easily coordinated and, if food is provided, will definitely attract many students. Popular topics may include the following: what a career in emergency medicine entails, residency application advice, a discussion of fellowship opportunities and specialized interests within emergency medicine (e.g., pediatrics, toxicology, hyperbarics, research, bioethics, public policy, disaster medicine, international emergency medicine), and current emergency medicine topics of national importance (e.g., emergency department overcrowding, EMTALA, medical liability, health care reform). Beyond the lunch lecture, many EMIGs view skills clinics or workshops as an easy way to garner early student involvement. Common skills clinics include suturing, casting/splinting, phlebotomy, intubation, and electrocardiogram and film reading. Clinics are generally taught by residents or attendings and coordinated in conjunction with your faculty advisor. To supplement workshops, there are many free instructional resources available on the Internet though Web sites such as www.emra.org.

It is a good idea for you and your EMIG to get in touch with the major state and national emergency medicine organizations, as they often have resources to benefit both you and your EMIG. Coordinating a group trip to one of the two national meetings, ACEP in the fall or SAEM in the spring, is a smart way for you to stay in touch on a national level while bonding with your fellow classmates. On a smaller, less-expensive scale, there are always local meetings at the regional or state level.

Financing Your EMIG

Running an EMIG can be surprisingly expensive. For example, it is not uncommon to spend a few hundred dollars per skills clinic. An important exercise to do at the beginning of the year is to create a detailed, itemized budget. The less "guesstimation" of workshop materials, the more likely you will be to stay financially on-target. A well-run EMIG should be keeping track of its receipts as the year progresses; the president and treasurer should do a detailed accounting of finances at the midpoint of the year, to see if any adjustment of activities in the second half of the year is necessary. Referring to financial records from previous years can also provide information on how much things cost and remind you of costs you have missed.

An EMIG may choose to offset costs by charging a small admission fee to its clinics; other EMIGs may prefer to not charge students and instead apply for grants and run fundraisers. Grants will typically need to be approved by your school prior to submission; examples of grants available to EMIGs include a $500 SAEM EMIG grant and a $500 EMRA local action grant (both applications available online). Examples of fundraisers may include raffles of emergency medicine textbooks donated by emergency medicine faculty, sale of used textbooks or scrubs, bake sales, or reaching out to school alumni who are currently emergency physicians. Finally, do not overlook your school itself as a source of funding—be sure to check with your Office of Student Affairs, the undergraduate college, graduate student office, and the emergency medicine department itself to see if you can procure a small source of fairly reliable, recurrent funding. Most schools reserve funds for groups like EMIG but require preapproval of purchases and a record of event attendance. For the financial stability of your EMIG, a good goal to have in mind (although not always feasible) is to set aside a small amount of savings in an account in addition to maintaining a stockpile of workshop materials equivalent to at least 1 year's worth of EMIG activities.

Looking to the Future—Setting Your EMIG up for Success

For an EMIG to stay healthy, it must not only concern itself with its present activities but also look to its past and to its future. For example, an EMIG should make an effort to stay in touch with its graduating seniors; not only are they a part of the EMIG community, but they can also contribute significantly during the interview process by offering assessment of residency programs and interview housing. As for looking to the future, special care should be given to identifying leadership in underclassmen and helping them to develop the skills they will need to run the organization. Each board should leave the next board well-equipped with lessons learned, so that the new board can create a better EMIG than the one they inherited.

Summary

Participation in an EMIG is a great way to gain a mature vision of emergency medicine and to get the training you will need to become a future leader in the field. Involvement in an EMIG should be a part of any serious emergency medicine candidate's medical school career.

chapter 69

Medical Student Leadership

Timothy Cheslock, DO, PA-C
St. Vincent Health Center

Jill Corbo, MD, RDMS
Director, Emergency Ultrasound Fellowship, Jacobi Medical Center
Associate Professor of Emergency Medicine, Albert Einstein College of Medicine

Travis Watson, MD
Penn State

While many emergency physicians are looked on as leaders within their department, they were not instinctively born to that role. Leadership is a trait that is developed and honed over time. Not only are clinical skills important to the emergency physician, but so is the ability to work well with others such that they look to you for leadership and guidance.

There are many opportunities for the aspiring emergency physician to start developing these crucial interactions and leadership skills as a medical student. There are student opportunities for leadership within your school and in many national emergency medicine organizations. By becoming involved early on in your medical school career, you will not only strengthen your CV and application but also develop an established pattern of reliability, integrity, and personal interactions that are all valuable skills sought by emergency medicine residencies.

Most new first-year students are more concerned about the next anatomy test or physiology exam, but it is important to realize that becoming involved in your school's clubs and extracurricular activities can be just as important. It may be all that separates you from the next candidate when competing for that coveted residency position. While you may not be able to run for office of a school club until the spring of your first year, you can be a project coordinator for a special event, or help organize a club fundraiser. Every activity where you stand out and take charge increases your exposure and helps to showcase your organizational abilities and leadership characteristics.

Emergency Medicine Interest Groups

Most medical schools have an emergency medicine interest group (EMIG), and if yours does not, it is a tremendous opportunity for you to start one. While the activity level varies from school to school, interest groups have speakers, workshops, and/or public service events throughout the year. Officer positions typically include a president, vice president, secretary, treasurer, and representatives to state and national organizations. Most school elections are held in the spring each year for the following year. Do not be discouraged, however, if you cannot become elected to one of the few positions available in your school's clubs. There are many positions available in organizations at the local, state, and national level, where experience and presentation are important in obtaining a position of leadership. School faculties are impressed with leadership outside the school as well, because you are acting as a representative of the school. In almost all cases, school club officers are usually second-year students. By the time the third and fourth years come, few students are close to campus and are extremely busy with clinical rotations and clerkships.

The Emergency Medicine Residents' Association

The Emergency Medicine Residents' Association is the largest organization of emergency medicine residents in the county. Their mission is simple: "EMRA promotes excellence in patient care through the education and development of emergency medicine residency trained physicians." The leadership of EMRA includes a board of directors composed of a president, president-elect, immediate past-president/treasurer, *EM Resident* Editor, ACEP representative, academic affairs representative, and technology coordinator; as well as a council speaker and vice-speaker. The medical student leadership of EMRA is the Medical Student Governing Council (MSGC) and Medical Student Council (MSC). The MSGC is composed of a chair, vice-chair, east and west coordinator, technology coordinator, and newsletter editor. The MSC is comprised of regional representatives, an osteopathic coordinator, international coordinator, and a mentorship coordinator. Interested student applications are submitted by March 1 with a term commencing annually in May.

The MSGC is responsible for coordinating the EMRA medical student forum at the ACEP Fall Scientific Assembly and assisting with the annual residency fair. Throughout the year, the MSGC and MSC promote emergency medicine in medical schools throughout the country via electronic newsletters and maintain frequent contact with school's EMIGs. A student-resident mentor program was initiated in 2006 whereby interested students are matched with an emergency medicine resident mentor. This opportunity can be valuable in exploring residency programs and also in preparing a personal statement and CV for the Electronic Residency Application Service (ERAS) application. Resident mentors offer a unique perspective on the application process and profession itself. As the newest members of the field, they are closest to students in that they were in your shoes just a short time ago.

The American College of Osteopathic Emergency Physicians Student Chapter

The goals of the American College of Osteopathic Emergency Physicians Student Chapter (ACOEP-SC) are to support the workings of the parent organization and to promote opportunities for osteopathic medical students interested in a career in emergency medicine. The student chapter has sponsored an Osteopathic Emergency Medicine Residency Expo at the last two ACOEP Fall meetings, where a majority of the osteopathic emergency medicine programs are represented. This will continue to be an annual event and has been well received by both students and program directors. The student chapter also hosts a student seminar at both the fall and spring ACOEP meetings. Seminar topics are designed to prepare students for an emergency medicine career via information of the application process and how to interview. Panel discussions with program directors have also been included. There are lectures and workshops on osteopathic techniques for the emergency department as well as an osteopathic manipulative treatment clinic hosted by the students, where emergency physicians in attendance can receive treatments from the students.

The ACOEP-SC provides a number of opportunities to osteopathic medical students to become involved in emergency medicine. The Student Chapter Officers consist of a president, vice president, secretary, treasurer, GME Committee chair, Convention Committee co-chairs (two), Public Relations Committee (two positions), and a constitution and bylaws chair. Applicants can self-nominate themselves for these positions, which are elected at the Fall ACOEP meeting, usually held in conjunction with the Annual American Osteopathic Association Meeting. Voting takes place at the student chapter meeting at the end of the business meeting. One vote can be cast per school by the student representative of that school for each of the positions being elected. Student members are also appointed to serve as student representatives to the various ACOEP committees, some being specialty committees such as pediatric emergency medicine, EMS, and undergraduate medical education. There are other administrative committees such as communications/publications, governmental affairs, and constitution and bylaws. Being a student representative to a committee allows the student to become a part of the workings of the college and is an opportunity to become exposed to the full spectrum of emergency medicine. Whatever your interest, there is a committee that will fit your needs. Students report back to the student chapters on the committee business and can bring student concerns forward as well.

American Medical Student Association

With a half-century history of medical student activism, American Medical Student Association (AMSA) is the oldest and largest independent association of physicians-in-training in the United States. Today, AMSA is a student-governed, national organization committed to representing the concerns of physicians-in-training. With a membership of more than 68,000 medical students, premedical students, interns, residents, and practicing physicians from across the country, AMSA continues its commitment to improving medical training and the nation's health. Membership is available to medical students enrolled in or on leave of absence from any LCME or AOA accredited or provisionally accredited North American allopathic or osteopathic training program.

There are many opportunities for students to get involved in the AMSA organization. One can join action committees and interest groups by adding your e-mail address to the list server. To get more involved, one would recommend attending their annual convention to learn more about this organization. There are many different positions with varying degrees of responsibilities and time commitments, including president, vice-president, treasurer, or action committee chair. Committees include advocacy, medical education, health policy, community and public health, global health action, and humanistic medicine.

American Medical Association

The American Medical Association (AMA) is a national organization made up of physicians with the mission "to promote the art and science of medicine and the betterment of public health." Membership in the AMA is open to medical students enrolled in an LCME or AOA accredited program. Medical students are represented in the AMA through their own democratic, policy-making body: the American Medical Association-Medical Student Section (AMA-MSS), which has nearly 50,000 members.

The AMA-MSS is dedicated to representing medical students, improving medical education, developing leadership, and promoting activism for the health of America. It has many levels of leadership spanning the local, state, and national levels. The Medical Student Section (MSS) Governing Council includes a chair, vice-chair, delegate, alternate delegate, at-large officer, speaker, vice speaker, and AMA trustee. In addition, AMA Councils provide another opportunity for medical student leadership. These include the Council on Constitution and Bylaws, Ethical and Judicial Affairs, Legislation, Long Range Planning and Development, Medical Education, Medical Service, and Science and Public Health.

The MSS Governing Council also appoints a number of standing and ad-hoc committees comprised entirely of medical students. There is a committee for essentially every area in which the MSS makes policy or carries out action. A complete list of the committees, contact information for the current members, and activities of each committee is available on the AMA-MSS Web site.

American Osteopathic Association

The American Osteopathic Association (AOA) has many opportunities for students to become involved its national organization. Osteopathic Students may serve as representatives on the many committees that are part of the AOA leadership. Applications are due to the AOA by January 15 of each year. Appointees are notified by mid July for the upcoming academic year. The AOA covers travel expenses to attend the committee meetings. A stipend is also provided to cover hotel and meals during the event. Osteopathic students are encouraged to participate at this level starting in their second year of school.

In Closing

Whether you participate in any of the above offerings or serve as a representative or officer in any of the numerous medical student groups, you will be gaining valuable experience that will help you in your future career as an emergency physician. Do not be afraid or intimidated by the prospect of responsibility. Even if you have never served in a leadership position before, you will receive guidance and direction as to how best approach the job. Physicians are eager to mentor students in the hopes of keeping them involved as they progress into residency and practice. The experience you gain and the networking you will participate in can open many doors for you in the future. Best of luck!

Emergency Medicine Professional Societies

chapter 70

Emergency Medicine Professional Societies: An Overview

John Moorhead, MD, MS, FACEP
Oregon Health and Science University

Debra Perina, MD, FACEP
University of Virginia

For a medical student considering a career in emergency medicine, understanding the specialty and how to make a successful career are very important. There are multiple emergency medicine and national organizations inside as well as outside the specialty that impact on the training and practice of emergency medicine. Understanding the missions of these various organizations can assist medical students in acquiring a broader knowledge of the specialty, more fully appreciate what it means to be an emergency physician, identify "away" electives, and provide opportunities for involvement in organized medicine and leadership development. Additionally, online communications with individuals associated with many of these organizations can provide advice and mentorship opportunities for students that complement their medical school faculty. The number of organizations and their acronyms often lead to confusion in deciphering the "alphabet soup" and understanding the mission and niche each organization represents. To help students gain a greater understanding of the organizations that interface closest with medical students, each organization along with its history and mission are discussed in the remainder of this chapter in alphabetical order. Each organization maintains its own Web site, which students are encouraged to visit for further information.

American Association of Medical Colleges

The American Association of Medical Colleges (AAMC: www.aamc.org) is an organization of U.S. medical schools that together with the AMA sponsors the Liaison Council for Medical Education (LCME), which accredits undergraduate medical education. The AAMC sponsors the medical student matching program, the journal *Academic Medicine*, and a national meeting of faculty and medical school administrators. Based in Washington, DC, the AAMC is very interested in medical student input and sponsors the Organization of Resident Representatives (ORR).

American Academy of Emergency Medicine

The American Academy of Emergency Medicine (AAEM: www.aaem.org) AAEM is the newest specialty society in emergency medicine, founded in 1992, and is an independent association of board-certified emergency physicians that promotes board certification as a credentialing standard and fair business practices. It is committed to improving the practice environment of emergency medicine specialists. AAEM sponsors annual educational activities, as well as a resident section. AAEM is associated with the *Journal of Emergency Medicine*. The Academy has a presence in Washington, DC, and meets with congressional leaders, the Health Care Finance Administration, and the Office of the Inspector General on issues of interest to emergency medicine.

American Board of Emergency Medicine

The American Board of Emergency Medicine (ABEM: www. abem.org) was incorporated in 1976 and is sponsored by three organizations: ACEP, SAEM, and the AMA. It is the twenty-third member of the American Board of Medical Specialties and is the organization that certifies emergency physicians. ABEM constructs and administers the annual resident in-service examination, the written qualifying and oral initial certification examination, and the maintenance of certification program to aid physicians in remaining current throughout their careers. ABEM verifies physician certification to licensing boards and other qualified inquiries. ABEM also conducts research within the specialty and maintains an ongoing longitudinal study that contains both resident and practicing physician cohorts to follow physician attitudes and changes during a lifetime of emergency medicine practice. ABEM is located in East Lansing, Michigan.

American College of Emergency Physicians

The American College of Emergency Physicians (ACEP: www.acep.org) is the oldest and largest of all the emergency medicine specialty organizations, founded August 16, 1968, by a group of eight emergency physicians in Lansing, Michigan, who banded together to create an organization of individuals who worked in emergency departments. This is considered the "founding of the specialty of emergency medicine." ACEP is the oldest and largest of all the specialty organizations. ACEP's mission is to represent emergency physicians through advocacy efforts and to provide member benefits including continuing medical education. Advocacy is organized on a national level through staff in a Washington, DC, office, and its headquarters is located in Dallas, Texas. ACEP sponsors the journal *Annals of Emergency Medicine*, which was the first specialty journal. ACEP also researches, creates, and publishes clinical policies concerning the appropriate management of emergency department patients with certain disease processes. A significant strength of ACEP is the organization of state chapters that focus efforts on regional educational programs and emergency physician advocacy at the state legislative level. Every ACEP committee has resident representation through EMRA. Most state chapters make efforts to involve residents and sponsor medical student interest groups. ACEP has a national educational meeting each Fall (*Scientific Assembly*) and many other educational offerings during the year. ACEP together with SAEM sponsors the Emergency Medicine Foundation (EMF), which awards annual research grants in various categories, including one specifically designated for medical student projects.

Accreditation Council for Graduate Medical Education

The Accreditation Council for Graduate Medical Education (ACGME: www.acgme.org) is responsible for setting the standards for all allopathic training programs, as well as conducting site visits, subsequent reviews, and accreditation of all training allopathic programs in the United States. The ACGME is headquartered in Chicago and maintains a Web site, where information pertinent to training requirements and accreditation status of training programs can be accessed, providing information to medical students considering specialty training. The ACGME is sponsored by the AMA.

American College of Osteopathic Emergency Physicians

The American College of Osteopathic Emergency Physicians (ACOEP: www.acoep.org), the specialty organization for osteopathic emergency physicians, began in 1975. It sponsors ongoing educational opportunities, curriculum and faculty development, research presentations and funding grants, and an annual Spring educational meeting in April. ACOEP is based in Chicago, Illinois.

American Medical Association

The American Medical Association (AMA: www.ama-assn.org) is the largest physician professional organization in the country, with its headquarters in Chicago. Formed in 1847, the AMA plays a major role in advocating for policy and reimbursement issues on behalf of all physicians. Since its inception, the AMA has been instrumental in raising the quality of medical care in the United states through its efforts in medical education and certification, medical ethics, publishing a highly rated journal (*Journal of the American Medical Association [JAMA]*), and political advocacy on behalf of physicians and patients. The policy-making body (House of Delegates) is composed on physicians representing state medical societies, medical specialties, and sections of the AMA. Opportunities are available for medical students (Medical Student Section) and residents/fellows (Resident and Fellow Section) to participate in the policymaking process, as well as gain opportunities for volunteer work and self-education in the nonclinical aspects of medicine. The medical student section represents nearly 60% of all medical students in the United States and is the largest medical student organization in the country. The section meets semiannually at the AMA meetings. ACEP organizes and sponsors the Section Council for Emergency Medicine that coordinates input from the specialty to the AMA policy-making process. The section council includes resident/fellow and medical student sections' representatives and emergency physicians who represent their state associations. Many leadership opportunities and scholarships to attend meetings are available to residents and students. The AMA also coordinates an on-line Fellowship and Residency Electronic Interactive Database (FREIDA), which allows medical student and resident physician members to view detailed information on all ACGME-accredited programs.

American Osteopathic Association

The American Osteopathic Association (AOA: www.osteopathic.org) is the professional organization of osteopathic physicians dedicated to advancing the philosophy and practice of osteopathic medicine. The AOA accredits osteopathic undergraduate and graduate training programs. The AOA sponsors the American Board of Osteopathic Emergency Medicine (ABOEM), which is the certifying body for osteopathic emergency physicians similar to the certification process by ABEM for allopathic emergency physicians. The AOA is affiliated with specialty colleges such as ACOEP and works jointly to provide physician reviewers to conduct accreditation surveys for all emergency medicine osteopathic training programs. The AOA also sponsors a separate affiliated association, the Student Osteopathic Medical Association, with its own governing committee and convention. The AOA is based in Chicago and also maintains a Washington office for lobbying congressional members to represent osteopathic physicians' interests.

Council of Emergency Medicine Residency Directors

The Council of Emergency Medicine Residency Directors (CORD: www.cordem.org) was established in 1990 whose membership is made up of program directors and associate program directors of emergency medicine residency programs dedicated to establishing and maintaining high standards of excellence in emergency medicine training programs. CORD is concerned with all matters related to resident training, medical student training electives, and the residency match in Emergency Medicine. CORD sponsors two educational meetings per year including a faculty development workshop open to residents beginning an academic career. CORD coordinates the annual resident CPC competition with the regional winner selected at the Spring SAEM meeting and the national winner selected at the Fall ACEP Scientific Assembly. CORD has worked closely with the medical student match process to ensure that it is efficient and ethical. CORD developed the Standard Letter of Recommendation (SLOR) to better assist medical students and programs in obtaining timely and more applicable candidate information to facilitate the application process. CORD also supports medical student interest groups and maintains a list server for medical student rotation coordinators to allow them to network nationally sharing ideas and concepts to create the best educational experiences for medical students. CORD also maintains a list serve for residency directors to allow them to share information of mutual interest, as well as, post open training slots to facilitate placement of students and transferring residents. CORD is based in Lansing, Michigan.

Emergency Medicine Residents' Association

The Emergency Medicine Residents' Association (EMRA: www.emra.org) was formed in 1974 as the first independent resident association and the second oldest organization in emergency medicine. Its headquarters is in Dallas, Texas. EMRA provides a unified voice for residents and fellows in training programs. It is the emergency medicine organization for residents and students run solely by residents and students. Member benefits include online and written communication vehicles for residents and students, educational meetings, and committee membership through appointment to the committees of ACEP and EMRA. EMRA is governed by a board of directors and has a representative council made up of one resident from each ACGME/AOA accredited emergency medicine residency program and one representative from the medical student section. This provides opportunities for students and residents to be involved in policy development, impacting issues that are pertinent to resident and medical students. EMRA also sponsors the Medical Student Committee, which is a section specific to the needs of medical students interested in a career in emergency medicine. EMRA meets regularly with other key emergency medicine organizations such as ACEP, ABEM, RRC-Emergency Medicine, AMA-ORR, CORD, EMF, and the National Consortium of Residents to ensure viewpoints of emergency medicine residents on pertinent issues are expressed. EMRA maintains a Web site that contains much useful information regarding wellness issues for residents and the job-seeking process. EMRA also publishes a newsletter, *EM Resident,* as well as other publications such as *EMRA Antibiotic Guide; Emergency Medicine's Top Clinical Problems; Career PlanningGuide* ; *Contract Issues for Emergency Physicians; and many others..*

Emergency Medicine Residents' Association Medical Student Committee

EMRA supports a medical student committee created in 1992 to give medical students a voice and national organization to promote information and contacts for medical students nationwide considering a career in emergency medicine (Emergency Medicine Residents Association Medical Student Committee [EMRA MSC: www.emra.org). The committee sponsors a medical student forum held in conjunction with the Fall ACEP Scientific Assembly meeting. Students can network with residents and national leaders to learn more about the specialty and become involved. Becoming a member of this organization also provides a free subscription to *Annals of Emergency Medicine.* This journal allows the student to read cutting edge research in emergency medicine making one more knowledgeable about emergency medicine, which can enhance interviewing for residency. The MSC is composed of 12 medical student members and a chair selected by the president-elect of EMRA. The organization also provides information on away clerkships, visiting speakers, research opportunities, and comparative information regarding residencies.

National Association of EMS Physicians

The National Association of EMS Physicians (NAEMSP: www.naemsp.org) consists of physician medical directors of EMS services as well as other interested parties promoting EMS training and operations and disaster management. The organization has reduced membership for residents and medical students. NAEMSP publishes a journal, *Prehospital Emergency Care,* and maintains an office in Lenexa, Kansas.

Organization of Resident Representatives

The Organization of Resident Representatives (ORR: www.ama-assn.org), is a resident group organized by the AAMC to develop recommendations for resident issues regarding postgraduate medical education. Each AAMC member organization appoints residents to a two year term on the ORR. Residents from all medical specialty training programs are represented.

Residency Review Committee for Emergency Medicine

The Residency Review Committee for Emergency Medicine (RRC-Emergency Medicine: www.acgme.org) is the ACGME committee that periodically reviews and accredits all emergency medicine programs as an arm of the ACGME (see earlier). The RRC-Emergency Medicine is composed of emergency physicians from the AMA, ACEP, and ABEM. It also has a voting resident member from EMRA sitting on the Committee as well. The RRC-Emergency Medicine maintains an office in Chicago.

Society for Academic Emergency Medicine

The Society for Academic Emergency Medicine (SAEM:www.saaem.org) was formed by the merger of two previous independent organizations, The Society of Teachers of Emergency Medicine, which had a primary education and teaching focus, and the University Association of Emergency Medicine, which had a primary research focus. SAEM is an association of academic faculty, fellows, residents, and medical students whose mission is to improve patient care by advancing research and education in emergency medicine. SAEM sponsors the journal *Academic Emergency Medicine,* and has an annual meeting each Spring showcasing cutting-edge research and promoting education and teaching skills for faculty and residents. Opportunities exist for residents and students to present research and participate in committees and interest groups. SAEM maintains a list of emergency medicine interest groups and contacts for "away" rotations that students can use to facilitate elective rotations, and it maintains a Web site with a "medical student home page" containing additional information. SAEM sponsors a medical student forum as part of its Spring Meeting. In addition, SAEM sponsors several regional meetings. It also sponsors an emergency medicine medical student interest group that provides educational grants to establish or support existing emergency medicine medical school interest groups. SAEM also has a medical student educators section that has developed an online "Virtual Advisor" mentorship program for students interested in emergency medicine. SAEM sponsors an "Excellence in Emergency Medicine" award that is given to each medical school for a senior medical student who has demonstrated excellence in the specialty. Recipients receive a free 1-year membership. SAEM is based in Lansing, Michigan.

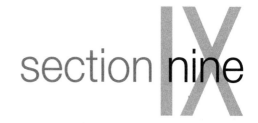

section nine

Preparation for a Shift in the Emergency Department

chapter 71

Important Emergency Medicine Books

Jeremy T. Cushman, MD, MS
Past President, EMRA
Director, EMS Fellowship, Division of EMS and Office of Prehospital Care
Department of Emergency Medicine, University of Rochester School of Medicine and Dentistry

Roopa Rashi Dhawan, BS
University of Alabama School of Medicine

Cristi N. Vaughn, MD
Brody School of Medicine, East Carolina University

There are hundreds of reference and review books in emergency medicine. What follows is a brief list of the more commonly used references for the medical student preparing for their emergency medicine clerkship. All have different formats, styles, and content, and the brief description is designed to help you determine which might be best for you.

Blackwell Underground Clinical Vignettes: Emergency Medicine

(Blackwell Underground Clinical Vignettes Series)
V. Bhushan, V. Pal, and T. Le
Lippincott Williams & Wilkins
Softcover: 128 pages; $19.95
Includes 50 vignettes emphasizing common clinical complaints in the emergency department. Underground Clinical Vignettes reinforces buzzwords in history taking, findings on physical exam, labs, imaging, and even pathological findings for each condition. The book also includes 73 "minicases," which are diseases followed by key facts meant for quick review for students. The book was developed to help students with the "prototypical" clinical scenarios encountered on USMLE Step 2 CK.

Blueprints Clinical Cases in Emergency Medicine

(Blueprints Clinical Cases)
C. Tsien, M. Filbin, and A. Caughey
Lippincott Williams & Wilkins
Softcover: 160 pages; $29.95
This book presents symptom based clinical cases followed by a short discussion and four or five questions regarding management. Features a 200-question mock exam at the end of the text. The included "thought question" boxes are meant to encourage critical thinking.

Blueprints Emergency Medicine

(Blueprints Series)
N. Mick, J. Peters, D. Egan, E. Nadel, and S. Silvers
Lippincott Williams & Wilkins
Softcover: 324 pages; $34.95
Blueprints covers the essential topics of emergency medicine in a systems-based approach. It includes many figures and tables and concludes with 75 board-format questions with explanations. Each topic is briefly summarized in two or three pages for quick reading. Key points boxes at the end of each section emphasize major concepts.

Case Files Emergency Medicine

(Lange Case Files Series)
E. Toy, B. Simon, T. Liu, and J. Trujillo
McGraw-Hill Medical
Softcover: 480 pages; $29.95
By presenting the most common clinical problems in emergency medicine and utilizing a case-based approach, this series of books has been popular among medical students. Clinical pearls, key terms and concepts, as well as USMLE-style questions and answers are included. This series often includes treatment algorithms, which are helpful both on rotation and for exams.

Clinical Procedures in Emergency Medicine

J. Roberts and J. Hedges
Elsevier Saunders
Hardcover: 1504 pages; $179.00
This is a comprehensive reference for procedures done in the emergency department. Gives clear instructions and provides information regarding equipment, technique, complications, and contraindications for each procedure. Numerous helpful tables assist in the interpretation of test results and assist in management decisions. Images and detailed diagrams are black and white.

Color Atlas of Emergency Department Procedures

C. Custalow
Elsevier Saunders
Hardcover: 205 pages; $145.00
This concise guide has clear diagrams and color photographs of many emergency department procedures. Each step provides a color photograph side by side with a diagram illustrating anatomy, landmarks, and other helpful information. The layout is suited for quick reference: chapters give a brief description of each procedure, and bulleted lists include clinical indications, potential complications, and essential equipment.

Emergency Medicine: A Comprehensive Study Guide

J. Tintinalli, G. Kelen, and J. Stapczynski
McGraw-Hill Professional
Hardcover: 2016 pages; $185.00
This book is highly acclaimed as the essential emergency medicine reference. While a comprehensive text might be beyond the average student budget, it is well worth referring to when seeking a more solid knowledge base. It is be widely available in medical libraries and emergency departments.

Emergency Medicine Manual

McGraw-Hill Professional
O. Ma, D. Cline, J. Tintinalli, G. Kelen, and J. Stapczynski
Softcover: 977 pages; $47.95
Also known as the "Baby Tintinalli," this manual is billed as the best-selling pocket reference in emergency medicine. It condenses the clinical content from the text: *Emergency Medicine: A Comprehensive Study Guide*. Thorough for a pocket guide, it includes color photos of dermatologic and ophthalmic conditions, pharmacologic considerations throughout, and tables of critical differential diagnoses.

Emergency Medicine Secrets

V. Markovchick and P. Pons
Mosby
Softcover: 650 pages; $41.95
Written in a question and answer format, this text is designed to help students prepare for "pimping" from attendings. Topics are organized in a systems based fashion. For each subject, references to current research are given. Online access to the complete text via studentconsult.com is an added bonus.

Emergency Medicine's Top Clinical Problems

G. Katz and H. Nayak
EMRA
Softcover: 170 pages; $19.95 list price, $14.95 member price
A rapid pocket reference and teaching tool that is free for students with EMRA membership. Each chapter starts with critical actions for various clinical situations, and then expounds on the problem with disease-specific information and presentation. This reference is extremely useful in the emergency department when you need information on the fly. It has been recently been updated with a quiz tool for each clinical problem.

EMRA Antibiotic Guide

B. Levine
EMRA
Softcover: 124 pages; $25.95 list prince, $15.95 member price
The *EMRA Antibiotic Guide* is designed to be a quick reference guide to antibiotic use in the emergency department. The contents are organized alphabetically by organ system, followed by sections on "Special Topics" to make reference quick and easy for a particular disease process. Each organ system and special topic section is color coded for quick reference and the guide is updated every few years.

First Aid for the Emergency Medicine Clerkship

(First Aid Clinical Clerkship Series)
L. Stead, S. Stead, and M. Kaufman
McGraw-Hill Medical
Softcover: 416 pages; $34.95
This text is written in an outline format that parallels the other First Aid books, with high yield facts about more common complaints seen in the emergency department. Like the other books in the series, it is written primarily for students by students. Outside margins include mnemonics, diagrams, exam, and ward tips. The book also features tear out pocket sized cards that may be helpful to students.

Rosen's Emergency Medicine

J. Marx, R. Hockberger, and R. Walls
Elsevier Saunders
Hardcover: 3-volume set, 2,766 pages; $225.00
This text is an important comprehensive reference that can be found in most emergency departments. Although the three-volume set is quite an investment for a student, it is a valuable resource. The newest edition includes full color illustrations and, for an additional fee, access to a continually updated online reference version of the text.

Tarascon Adult Emergency Pocketbook

S. Rothrock
Tarascon Publishing
Softcover: 208 pages; $14.95
From the makers of the pocket pharmacopoeia, this is a compact reference of lists, figures, and tables organized in a handy pocket guide. It includes expert commentary and numerous journal references on current academic controversies within the field. It provides convenient reference sections on topics such as dysrhythmia protocols, emergency drug infusions, antibiotic therapy, rapid-sequence intubation, toxicology, trauma care, and burns. There is also a newly revised and expanded pediatric version.

chapter 72

PDA Technology in the Emergency Department

Robert Blankenship, MD, FACEP
Madigan Army Medical Center

Palmtop computing has exploded and personal digital assistants (PDAs) are readily available at reasonable prices. It seems impossible to go anywhere without seeing someone tapping away on a thumb-sized keyboard or writing with his or her stylus on the latest handheld model to arrive to market. Even in medicine, a field steeped in tradition and filled with individuals typically regarded as conservative, PDAs have quickly made an imprint. Many physicians and medical students are now using PDAs; a recent estimate pegged usage by physicians between 45% and 85%.[1] Although a variable number of physicians are using PDAs, only about half those polled use them as an integral part of their medical practice. Drug reference software is, by far, the group of applications most used by physicians, but clinical reference material, medical calculators, automated prescription preparation, and tools designed to allow easier access to evidence-based medicine are also extremely popular.

To the newly initiated, the world of PDAs can be both bewildering and a little frightening. There are seeming infinite arrays of choices that a user interested in palmtop computing must make before they can even begin to reap the benefits afforded by PDAs. Like most of the computer industry, the hardware and software choices are constantly changing and prices are perpetually in flux; this makes comparisons regarding ease of use, functionality, and "value" extremely challenging. It is our goal to provide a roadmap that a PDA initiate may follow when considering a new handheld computer purchase, to discuss how hardware choices can affect the utility and functionality of PDAs, and to make users aware of some of the basic medical software that is available. The reward for making careful selections can be a revolution in your practice of medicine.

Choosing a PDA

To select a suitable PDA for your practice, it is important to take a moment and decide which features best suit your needs. All PDAs let you track and manage your schedule, contacts, notes, and tasks; not all PDAs, however, have wireless capabilities, can double as a cellular phone, or can play videos or MP3s. There is an "alphabet soup" of industry acronyms and these can make selecting a PDA may seem like a daunting task—but it need not be. We present a stepwise approach for selecting your first (or next) PDA.

Step 1: Selecting an Operating System

When choosing a PDA, the first step is to decide which operating system (OS) to use. Fortunately, there are only two main PDA operating systems: Palm OS and Windows Mobile (formerly known as Pocket PC or Windows CE).

Palm OS has been the industry leader. Its success is due to many factors:

1. It has been used for the longest period of time, so its customer base is larger.

2. It is very stable (has few crashes) and small in size.
3. Most users find it to be relatively simple and easy to use.
4.. Given the large number of users, the vast majority of software developed for PDAs was built to run on this OS. In fact, a survey from 2001 revealed 97% of the software titles sold was for the Palm OS.

Windows Mobile is the latest PDA OS built by Microsoft as a successor to both the Windows CE and PocketPC operating systems. This is a visually stunning OS that is very similar in look and feel to Microsoft's Windows desktop OS. Many users find this familiarity helpful as they begin to use a PDA. In years past, the Windows Mobile PDAs were more expensive, heavier, and lacking in software, making them much less attractive to the health care professional. However, in the past few years, Windows Mobile devices have evolved remarkably.

So, here are its advantages:

*   It is a relatively inexpensive device with speedy processors and large amounts of storage space. This combination has spurred companies to develop much more software for Windows Mobile devices, including popular medical software such as Epocrates.
*   Recently released software finally allows Windows Mobile PDAs to synchronize with Apple Macintosh computers—a long-needed fix.

Due to these changes, Windows Mobile can now be heartily recommended to medical providers. In fact, the latest data suggest that Microsoft and Palm are in a dead heat, with each operating system capturing 40% of the market share.

Either type of system would be a viable option for your medical practice, but one of them will be more likely to suit your particular practice. To determine which one to purchase, you really need to know the following:

*   Which platforms are your colleagues using (so that you can exchange information more easily)?
*   Which platform does your health care system prefer (so that your operating system will be compatible with medical applications the health care system implements)?
*   What is your personal preference? Windows Mobile looks similar to and interfaces well with Windows and other Microsoft products. This familiarity can be comforting as you learn to use a PDA.

Step 2: Memory Selection

Memory on a PDA refers to the random access memory (RAM) and any storage/expansion slots of the device. RAM on a handheld computer is similar to a hard drive on a desktop computer; it is where the device stores information for later retrieval. All of the latest devices for both Pocket PC and Palm have a minimum of 32 MB of RAM with most devices having 64 MB of RAM or more. Having 32 MB might suffice for the new PDA user, but I recommend at least 64 MB for Palm OS and 64-128 MB for Windows Mobile.

Another way to increase your memory storage potential is to purchase a PDA with an expansion slot. Most of the newer PDAs have expansion slots, but there is no universal standard on the type of memory cards used by PDA manufacturers. Most memory storage types are similar in function and price per megabyte. Some things you will want to consider when selecting an expansion port are

*   Do any of your friends/colleagues have a similar slot that will allow you to share files?

- Do you have any other digital equipment that uses a particular type of memory (i.e., digital camera, MP3 player, or computer)?

In the absence of any overriding factors (such as those mentioned above), you should strongly consider purchasing a PDA that offers secure digital (SD) expandability as SD is the most ubiquitous in recent PDAs.

Step 3: Selecting a Screen

Because almost all new PDAs have color screens, the screen choice is no longer a big issue. If you plan to use your PDA outdoors, you may want a device with a *transflective* display.

Step 4: Powering Your Device

To use your PDA more than four continuous hours while on shift, you will need one that allows you to change batteries easily or one with an extended battery. If this is not a concern, do not worry about it.

Step 5: Selecting Convergence Features

The recent trend for some PDA manufacturers is to build a PDA with wireless capabilities, telephones, cameras, and many other features. Along with these enhancements can come a hefty price tag, which begs the question: What do you really need?

A good number of the latest-generation Palm and Windows Mobile PDAs come with either Bluetooth or WiFi (Ethernet 802.11a/b/g) wireless capabilities. These technologies allow you to connect to wireless area networks (WANs). You could, for example, perform a Web-based search on a particular medical condition at the patient's bedside without being physically connected to a computer. You could also transmit a patient's prescription to the pharmacy before you leave the room, negating the need for a paper script or walking to a computer terminal to enter the prescription. If your hospital has WiFi or Bluetooth integration, this is a feature to consider buying.

For the past few years, PDA makers have been working to develop a telephone-PDA combination that did not sacrifice the functionality of either device. They have accomplished that goal, but these convergence devices do not come cheap. There is not only an additional cost for the device, but you have to pay extra monthly for your data service.

Step 6: Hold the PDAs in Your Hand

The last step is actually the most important: Sample the different PDAs. Personal taste varies on the size and weight you are looking for, so there is no substitute for actually holding these devices before one is purchased. You might also ask a friend with a PDA to borrow it for an hour on shift.

Now that you have purchased your PDA, we would like to assist you in findings some great software. Unfortunately, we could never cover all the great software currently available for medical students in the space we have for this chapter. Nevertheless, we will do our best to review some of the most commonly used software available for medical students.

Clinical Drug References: Epocrates Rx and Tarascon Pocket Pharmacopoeia Deluxe

Epocrates (http://www.epocrates.com) Drug databases are among the most popular programs used by health care providers, and perhaps none is more popular than Epocrates, with over 850,000 registered health care professional users.[2] Epocrates Rx was released several years ago as a free application that featured a comprehensive, regularly updated drug database. Since then, the program has grown substantially in functionality, and the number of users has increased tremendously. Epocrates Rx offers information on over 3,300 brand and generic drugs, everything from adult and pediatric doses to contraindications, drug interactions, and adverse reactions.[3] Another useful feature of this software is MultiCheck, which allows one to look up potentially harmful interactions between two or more prescription drugs. Epocrates also has a formulary function, which allows the provider to access up-to-date formulary information from multiple health plans and hospitals on a PDA. Physicians and other health care professionals can download the formularies they use most often, quickly check which drugs are covered, and find plan-specific details on co-pay tiers, prior authorization requirements, and quantity limits. Over 70 health care organizations representing 95 million subscribers currently host their formulary information with Epocrates. DocAlert Messaging is another powerful Epocrates feature. DocAlerts are concise clinical, health or product related messages delivered to your handheld device after you perform a HotSync operation while connected to the Internet. The DocAlert messages include safety alerts from the FDA, the ISMP (Institute for Safe Medication Practices), and the CDC (Centers for Disease Control and Prevention), treatment guidelines from the CDC and Agency for Healthcare Research and Quality (AHRQ), notification of recent Epocrates database updates (new drugs, formularies, tables, etc.), evidence-based medicine news from leading medical journals (POEMS) and institutions, Reuters health and medical news, among others. Due to the success of DocAlert messages in getting critical information to health care professionals, the HHS (United States Department of Health and Human Services) is considering using the DocAlert system to notify front-line health professionals in the event of a bioterrorist attack.[4]

All of these listed functions are available in the free version of Epocrates Rx. Currently, the free version is only compatible with Palm OS devices used with Windows computers; however, most individuals will want to pay the subscription fee to receive the additional features of the premium version, Epocrates Rx Pro. Included in this version is comprehensive information on over 400 of the most commonly used alternative medications, including reported uses, doses, cautions, drug interactions, and adverse reactions. It is also possible to check for interactions between alternative and prescription medications. Also included in Epocrates Rx Pro is Epocrates ID. Epocrates ID is an infectious disease guide that lets you examine the treatment of infectious diseases by diagnosis, organism, or medication regimen. This program is tightly integrated with the core Epocrates Rx drug program, allowing you to quickly reference all the drug information with only a few clicks. Last, the professional version also offers over 50 tables and clinical guidelines, the MedMath medical calculator, and an integrated weight-based dosing calculator.[2]

Epocrates Rx was previously available only for Palm OS, but as of April 4, 2003, Epocrates Rx Pro became available for Windows Mobile as well. This version of Epocrates Pro offers comprehensive information on over 3,000 drugs, alternative medicines and interactions with prescription drugs, clinical tables and guidelines, formulary information, auto update, Epocrates ID, and DocAlert messages. For those who do not feel they need the features that come with the Pro version, a free edition of Epocrates Rx is now available for Windows Mobile devices.

Critics of this program claim Epocrates tracks which drugs and classes are referenced most often and sells that information to drug companies, managed care organizations, or other third party companies. While Epocrates admits to tracking which drugs and classes are referenced most often, it does not sell the information to any outside parties. Rather, the aggregate data it collects help the Epocrates clinical editors prioritize which drug monographs to enhance with additional content such as pediatric and renal dosing information. A full disclosure of their practices can be found in their comprehensive privacy policy at http://www.Epocrates.com/company/privacy.cfm. A free 30-day trial of Epocrates Rx Pro is available from their Web site; try it for yourself.

Tarascon Pocket Pharmacopoeia Deluxe (http://www.tarascon.com). The Tarascon Pocket Pharmacopoeia is the leading portable drug reference, and in a 1999 survey published in *Annals of Internal Medicine,* the Pocket Pharmacopoeia tied with the stethoscope as the most essential item in resident physicians' white coat pockets.[5] It should be no surprise that its PDA version (Tarascon Pocket Pharmacopoeia) is another common program used by providers as a drug reference.

The graphical user interface for the Tarascon Pocket Pharmacopoeia Deluxe PDA Edition is very similar to that used in the text version making it easy for clinicians to migrate to the PDA version. This program contains comprehensive information on over 4,000 drugs to include adult and pediatric dosing, packaging information, dosage forms, and warnings. The Tarascon Pocket Pharmacopoeia Deluxe PDA Edition also contains a fully integrated "Herbal & Alternative Therapy" section. You can search for medications by name, class, or category or by those selected by the user as commonly used drugs. It will allow you to check for potentially harmful interactions between two or more prescription drugs, as well as alternative medications. A new feature is a notation for each drug (under "cost") as to whether a patient assistance program is available, using data supplied by www.needymeds.com. Last, the drug content can be updated every time your PDA hot syncs and is connected to the internet ensuring you have the most up-to-date information.

In many ways, the Tarascon Pocket Pharmacopoeia Deluxe PDA Edition and Epocrates are similar; however, Tarascon does not have an integrated infectious disease companion piece and it does not offer a DocAlert system. Tarascon has concerns that some of the DocAlerts from Epocrates are sponsored by pharmaceutical companies so Tarascon has chosen to not mirror the DocAlert approach in an effort to remain independent of all forms of advertising.

While some may see the above as limitations of the Tarascon program, there are some benefits of Tarascon over Epocrates. Perhaps the most significant advantage is Tarascon supports most extended memory cards allowing the program to be stored and run from the memory card. Another advantage of Tarascon is it offers a rich array of off-label pediatric dosing. For those concerned with Epocrates collection of aggregated data on how Epocrates users are using ePocrates software[6] Tarascon's privacy policy clearly states they do not track customer usage of the product or sell their personal information to others in any form. Last, Tarscon's subscription price is approximately half the price of Epocrates.

Both of these listed pharmacology reference programs are very useful and will serve you well. Which one you will like depends on individual preferences. Both vendors offer free trial versions of their software, so you can decide which one you like better before you pay any money.

Antibiotic Guides

There are three main antibiotic guides available for PDA: the Sanford Guide ($27.50), the Johns Hopkins Guide (free, Palm OS only), and the EMRA Antibiotic Guide ($15.95 for EMRA members, $25.95 for nonmembers). They differ in price, frequency of updates, and organization.

Sanford Guide (www.sanfordguide.com). The Sanford Guide is the best-established antibiotic guide. The PDA version includes all of the content of the print edition, although some of the antibiotic sensitivity tables are much more difficult to read on a PDA. The PDA version is also roughly three times the price of the pocket edition. The Sanford Guide has the most complete coverage of pediatric dosages, and includes a creatinine clearance calculator for renal dosing. It is the most expensive guide, and requires a new purchase with each yearly update.

Johns Hopkins Guide (http://hopkins-abxguide.org). This free guide can answer most of the antibiotic questions a medical student will face. Pediatric dosing information is somewhat limited, but most of the major pediatric infectious diseases are covered. The guide can be viewed by diagnosis, pathogen, or antibiotic and includes clinical pearls. It is updated when the PDA is synchronized with an Internet-connected computer. Only generic drug names are used. This program is only available for Palm OS.

EMRA Antibiotic Guide (http://www2.acep.org/bookstore/index.cfm?go=product detail&id=10160). The only antibiotic guide tailored for the emergency department, the EMRA Antibiotic Guide is concise and clear. It is organized by organ, diagnosis, organism, or topic. Students would need to supplement this guide for general medical or surgical rotations.

One of the authors of this chapter is involved with programming the EMRA Antibiotic Guide.

PreTest for Palm OS (www.brainglue.com). Many books in the PreTest series are now available for Palm OS. (Emergency medicine, unfortunately, is not available at this writing.) These programs include the same content as the print editions, and will also give a running tally of your score in given chapters. The test questions do not shuffle well, but these are the best available option for doing test questions on a Palm.

McGraw-Hill's Diagnosaurus (http://books.mcgraw hill.com/medical/diagnosaurus/index.html). McGraw-Hill's Diagnosaurus is a free reference program for both the Palm and Pocket PC, boasting over 1,000 differential diagnoses. Diagnosaurus's best feature is that it allows users to search for a differential by disease, symptom, or organ system. Although Diagnosaurus provides a well thought out differential, it lacks treatment information. If users are unfamiliar with a specific disease process they then need to go elsewhere for treatment options. Nevertheless, Diagnosaurus can be an invaluable supplement that students may want to have at hand.

MedCalc (http://www.med-ia.ch/medcalc/). This program is one of the most commonly used medical calculators for Palm OS. It is useful for calculating a number of clinically useful parameters such as the A-a gradient, electrolyte corrections, likelihood ratios, etc. It also has an EDC calculator, so you can get rid of your pregnancy wheel. The user interface is wonderful. It allows you to look through its over 70 formulas based on the category, or you may specify those you use most often in a "custom" list for easy access. Unfortunately, this program is currently only available for Palm.

In summary, a PDA can be an excellent resource to you as a medical student. While there are a wide variety of devices and operating systems available you can easily follow the above advice to select a great PDA that fits your needs and make you a more effective clinician.

References

1. Garritty C, El Emam K. Who's using PDAs? Estimates of PDA use by health care providers: a systematic review of surveys. Available at http://www.jmir.org/2006/2/e7/. Accessed July 30, 2006.
2. Broida R. Epocrates Rx Pro. *Handheld Computing.* 2003;6:56.
3. Larkin M. Technology and public health. *Lancet Infect Dis.* 2003;3(5):314-315.
4. Lynn LA, Bellini LM. Portable knowledge: a look inside white coat pockets. *Ann Intern Med.* 1999;130:247-250.
5. Copeland J. Letter to the editor. *JAMC 2003*; 168(12):1526.
6. Cameron S. Infectious disease guides. For users of hand-held computers. *Can Fam Physician. 2002*;48:1507-1508.

chapter 73

Checklist for a Shift in the Emergency Department

Joshua Moskovitz, MD, MPH
University of Maryland

Jeremy Sperling, MD, FACEP
Weill Medical College of Cornell University; New York-Presbyterian Hospital

Just like any other clerkship in medical school, preparing for the first day of an emergency medicine rotation is essential. Whether it is as simple as knowing where to report and what to wear the first day or making sure you have all the essential tools for your first emergency department shift, preparation is the key to success. Emergency medicine can be unpredictable, complex, and fast paced, so carefully think ahead of time what you will need to hit the ground running.

Tools of the Trade

No two emergency departments are alike. While some will have plasma TVs in every patient room, others might not have working ophthalmoscopes available. Fellow classmates who recently finished the same emergency medicine clerkship are a great source for finding out what equipment will be available to you and what you must provide for yourself. Below is a list of items you might need during an emergency department shift divided into categories of necessity. Also listed are items you will use often and may help expedite your patient care. Do not purchase any of the disposable items. Be careful when bringing anything valuable to the emergency department, as emergency departments are public places and security can be a concern.

Highly Recommended

- Identification badge
- Stethoscope
- Pocket medication guide (e.g., Tarascon Pocket Pharmacopoeia)
- Antibiotic guide (e.g., EMRA Antibiotic Guide, Sanford Guide or Epocrates)
- Pens
- Pen light
- Trauma shears
- Passwords for computer programs commonly used in the emergency department (consider putting all on one index card or in your PDA and sending yourself an e-mail with all this information as backup)
- List of all commonly used beeper and phone numbers for the department (some emergency departments may have a reference card).

Recommended

- ECG calipers (can double for two-point discrimination)
- Pocket emergency medicine clinical guide (e.g., Top 30 Clinical Problems, Tarascon Adult Emergency Pocketbook)
- PDA (see Chapter 72)
- Snack or bag lunch
- Guaiac cards and developer (when found, hold onto the developer; certain hospitals are notorious for always running out of developer)

Optional

- Ophthalmoscope/otoscope
- Reflex hammer
- Pocket pulse oximeter (expensive item, but if you have one and it can be stored safely in your white coat, it can be quite helpful at times in a busy emergency department)
- Plastic safety goggles (for traumas or wound irrigation)
- Steri-Strips (might be time-saving to find some and carry with you)
- Digital camera (Always ask the emergency department attending and get informed consent from the patient before using any photographs. If you can keep one safely stored in your bag and you see a fascinating case, this could be your opportunity to write up a care report or use a picture for a lecture.)
- Index cards for patient tracking (some emergency medicine rotations make patient and procedure tracking mandatory)
- Emergency medicine articles or small textbook for downtime

Work Attire

Every emergency department has its own expectation of student and resident attire. Some departments/faculty prefer students and residents to be more formal, while others have no preference. Always ask the clerkship director the first day of the rotation what the preferred student dress is. This may even vary between different hospital sites within the same emergency medicine residency program (e.g., private community hospital versus county hospital) and different attendings within the same emergency department. To obtain this information before the first day of the rotation, the residency administrator or the emergency medicine chief residents are excellent sources for this information and other questions you may have.

While working clinically in the emergency department, many institutions require students to wear a short white coat and residents to wear a long white coat at all times. The pediatric emergency department is the one setting where white coats may be discouraged, as they may be seen as intimidating to little children.

Scrubs tend to be the standard apparel, but some emergency departments prefer more formal attire. If you are going to wear scrubs, make sure they are clean, neat, and match! First impressions are everything to both the patient and the attending. Be careful about wearing scrubs that display another institution's name or colors as some hospitals have policies against this. Avoid wearing tee-shirts, sweat shirts, jeans, or open-toed shoes even if you observe residents in them. Do not wear outfits that allow skin or undergarments to be seen (e.g., do you want to know the color of your physician's underwear or see their naval piercing?). In addition, do not wear anything with political messages (e.g., a pin that names a presidential candidate).

Make sure to have an ID badge and wear it all times. Certain institutions will want institution-specific IDs and may require you to get one on the first day. Also, some hospitals require an ID (usually with a swipe mechanism) to pass through certain doors;

these doors may allow you to gain access to supply rooms, clean bathrooms, break rooms, or even the emergency department itself.

At times when you will not be working clinically (e.g., orientation, lecture days), consider wearing business casual clothing rather than scrubs. If you are going to give any form of presentation to the group, dressing more formally (e.g., shirt and tie) is always considered appropriate. If an EMS ride along is part of the rotation, make sure you know specifically what EMS expects you to wear because white coats and scrubs are generally not appropriate for ride-alongs.

Directions

A sure way to quickly draw unwanted attention to yourself in emergency medicine is to be late. Make sure you have correct directions to the emergency department and know where and when you are supposed to meet. Your behavior during medical school is highly predictive of your behavior during residency; students who come early and prepared to work hard will be highly appreciated by the faculty.

chapter 74

Emergency Medicine Documentation and Charting

Steven Kaplan, MD
Associate Director, Emergency Medicine Operations, Weill Medical College of Cornell University
New York-Presbyterian Hospital

Documentation of the medical record is an often discussed but only minimally taught skill that has widespread impact throughout a physician's medical career. Physicians are constantly reminded of the importance of complete and accurate charting but only rarely are time and attention paid to review and improvement of medical documentation. The emergency department is one of the most active patient care areas with competing needs for time and attention. The environment is characterized by noise, high levels of acuity, frequent distractions, and often-limited resources, all interfering with the physician's ability to focus on documentation. In this chapter I hope to describe the importance of accurate documentation and provide some hints on how to improve this often neglected skill.

Why Is Documentation So Important?

There are many reasons why complete and accurate emergency department record documentation is important. Many physicians believe that the medical record must be complete for medical-legal reasons. Others believe that the documentation is necessary for billing needs. Still others believe that the medical record is a communication tool. They are all correct. The medical record serves many purposes but the single most important reason for complete and accurate documentation is that the medical record should accurately reflect the care that was provided in the emergency department, the decision making that was involved in that care, and any interventions, procedures, medications administered, adverse incidents, and responses to treatment that occurred. Simply put, the record should accurately describe exactly what happened to the patient while he or she was in the emergency department.

Where to Begin

All entries in the medical record should begin with the date and time. Whether you are documenting in an electronic medical record (EMR) that will automatically time-stamp new entries or a paper chart, each note should begin with the date and time. Time is often the absent key element. Without a documentation of time, it is often impossible to accurately understand the sequence of events that occurred during patient care in the emergency department. Nursing records, with their ongoing narrative of care, are an excellent example of well-timed documentation. A dilemma frequently encountered by physicians as they document care is how to time a note that is written after the care is provided. Ideally the chart should reflect the time that the care was provided. There are several solutions to this problem. The note can be dated followed by "Time Patient Seen:" with the time entered to reflect the time the patient was seen. Alternatively the note can be dated and timed when written and in the body of the note indicate the time that the care was provided. "I saw Mr. X at 4PM. He is a . . . ." The latter method is important for use with an EMR as the time stamp of an EMR will be the time that the entry is made. If you are involved in the creation of your department's emergency department record you can be instrumental in creating spaces or electronic prompts for documentation of the actual time of care. Whereas all notes should be started with a date and time, all notes must be completed with a signature. Not only should each and every note be signed, but the signature must be legible or in some manner easily identify the physician providing the care and doing the documentation.

Comprehensive Documentation

Documentation of an emergency department encounter includes much more than the initial history and physical examination. Comprehensive documentation includes a triage assessment, registration information, a physician history and physical examination, nursing assessments, and discharge instructions. Additionally, the documentation of an emergency department encounter may include follow-up encounter notes; procedure notes; documentation of responses to therapies or procedures; laboratory, ECG and radiology test results; notes by consultants, social workers, and other care providers; incident reports; transfers of care; and any other expected or unexpected aspects of the patient's care. Remember, the ultimate goal of the documentation is to accurately and chronologically reflect what happened to a patient throughout the course of the emergency department visit and to document recommended plans for follow-up care.

Discharge Instructions

Documentation of comprehensive and legible discharge instructions is critical to excellent emergency department care, safe patient care, and improved patient satisfaction. Even if the patient was given detailed verbal instructions, the circumstances of the emergency department visit, fear, injury, fatigue, or medications might prevent the patient from fully understanding or remembering the conversation. Thus, the value of legible, comprehensive, understandable discharge instructions cannot be overemphasized. At a minimum discharge instructions should include a diagnosis; a treatment plan appropriate for that diagnosis; appropriate and realistic follow-up instructions; and instructions to return to the emergency department for new or worsening symptoms, specific symptoms related to the primary diagnosis, or any acute problems. Many emergency departments are using detailed preprinted or computerized discharge instructions. These instructions are valuable because they are comprehensive, uniform, standardized, and legible. Additionally they can provide educational information to patients about their medical conditions.

Additional Words of Wisdom

Registration Issues. It is important to confirm the accuracy of registration and contact information. It is not unusual that emergency department staff need to contact a patient after the patient has been discharged from the emergency department. Patients may be called for changes in radiology reports, unexpected laboratory findings, positive culture results, or a variety of other indications. If the contact information is not accurate, patient safety and best care may be compromised.

AMA. When a patient leaves the emergency department against medical advice, you will commonly see a document signed by the patient acknowledging that he or she understands the risks of leaving against medical advice (AMA). Documentation should be added by the physician to clarify the circumstances of the AMA discharge, noting the patient's capacity to truly understand the potential risks of leaving AMA. Additionally, patients leaving AMA should not be "punished" by withholding prescriptions or other treatments. Patients' discharge instructions should be clear and comprehensive, treatment should be maximized despite the AMA discharge, and patients should be clearly advised that they are welcome to return to the emergency department as necessary.

Refusal of Care. Patients should be included in the decisions made about their care and may choose to decline individual recommended tests or treatments. Documentation should reflect any discussions that occurred and indicate that a patient has made an informed refusal of a particular part of his or her care. Again, the patient should not be punished

Informed Consent. Informed consent is extremely important and often poorly executed. A patient must truly understand any procedure for which he or she is asked to sign permission. The patient must understand why the procedure is being performed, the risks and benefits of the procedure, any alternatives to the procedure and what to expect during and after a procedure. The physician or health care provider obtaining the informed consent must be exquisitely familiar with the procedure and should be able to answer any and all questions that the patient may have about the procedure. Only after this detailed conversation has occurred can a patient truly provide informed consent. Of course, this conversation with the patient should be documented in detail in the medical record.

Arguments. The medical record should never be a place where health care providers argue over or vent about differences of opinion. The record should accurately and objectively include only that information that is relevant to the care of the patient.

Corrections. It is a fact of human behavior that documentation errors will occur. Correction of errors may be made but should be made in a way that clearly reveals that an error is being corrected and should not appear to be hiding or altering information contained in the record. Corrections should be made by drawing a single line through the incorrect information. The correction should be dated and timed and signed in the standard manner.

HIPAA. Remember that the medical record is a confidential document. No information regarding a patient's care in the emergency department should be shared without the explicit consent of the patient.

In conclusion, documentation is an important part of medical care and the value of doing it well cannot be emphasized enough! The chart should not be documented primarily for billing purposes or for medical-legal purposes but rather to objectively document the care that a patient received on a particular encounter with the health care system. Excellent documentation is a skill that will improve over time when attention is paid to doing it accurately and carefully.

Appendix

chapter 75

Important Website Resources

Julian Jakubowski, DO
St. Barnabas Hospital

Zach Patrick, DO
Des Moines University, College of Osteopathic Medicine

Emergency Medicine-Based Organization Websites

American Academy of Emergency Physicians (AAEM)
http://www.aaem.org/
http://www.aaemrsa.org/index.php (Student Section)
611 East Wells Street, Milwaukee, WI 53202
Telephone: (414) 276-7390 or (800) 884-AAEM Fax: (414)272-6070
Representation through AAEM Political Action Committee the political action
committee of AAEM, subscriptions to *The Journal of Emergency Medicine* and *Common
Sense* residency catalog and Job Bank.

American Board of Emergency Medicine (ABEM)
http://www.abem.org/
3000 Coolidge Road, East Lansing, MI 48823-6319
Telephone: (517) 332-4800 Fax: (517) 332-2234
ABEM certifies qualifying physicians who specialize in emergency medicine.

American College of Emergency Physicians (ACEP)
http://www.acep.org/
1125 Executive Circle, Irving, TX 75038-2522
Telephone: (800) 798-1822 Fax: (972) 580-2816
ACEP is one of the leading advocates for emergency physicians, their patients, and the
public. Its membership consists of more than 23,000 emergency medicine specialists,
including academicians, clinicians, researchers, residents, and students.

American College of Osteopathic Emergency Physicians (ACOEP)
http://www.acoep.org/
http://www.acoepsc.org/ (Student Section)
142 East Ontario Street, Suite 550, Chicago, IL 60611
Telephone: (312) 587-3709 or (800) 521-3709 Fax: (312) 587-9951
ACOEP exists to support high-quality emergency care, promote and protect the interests
of osteopathic emergency physicians, ensure the highest standards of postgraduate
education, and provide leadership in research through the Foundation for Osteopathic
Emergency Medicine.

American Osteopathic Board of Emergency Medicine (AOBEM)

http://www.aobem.org/
142 East Ontario Street, Chicago, IL 60611
Telephone: (312) 335-1065 Fax: (312) 335-5489
Members of the American College of Osteopathic Emergency Physicians (ACOEP),
which established residency training programs in osteopathic emergency medicine.

Council of Emergency Medicine Residency Directors (CORD)

http://www.cordem.org/
901 North Washington Avenue, Lansing, MI 48906
Telephone: (517) 485-5484 Fax: (517) 485-0801
To improve, establish, and maintain high standards of excellence in emergency medicine
training programs. Developed the Standard Letter of Recommendation (SLOR) used in
the residency application process.

Emergency Medicine Foundation (EMF)

http://www.emfoundation.org/
1125 Executive Circle, Irving, TX 75038-2522
Telephone: (800) 798-1822 Fax: (972) 580-2816
An organization that supports and funds initial research in the field of emergency
medicine.

Emergency Medicine Residents' Association (EMRA)

http://www.emra.org/
1125 Executive Circle, Irving, TX 75038-2522
Telephone: (800) 798-1822 ext. 3298 Fax: (972)580-2829
EMRA is the largest, oldest, and only independent resident organization in the world with
a membership of more than 7,000 residents, fellows, medical students, and alumni. In
addition to advocacy, EMRA offers its members a comprehensive list of resources
including free publications for students and residents.

Society for Academic Emergency Medicine (SAEM)

http://www.saem.org/
901 North Washington Avenue, Lansing, MI 48906-5137
Telephone: (517) 485-5484 Fax: (517) 485-0801
SAEM promotes and supports the pursuit of research in emergency medicine. The site has
a residency guide for students as well.

chapter 76

Organization Websites

2006-2007 EMRA Medical Student Committee

Association of American Medical Colleges (AAMC)
http://www.aamc.org/
2450 North Street NW, Washington, DC 20037
Telephone: (202) 828-0400 Fax: (202) 828-1125

American Academy of Clinical Toxicology (AACT)
http://www.aactox.org/
777 East Park Drive, PO Box 8820, Harrisburg, PA 17105-8820
Telephone: (717) 558-7750 Fax: (717) 558-7845

American Association of Poison Control Centers (AAPCC)
http://www.aapcc.org/
3201 New Mexico Avenue, Suite 310, Washington, DC 20016
elephone: (202) 362-7217

American Board of Medical Specialties (ABMS)
http://www.abms.org/
1007 Church Street, Suite 404, Evanston, IL 60201-5913
Telephone: (847) 491-9091 Fax: (847) 328-3596

Accreditation Council for Graduate Medical Education (ACGME)
http://www.acgme.org/
515 North State St, Suite 2000, Chicago, IL 60610
Telephone: (312) 464-4920 Fax: (312) 464-4098

American College of Medical Toxicology (ACMT)
http://www.acmt.net/
777 East Park Drive, PO Box 8820, Harrisburg, PA 17105-8820

American College of Sports Medicine (ACSM)
http://www.acsm.org/
401 West Michigan Street, Indianapolis, IN 46202-3233
Telephone: (913) 637-9200

American Hospital Association (AHA)
http://www.aha.org/
One North Franklin, Chicago, IL 60606
Telephone: (312) 422-3000 Fax: 312.422.4796

American Medical Association (AMA)
http://www.ama-assn.org/
515 North State Street, Chicago, IL 60610
Telephone: (312) 464-5000

Air Medical Physicians Association (AMPA)
http://www.ampa.org/
383 F Street, Salt Lake City, UT 84103
Telephone: (801) 408-3699 Fax: (801) 408-1668

American Medical Society for Sports Medicine (AMSSM)
http://www.amssm.org/
11639 Earnshaw Overland Park, KS 66210
Telephone: (913) 327-1415 Fax: (913) 327-1491

American Osteopathic Association (AOA)
http://www.do-online.osteotech.org/
142 East Ontario Street, Chicago, IL 60611
Telephone: (800) 621-1773 Fax: (312) 202-8200

American Osteopathic Academy of Sports Medicine (AOASM)
http://www.aoasm.org/
7600 Terrace Avenue, Suite 203, Middleton, WI 53562
Telephone: (608) 831-4400 Fax: (608) 831-5185

American Orthopaedic Society for Sports Medicine (AOSSM)
http://www.aaos.org/
6300 North River Rd, Suite 200, Rosemont, IL 60018
Telephone: (847) 292-4900 Fax: (847) 823-8125

American Public Health Association (APHA)
http://www.apha.org/
800 I Street NW, Washington, DC 20001-3710
Telephone: (202) 777-APHA Fax: (202) 777-2534

Council of Medical Specialty Societies (CMMS)
http://www.cmss.org/
51 Sherwood Terrace, Suite M, Lake Bluff, IL 60044-2232
Telephone: (847) 295-3456 Fax: (847)-295-3759

National Association of EMS Physicians (NAEMSP)
http://www.naemsp.org
PO Box 15945-281, Lenexa, KS 66285
Telephone: 800.228.3677 Fax: (913) 541-0156

National Residency Matching Program (NRMP)
http://nrmp.aamc.org/
2450 North Street NW, Suite 201, Washington, DC 20037-1141
Telephone: (202) 862-6077

Undersea and Hyperbaric Medical Society (UHMS)
http://www.uhms.org/
10531 Metropolitan Avenue, Kensington, MD 20895
Telephone: (301) 942-2980

chapter 77

Acronyms

AACEM	Association of Academic Chairs of Emergency Medicine
AACOM	American Association of Colleges of Osteopathic Medicine
AACT	American Academy of Clinical Toxicology
AAMC	Association of American Medical Colleges
AAPCC	American Association of Poison Control Centers
ABEM	American Board of Emergency Medicine
ABMS	American Board of Medical Specialties
ACEP	American College of Emergency Physicians
ACGME	Accreditation Council for Graduate Medical Education
ACLS	advanced cardiac life support
ACMT	American College of Medical Toxicology
ACOEP	American College of Osteopathic Emergency Physicians
AHA	American Hospital Association
AMA	American Medical Association
AOA	American Osteopathic Association
	Alpha Omega Alpha Honor Society
AOBEM	American Osteopathic Board of Emergency Medicine
ATA	atmospheric absolute
ATSDR	Agency for Toxic Substances and Drug Research
BLS	basic life support
BOS	Bureau of Osteopathic Specialists
CAQ	certification of added qualifications
CDC	Centers for Disease Control and Prevention
CFR	certified first responder
CIR	Council of Interns and Residents
CME	continuing medical education
CMSS	Council of Medical Specialty Societies
COBRA	Consolidated Omnibus Budget Reconciliation Act
COPT	Council of Postdoctoral Training
CORD	Council of Emergency Medicine Residency Directors
COSGP	Council of Osteopathic Student Government Presidents

CPR	cardiopulmonary resuscitation
CT	computed tomography
CV	curriculum vitae
DMATs	Disaster Medical Assistance Teams
ECCOPT	Executive Committee of COPT
ECG	electrocardiogram
ECMO	extracorporeal membrane oxygenation
ED	emergency department
EM	emergency medicine
EMF	Emergency Medicine Foundation
EMIG	emergency medicine interest group
EMS	emergency medical services
EMT	emergency medical techniciation
EMTALA	Emergency Medical Treatment and Labor Act
EMT-B	emergency medical technician – basic
EMT-P	emergency medical technician – paramedic
EP	emergency phician
ERAS	Electronic Residency Application System
FAEM	Foundation for Academic Emergency Medicine
FDA	Food and Drug Administration
FOEM	Foundation for Osteopathic Emergency Medicine
FREIDA	Fellowship and Residency Electronic Interactive Database
FSMB	Federatiopn of State Medical Boards
GME	graduate medical education
GMEC	Graduate Medical Education Committee
GPS	Global Positioning System
HBO2	hyperbaric oxygen
HCFA	Health Care FinancingAdministration
ICU	intensive care unit
IR	institutional requirements
IRC	Institutional Review Committee
ISP	Internet service provider
JCAHO	Joint Commission on Accreditation of Healthcare Organizations
LCME	Liaison Council for Medical Education
LREC	Liaison Residency Endorsement Committee
MSC	Medical Student Committee
MSS	Medical Student Section
NACCT	North American Congress of Clinical Toxicology
NASA	National Aeronautics and Space Administration
NDMS	National Disaster Medical System
NIH	National Institutes of Health

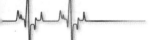

NP	nurse practitioner
NRMP	National Residency Match Program
OEMR	Osteopathic emergency medicine residency
OIG	Office of Inspector General
OPTI	Osteopathic Postdoctoral Training Institute
ORR	Organization of Resident Representatives
PA	physician assistant
PALS	pediatric advanced life support
PIF	program information forms
RN	registered nurse
RRC-EM	Residency Review Committee for Emergency Medicine
SAEM	Society for Academic Emergency Medicine
SEMPA	Society of Emergency Medicine Physician Assistants
SLOR	standard letter of recommendation
SOMA	Student Osteopathic Medical Association
STEM	Society for Teachers of Emergency Medicine
UA/EMS	University Association for Emergency Medical Services
UAEM	University Association of Emergency Medicine
USAR	urban search and rescue
USMLE	United States Medical Licensing Examination